Computational Vision

Information Processing in Perception and Visual Behavior

Hanspeter A. Mallot

translated by John S. Allen

A Bradford Book

The MIT Press

Cambridge, Massachusetts

London, England

Library of Congress Cataloging-in-Publication Data

Mallot, Hanspeter A.
   [Sehen und die Verarbeitung visueller Informationen. English]
   Computational vision : information processing in perception and visual
   behavior / Hanspeter A. Mallot : translated by John S. Allen.
      p.   cm.   —(Computational neuroscience)
   "A Bradford Book."
   Includes bibliographical references and index.
   ISBN 0-262-13381-4 (alk. hc)
   1. Vision—Computer simulation. 2. Computational neuroscience. 3.
Visual cortex—Computer simulation. I. Title. II. Series.
QP475 .M23   2000
612.8'4'0113—dc21   00-030381

When we realize that the objects are phenomena owing their appearance to a perceiving subject, we rest on old, secured ground which was prepared in a unique way by Kant to carry the edifice of all science. Kant has distinguished man as a subject from the objects and has discovered the principles by which the objects are reconstructed in our minds.

Biology has the responsibility to extend Kant's results into two directions: 1. to take into account the role of our body, in particular of our sense organs and our central nervous system and 2. to investigate the relations of other subjects (i.e., animals) to the objects.

—"Theoretische Biologie"
Jakob von Uexküll, 1928
(translation by HAM)

Contents

V   Appendix   243

Preface

Our knowledge of the world surrounding us is mediated by our senses. In visual perception, we sense the light emanating from objects in the environment and infer from this light a wealth of information about the environment. We are able to "see" depth and shape of objects, the color of surfaces, the segmentation of the scene into distinct objects, or the mood of a partner in a conversation. All this is based on images, i.e., two-dimensional distributions of intensities, which as such do not at all contain depth, shape, or moods. The fact that we are able to see all this is among the most amazing and fascinating abilities of our brain.

In this book, the performance of the perceptual apparatus is discussed on the level of information processing. Contributions from psychophysics and computational neuroscience are given equal weight as theories and algorithms developed for machine vision and photogrametry. Indeed, this combination is the very idea of *computational* vision. In the tradition of Bela Julesz and David Marr, most of the book is devoted to early vision, i.e., stages of visual processing that do not require top-down inferences from "higher" stages. However, in biological organisms as well as in robots, vision has to serve a purpose. Aspects of behavior-oriented vision covered in the book include eye-movement and visual navigation.

The book is based on courses given since 1987 at the universities of Mainz, Bochum, and Tübingen. I tried to keep it readable for students of psychology and the neurosciences as well as for students with a physics or computer vision background. The mathematical material is selected such as to give a survey of the various techniques employed in computational vision. Most of the ideas are introduced simultaneously as "prose" text, by formal equations, and in figures. As an additional refresher of college mathematics, a glossary of mathematical terms has been compiled.

I am grateful to my colleagues and students at the Max-Planck-Institut for Biological Cybernetics in Tübingen and the Department of Neural Computing at the Ruhr-Universität Bochum who have supported this work in many ways. Gerd–Jürgen Giefing, Walter Gillner, Holger Krapp und Roland Hengstenberg have provided figures that are included in the book. Valuable comments on the draft have been given by Matthias Franz, Karl Gegenfurtner, Sabine Gillner, Heiko Neumann, by the translator, John S. Allen, and by my wife, Bärbel Foese-Mallot.

Tübingen, April 2000
Hanspeter Mallot

Computational Vision

Part I

Fundamentals

Among the many possible definitions of the concept of "vision," the present text concentrates on information processing; that is, on the reconstruction of the characteristics of the environment from images. The first chapter is intended to establish a conceptual framework: vision does not occur simply because we open our eyes and turn them toward the world. Rather, vision is an active process, similar in many ways to the testing of hypotheses using data provided by the senses. A series of demonstrations will show that the relationship between what is present and what is seen is not a simple one.

Before we turn to the active aspects of seeing and the related processing of information in the later parts of the book, we will (in Chapter 2) examine the most important characteristics of the generation of images. Clearly, the nature and properties of the available data, that is, of the images, is of great importance to its subsequent interpretation. Camera analogies and perspective are very important here, but reflections from surfaces and eye movements will also be discussed.

Chapter 1

Introduction

1.1 Biological information processing

1.1.1 The perception-action cycle

Living beings relate to their surroundings in many kinds of ways. The interactions may be considered physically and chemically and may be studied as exchanges of matter and energy. Although all life forms have this type of energetic and material basis, such an approach falls short in the study of sensory and effector processes. For example, the physical nature of the sensation of light from a printed page is related only very indirectly to the text: the wavelength, the contrast, the size and the intensity—in fact, all of the physically relevant quantities—can be varied within wide limits without changing the meaning of the stimulus for the reader. Based on observations of this type, a perception-action cycle characterized by the flow of information rather than a flow of material or energy, is considered to be an essential characteristic of behaving organisms, or "agents" (see Figure 1.1). The idea that perception and action are coupled via an accessible part of the world called the *environment* dates back to Jakob von Uexküll (1926). The relationship between perception and behavior also plays an increasing role in computer vision and robotics (Brooks 1986); to make clear the distinction from older approaches which are directed only toward perception, the term "behavior-oriented approach" is used.

The concept of information used in this book is closely related to that of the action-perception cycle: information is what is transported along the paths indicated by arrows in Figure 1.1 (Tembrock 1992). The meaning of a stimulus is ultimately determined by the behavior which it elicits in the organism, that is, by the role of that stimulus in the perception-action cycle (von Uexküll 1926, Gibson 1979, Dusenbery 1992). In this framework, therefore, information has a meaning which is to some extent independent of the quantity of information as measured by Shannon's (1948) theory of communication. Very meager quantities of information, as measured according to Shannon's theory, can be sufficient to generate and guide complex behaviors.

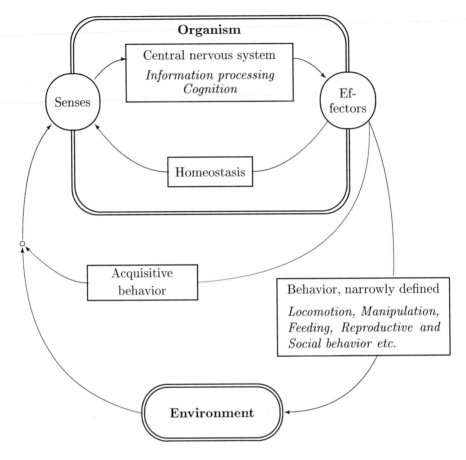

Figure 1.1
The perception-action cycle and the associated transfer of information. The senses (vision, hearing, smell, taste, touch, posture and balance as well as proprioception) provide information about the outside world and about the inner conditions of the organism. Through the effectors (motor system, glands) and the behaviors which they generate, the organism enters into a relationship with the environment. The effectors are related to the senses by three feedback loops: through internal regulation (homeostasis), sensory-motor and acquisitive behavior (for example, eye movement), and through alterations to the environment, which are effected through other behaviors.

This is demonstrated, for example, by the thought experiments of Braitenberg (1984), which examine the behavior of small wheeled vehicles with two point sensors, and two wheels driven or braked depending on the sensory input. Depending on whether the sensors are connected to the motors on the same or the opposite sides, and whether the sensory signal drives or brakes the motors, different "behaviors" can be generated, which appear to the outside observer to be based on significant amounts of information processing. The relationship of the behavior of such vehicles to their internal circuits has been intensively studied in what is called artificial life research, using simulated and real robots (cf. Langton 1995).

The concept of information processing, as introduced here for biological vision, is applied in entirely similar ways in robotics and in computer vision (Marr 1982, Ballard & Brown 1982, Horn 1986). The present description will therefore give technical and biological problems equal weight.

The central organ of information processing is the brain. Before we examine vision, the central subject matter of this book, we need to summarize the major tasks of the brain. These tasks define the areas of study in biological information processing.

Sensation and Perception: The brain interprets and integrates all sensory modalities (vision, hearing, smell, taste, touch, posture and balance, proprioception). Disturbances to the senses can occur as a result of poor brain function, even if the sense organs are perfectly normal. Examples of such disturbances include amblyopia and various agnosias.

Behavior: With the assistance of effectors (muscles, glands), the brain controls the behavior of the organism and regulates its internal conditions. Behavior is linked via the environment to the sense organs, and so a feedback loop arises. The brain serves as the control device in this loop. For experiments into perception, the presence or absence of feedback via the perception-action cycle is generally of great importance (open vs. closed-loop experiments, for example in navigation using visual cues).

Memory: Most researchers distinguish short-term or working memory, which holds information needed during processing, from long-term memory. One subdivision of long-term memory serves to store explicit items such as events, faces and objects, or rules ("declarative memory"). Another subdivision, called "procedural" or "non-declarative memory" contains implicit knowledge supporting associations, habits and skills.

Higher functions (cognition, motivation): The concept of cognition comprises abilities which require internal models or representations of the environment. Examples are latent learning (playful, non goal-directed learning of facts and regularities which are used later) and problem solving. Behavior guided by cognition is not organized in stereotypes of stimulus and reaction but also depends on the organism's current goal. The knowledge needed to realize these goals is stored in a declarative memory.

The study and description of these abilities as information processing tasks is the aim of theoretical neurobiology. The present book discusses mainly perception: that is, more or less, the upper left part of the information flow diagram of Fig. 1.1. Two aspects of visually guided behavior covered in this book are eye movements (Section 2.4) and visual navigation (Chapter 11).

1.1.2   How is information processing studied?

The biological sciences employ a number of quite different types of explanations.
In the context of this book, it is important to distinguish between the anatomy of
the central nervous system, and the behavioral and perceptual competences which
it supports. Even when physiological explanations are not available, inquiry into
the information sources used and into the logic of their evaluation and integration is
appropriate and fruitful. This type of explanation is called the *computational theory
of competence*; it has been pioneered by David Marr (1982). In order to provide a
framework for the information processing approach, we will summarize and slightly
extend the approach developed by Marr (1982).

1. *"Hardware" implementation:* This level primarily concerns itself with the anatomy and optics of the eye, as well as the anatomy of the visual pathways
   and related neural networks. In the study of artificial systems, it is usually
   assumed that the hardware is general and can be applied to any type of task.
   In biological systems, on the other hand, evolutionary adaptation has led to an
   interdependence between structure and function. Therefore, it is in principle
   possible to infer function from structure, as is attempted in neural network
   research (cf. Arbib 1995).

2. *Representation and algorithms:* How are images (i.e., distributions of intensity
   or neural activity) and the information derived from them represented, and
   which available neuronal operations can be interpreted as "computation"? The
   experimental approach to the study of these questions is primarily that of elec-
   trophysiology.

3. *Computational theory of competence:* This is information processing in the narrow sense. The central issue is of what must be calculated in order to derive the
   desired information from the spatio-temporal stimulus distribution. The definition of vision as inverse optics which will be presented in what follows has taken
   root here. On the level of computational theory, the brain and the computer
   are confronted with the same problems.

4. *Behavioral approach:* The computational theory of competence does not, for the
   most part, examine to what ends certain information is derived from the data.
   Rather, the goal of information processing is assumed to be the reconstruction
   of the most complete possible description of the scene being viewed. In biology,
   as also in robotics and computer vision, this assumption is usually not at all
   correct. Rather, the primary interest is in information which is relevant to behavior; that is, information which is actually required in order to function in a
   given environment (von Uexküll 1926). The "ecological" approach of J. J. Gibson (1950) expands on this concept, though it is not highly formalized. In the
   fields of behavioral and sensory ecology, an attempt is made to quantify the advantage of information processing competences in terms of evolutionary fitness
   or reproductive success that an organism gains from a particular perceptual or
   behavioral competence (Krebs & Davies 1993; Dusenbery 1992).

The levels listed above are not completely independent. It is nonetheless useful for heuristic purposes to distinguish them from one another. This book stresses the computational theory approach, which is very similar for computer and biological vision.

1.2 Information in images

1.2.1 What information can images contain?

In order for information to be acquired through the sense of vision, the light which emanates from a light source must itself contain such information. The following possibilities exist in principle:

1. *Light source:*
   The presence or disappearance of light sources provides very simple, though biologically very important information. Mussels close their shells when a shadow is cast on them, fireflies and deep-sea fishes have developed their own bioluminescent light sources to attract mates or prey, and honey bees navigate according to the position of the sun. Directional point sensors used in many robots are sufficient for detecting light sources and determining their direction.*

2. *Physical interactions of a ray of light with the visible world attach certain information about the world to the ray.* We first consider only a single ray of light.

   (a) *Opaque surfaces: reflection.* The light returned from a surface contains information on surface properties such as reflectivity ("color"), albedo ("brightness") or smoothness ("glossy" or "dull") as well as on the orientation of the surface.

   (b) *Transparent media: scattering.* Scattering can reveal physical characteristics of the medium or the position (distance) of the light source. As an example, consider "aerial perspective", i.e. the bluish appearance of mountain ranges at great distances.

   (c) *Boundaries between optical media: refraction.* Refraction is of minor importance as a source of information, but plays a very important role in generation of images.

---

*Darwin (1859, Chapter 6) suggested that such "point sensors" are actually the starting point of the evolution of eyes: "... I can see no very great difficulty (...) in believing that natural selection has converted the simple apparatus of an optic nerve merely coated with pigment and invested by transparent membrane, into an optical instrument as perfect as is possessed by any member of the great Articulate class." See also Halder et al. (1995) for recent evidence on the evolution of different eye types from one common ancestral organ.

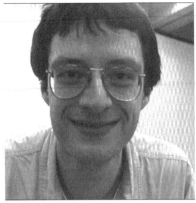
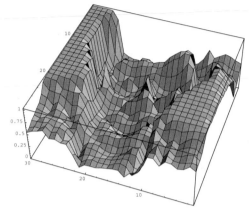

| Image | Intensity distribution $I(x,y)$ |

Figure 1.2
Images are two-dimensional distributions of intensities or gray values. **Left**: Gray scale image. **Right**: Representation of the same image as a gray scale "landscape."

  3. *Information in the distribution of incident rays of light*

   (a) *Temporal:* Information on movements of the observer (egomotion), on movements of objects, changes in the light source, etc. is conveyed by temporal, or spatio-temporal distributions of intensities.

   (b) *Spatial:* All rays of light incident on a given point are called the ambient optical array of this point (Gibson 1950). In a sense, the optical array characterizes the image which ideally could be observed at the point. Additional information is available with binocular vision.

Spatio-temporal distributions of the intensity of light, i.e. sequences of images, represent by far the most important source of visual information. They make it possible to see forms and movements. The representation of images as intensity maps (or "landscapes") is illustrated in Fig. 1.2. Image and intensity distribution contain exactly the same information (up to the limit of the pixel resolution, which differs in the two parts of Figure 1.2). Our perceptual system nonetheless is much better able to interpret the image than the intensity landscape. Attempting, to envision, by examining the intensity landscape, the object which is "visible" without effort in the image, gives an idea of the complexity of the problem which must be solved in visual information processing. This is the problem of computer vision.

1.2.2   What information can be derived from images?

The sources of information which have been described are confronted with a set of "perceptual needs" which the human visual system can generally satisfy. A few examples are given in what follows:

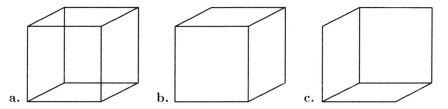

Figure 1.3
Necker's inversion of the cube shows the ambiguity of the three-dimensional interpretation of line drawings. The complete cube **a.** can be perceived as in **b.** or in **c.** Neither of the two interpretations can be maintained at will for any length of time.

Surface colors. Reflectivity (that is, color as a surface property) and albedo (brightness of the surface) are usually perceived independently of the spectral content and intensity of the light source. Perceiving surfaces unchanged under a wide range of different illuminants is an example of a perceptual constancy,* a very common but often unnoticed phenomenon of perception. If photographs are taken under artificial light using daylight-balanced color film, the resulting yellowish colors are not incorrect in terms of the physical spectra of the photographed light. If yellow predominates in the illuminant, the light reflected from the surfaces will also have more yellow components than under white illumination. A human observer, however, does not see this. Unlike the photographic process, the visual system can adapt to the spectrum of the light source, and can therefore see the same colors under different lighting conditions. The word "color," then, describes a perception which corresponds more closely to the properties of the surface than to the physical spectrum of the light reflected from that surface (cf. Chapter 5). The distinction between dull and glossy reflections is similarly made independently of the angular extent of the light source.

Depth. An important task of vision is to discern the distance of individual points from the observer, as well as the shape of surfaces and objects from their images. A large number of depth cues can make this possible, some of which will be discussed in detail in the course of this work. Besides stereopsis and motion parallax, which depend on there being more than one image, there are also depth cues in individual images, called "pictorial" depth cues. Examples are the three-dimensional interpretation of line drawings as wire-frame objects (Figure 1.3), shadows and shading (Figure 1.4), texture gradients (Figure 8.1) and occlusion. Many of these cues, each taken alone, allow no unambiguous perception of depth. The visual system therefore uses "plausible" assumptions about the environment; if these prove to be false, optical illusions occur.

---

*A constancy is the perception that an object remains unchanged when viewed from different positions or under different illuminations. In addition to color constancy, there is also constancy of perceived size and form in spite of perspective changes in the image. The term "constancy" is related to the notion of "invariance" used in the pattern recognition literature. It is distinguished from "invariance" in that changes are not simply ignored, but are taken into account.

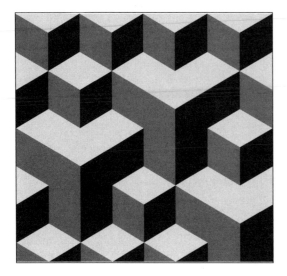

Figure 1.4
Perception of depth through shading alone is always subject to the concave/convex inversion. The pattern shown can be perceived as stairsteps receding toward the top and lighted from above, or as an overhanging structure lighted from below. Just as with Necker's cube, the two interpretations give way to each other. The well-known painting "Concave and Convex" by M.C. Escher (see Ernst 1976) provides an artistic example of convex-concave inversion.

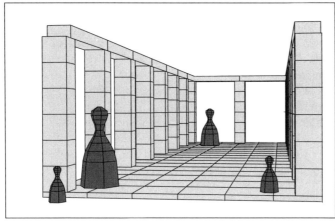

Figure 1.5
The corridor illusion. The second and third figure from the left have the same size in terms of the depicted three-dimensional environment. The sizes of the images of all but the second figure from the left are exactly the same.

Size and subtended angle.   In order to see the true size of an object, its distance as well as the angle it subtends must be known. Mistakes in evaluating the distance lead immediately to mistakes about size such as are visible, for example, in apparent changes in size as the Necker cube inverts. The relationship known as Emmert's law is roughly valid: perceived size ≈ subtended angle × apparent distance. It is another instance of perceptual constancy. A well-known example is the corridor illusion (Fig. 1.5).

An additional, very impressive demonstration of Emmert's law makes use of the so-called afterimage, which occurs due to local bleaching of the visual pigment. After looking monocularly (i.e., with one eye closed or covered) at a bright, sharply-defined light source* while moving the eye as little as possible, an afterimage is generated

---

*The light source should not be too strong in order to avoid injury.

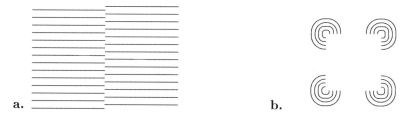

Figure 1.6
Subjective contours. **a.** An edge can be perceived at the boundary between the two hatched regions. **b.** The "missing" segments of the circles appear to be concealed by a square which lies on top of them. The sides of the square can be perceived as "subjective contours" even though they are not physically present in the image. For additional examples, cf. Kanizsa (1979).

on the retina. The afterimage may be made clearly visible by blinking. The area of the retina which is affected defines the angle subtended by the afterimage. Still, the perceived size of the afterimage can change considerably, since the afterimage is always perceived as attached to the surface at which the eyes are directed. When looking at a nearby object (for example, one's own hand), the afterimage appears much smaller than when gaze is directed at a more distant surface such as a wall.

Perceptual organization. Images have to be segmented into regions corresponding to various objects (image segmentation, figure/ground segregation). The existence of such regions (and objects) is not inferred from the image but is assumed by the visual system. Image segmentation works even when objects are only partially visible; an understanding of occlusion relations between objects defines a depth ordering which is an important monocular cue to depth. Large numbers of demonstrations of segmentation and grouping have been presented and studied in Gestalt psychology (Metzger 1975). They are often related to perceptual hysteresis (cf. Figures 1.6 – 1.8).

Perceptual organization not only assembles parts of the image into a perceived whole, but also determines the spatial interpretation of line drawings such as the Necker cube (Fig. 1.3). Perceptual organization is therefore more than just grouping, or "binding" of parts into a whole.

Motion. Motion is a specific type of change in the image. Changes which should not be interpreted as motion occur, for example, through dimming of the light source or due to a searchlight's turning away from a scene. In actual motions, on the other hand, parts of the image move coherently. Detecting motion therefore requires a simultaneous evaluation of temporal and spatial changes to the image. Movements accompanied by changes in shape present an especially difficult problem. For example, a rotating, elliptical figure can be seen as a pulsating circle (see page 194).

Movements of the observer lead to motion patterns covering large parts of the field of view ("optical flow"), which contain information about the egomotion of the

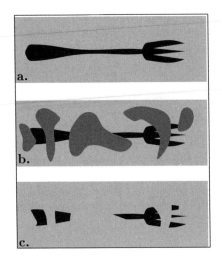

Figure 1.7
Perceptual grouping of parts separated by partial occlusion. The pieces of a fork in **b.** are exactly the same as in **c.** Grouping and completion are apparent only in **b.** where the interrupting lines can be seen to belong to an occluder rather than to the fork itself. They do therefore not divide the fork into pieces. Cf. Metzger (1975), page 420.

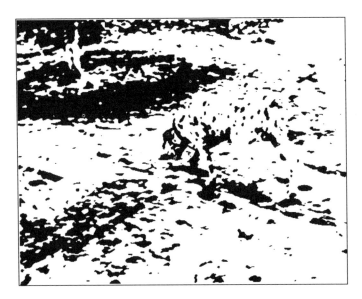

Figure 1.8
Segmentation of this image is difficult, but still possible. A Dalmatian dog (right center) and a tree trunk are recognizable. After R. C. James in Marr (1982).

observer and also about the three-dimensional structure of the surrounding world. The visual system is particularly sensitive to discontinuities of the motion field, both in space (usually caused by discontinuities in depth) and in time. Increased sensitivity to change is achieved by local spatial and temporal adaptation, which in turn results in aftereffects such as the so-called waterfall illusion.

Object and pattern recognition.   This is the classification of objects based on a prior image segmentation and certain characteristics of the observed regions. Classification by invariant object descriptions ignores irrelevant characteristics of the objects

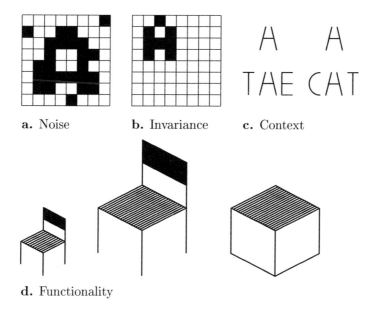

a. Noise   **b.** Invariance   **c.** Context

d. Functionality

Figure 1.9
Types of pattern recognition problems. **a.** Statistically noisy pattern (letter A). **b.** Size and positional invariance. **c.** The same patterns (above) must be classified in context (below). **d.** Objects as "utensils" for behavioral application. Size invariance leads to identification of the left and middle objects (doll's chair, chair), though only the middle and right ones are suitable for sitting.

such as size (Fig. 1.9). From the point of view of visually guided behavior, it makes sense to base the classification on possible functions that the object may have in an intended behavior. An extreme example for behavior-oriented recognition is provided by trigger stimuli in behavioral biology.

The list of "visible" information types could be extended. In the context of this book, we will, however, limit ourselves to the ones described above. They belong, above all, to the category of "early vision."

1.3 Vision as information processing

1.3.1 Theories of perception

In this book, we adopt the definition of Poggio et al. (1995) who characterize "vision" as "inverse optics," i.e., as the processing of visual information resulting in a description of the environment. This problem is indeed an inverse one, since optics itself explains the generation of images from three-dimensional descriptions of scenes.

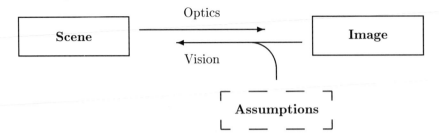

Figure 1.10
Vision as inverse optics

Obviously, images do not contain all information about the imaged scene, and inversion is therefore not generally possible without ambiguity. It is therefore necessary to draw on prior knowledge or assumptions about the environment in order to arrive at meaningful solutions. Many so-called illusions have to do with false assumptions. Despite this, "illusory" information is often the best which can be derived from a given image. Such illusions are therefore not to be regarded as interesting oddities of the visual system, but rather, they offer insight into the heuristics used by the system as it functions normally.

The concept of vision as "inverse optics" originated in computer vision, but also can be thought of as a theory of perception. It describes vision (and perception in general) as an active process, through which the environment is, in a certain way, constructed. The thought that sensory impressions do not correspond in a naïve way to perception underlies other approaches as well. For example, the "judgment theory" of perception proceeds from the concept that vision is a type of unconscious inference (Hermann von Helmholtz 1909-1911), while Gestalt theory assumes that sensory impressions organize themselves into a perception according to a set of "Gestalt rules" (cf. Metzger 1975, Westheimer 1999). The concept of information processing does not come down on the side of a cognitive (judgment theory) or neurophysiological (Gestalt theory) nature of the active component of perception, and so allows a consistent description of its rules.

1.3.2   Levels of complexity

As is already clear from the list of needs for information which perception can serve, the problem of visual perception includes many parts of differing complexity. Although it is difficult to categorize these, the following list is commonly used. Steps 1 through 3 are based on the idea of inverse optics, while steps 4 and 5 arise out of behavioral biology and psychology. These two steps are gaining increasing attention in the field of robotics as well.

1. *Early vision:* (Julesz 1971, 1991; Marr 1982) More or less local operations which generate "maps," that is, point-by-point distributions of values of various

quantities. Examples: maps of local edge elements, fields of local motion or displacement vectors, depth maps, color constancy.

2. *Middle vision and integration:* Assembly of the local information from different parts of the image, or from different operations carried out on the same location in the image. For example, image segmentation and contour completion, integration of depth cues. The goal is the reconstruction of visible surfaces and their characteristics.

3. *Scene analysis:* Recognition of the objects in a scene. Simple control of behaviors such as steering and obstacle avoidance.

4. *Active vision:* (Bajcsy 1988, Ballard 1991, Blake & Yuille 1992) Making optimal use of the available resources (such as image resolution or computing power) by means of eye movements and exploratory behavior. The simplest case of active vision is the adjustment of the sensor to depth and movement of a viewed object by accommodation, convergence of the eyes, and pursuit eye movements.

5. *Goal-directed vision:* Control of behaviors based on visual information. While the idea of inverse optics is closely connected with that of the complete reconstruction of the scene, a few selected items of information are often sufficient for the purpose of carrying out particular actions. This is especially advantageous when the needed information can be obtained directly; that is, bypassing the systematic pathway of points 1 through 3. Fig. 1.9d illustrates the difference between invariant image processing and goal directed vision. Further examples of goal-directed vision are discussed in Chapter 11.

Chapter 2

Imaging

Chapter 1 defined vision as inverse optics, that is, as an inversion of the process of the optical imaging of a scene on the retina. In order to understand this inversion, it is necessary to examine somewhat more closely how the image is generated. The problem is, firstly, of the assignment of gray levels or color values to each individual element of the "optical array" (intensities, section 2.1), then secondly of the geometric arrangement of these elements (imaging systems, section 2.2) and finally, of the consequences of this imaging for the structure of the image (perspective, Section 2.3). At the end of this chapter (Section 2.4), we will briefly examine eye movements.

2.1 Intensities

2.1.1 Physical quantities

The gray value at a given point in an image is determined by the intensity of the light which strikes the image plane at this point. This intensity is, in general, determined by the physical power of the light radiation, divided either by the area irradiated or by the spherical angle into which the power is radiated, depending on what physical entity is to be measured. Physically relevant quantities which do not make distinctions between different colors of light are:

1. *Radiant flux* Φ is a physical power measured in watts.
2. *Radiant intensity* is the power emitted into a cone with its apex at the light source and a solid angle Ω. The solid angle of a cone is defined as the area cut out of a unit sphere centered at the cone's apex. The unit of measurement is called the "steradian" (sr) and the entire sphere encompasses 4π sr. Radiant intensity is measured in watts per steradian.
3. *Irradiance:* This is the power incident on an area A.

$$E = \frac{d\Phi}{dA}, \ [E] = \frac{\mathrm{W}}{\mathrm{m}^2}. \tag{2.1}$$

Irradiance determines, for example, the stimulus to a photo-receptor in the retina or the darkening of photographic film. Irradiance can describe the intensity of an image, as well as the illumination of a surface by a light source.

4. *Radiance:* This is the power emitted from a surface patch of area A into a cone with a solid angle Ω in a given direction. The angle between this direction and the surface normal is ϑ. In contrast to irradiance, which is a scalar, radiance has a direction:

$$L = \frac{d^2\Phi}{\cos\vartheta \, d\Omega \, dA}, \quad [L] = \frac{W}{m^2 sr} \quad (\text{sr} = \text{steradians}). \tag{2.2}$$

Each of these quantities has a psychophysical counterpart, in which the power is weighted according to the spectral sensitivity of the human eye. The spectral sensitivity curve for a light adapted eye is shown in Fig. 5.6a as $\bar{y}(\lambda)$; it reaches its maximum at a wavelength of 555 nm. For the dark adapted eye, the curve is shifted to shorter wavelengths with a maximum at 507 nm. For both light and dark adapted eyes, the perceived brightness (luminous intensity) of a monochromatic light of wavelength 555 nm and radiant intensity of 1/683 watt per steradian is defined to be one candela. Table 2.1 lists physical and psychophysical quantities.

When calibrating a monitor, e.g. for psychophysical experiments into contrast perception, the relevant quantity to measure is luminance, given in candelas per square meter on the screen. The intensity of light actually meeting the retina is an illuminance, measured in lumen per square meter. Since retinal illuminance is hard to measure, it is often replaced by the "conventional retinal illuminance" or Troland value which is defined for each visual direction as the luminance in that direction multiplied by the foreshortened pupillary area as seen from that direction (cf. Wyszecki & Stiles 1982). The Troland value does not take into account the absorption of light by the optic media in the eye. It is measured in *troland*, where 1 troland equals 1 candela per square meter per square millimeter pupillary area.

Table 2.1

Important photometric quantities and the units in which they are measured (cf. Wyszecki & Stiles 1982, Pokorny & Smith 1986).

Physical: radiation		Psychophysical: light	
Quantity	Unit	Quantity	Unit
radiant flux	watts = W	luminous flux	lumen = lm
radiant intensity	W / sr	luminous intensity	lm/sr = candela = cd
irradiance	W / m²	illuminance	lm/m² = lux = lx
radiance	W / (m² × sr)	luminance	lm/(m² × sr)
			= candela / m²

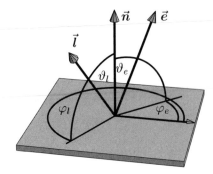

Figure 2.1
The reflectivity of a surface whose normal vector is $\vec{n}$ is generally a function of the direction of incidence of the light $\vec{l}$ and the direction of the reflected light $\vec{e}$. These directions are best given in spherical coordinates relative to the normal $\vec{n}$. (Eq. 2.3). In order to define the azimuth angles φ_l and φ_e, an x axis on the plane must be defined.

2.1.2   Geometry of reflection

In surface reflection, the irradiance which impinges on a surface is at least in part returned as radiance. The following are major factors which determine the radiance:

1. *Illumination (irradiance):*

   (a) Light source (strength, spectral composition, angular extent, e.g., point source vs. bright sky)

   (b) Obstruction by other objects (cast shadows)

   (c) Orientation of the surface with respect to the light source (shading)

2. *Reflectivity of the surface:*

   (a) Albedo (fraction of light reflected) and surface color (pigmentation)

   (b) Surface smoothness (dull, glossy, specular)

   (c) Orientation of the surface relative to the observer

Radiance and image intensity are proportional to irradiance:

$$\text{intensity} = \text{irradiance} \times \text{reflectivity}.$$

The ratio which is reflectivity depends on the properties of materials, and also on the orientation of the light source and observer in relation to the imaged surface. Let us establish a coordinate system whose origin is a fixed point on the surface, and whose z axis is the normal $\vec{n}$ to the surface at this point (Fig. 2.1). The normal should be chosen so that it has a positive component in the direction of the observer, and so, $\vartheta_e < 90°$. We can then identify a direction in space using the azimuth φ and the angle ϑ relative to the surface normal $\vec{n}$. (Note that $90° - \vartheta$ is the elevation in spherical coordinates.) For the vectors described in Figure 2.1, $\vec{l}$ (light source, direction of incident light) and $\vec{e}$ (eye, direction of reflected light), we then obtain:

$$\vec{l} = \begin{pmatrix} \cos\varphi_l \sin\vartheta_l \\ \sin\varphi_l \sin\vartheta_l \\ \cos\vartheta_l \end{pmatrix} ; \quad \vec{e} = \begin{pmatrix} \cos\varphi_e \sin\vartheta_e \\ \sin\varphi_e \sin\vartheta_e \\ \cos\vartheta_e \end{pmatrix} ; \quad \vec{n} = \begin{pmatrix} 0 \\ 0 \\ 1 \end{pmatrix}. \qquad (2.3)$$

If the angular extent of the light source is large, light from many directions falls on each point of the surface; the illumination of the surface is then given by an irradiance distribution $E(\vartheta_l, \varphi_l)$. If light arrives only from a point source in the direction (ϑ_l, φ_l), then E is zero for all other directions. The radiance which the surface emits is also described by a function, $L(\vartheta_e, \varphi_e)$. More generally, then, reflection is described by the so-called "bidirectional reflectivity function" f, which depends on the angles from which light is received and those in which it is emitted:

$$f(\vartheta_l, \varphi_l; \vartheta_e, \varphi_e) = \frac{L(\vartheta_e, \varphi_e)}{E(\vartheta_l, \varphi_l)}. \tag{2.4}$$

There are a number of simplifications and special cases of this most general formulation:

1. *Symmetry:* As a result of the reversibility of the path of a ray of light, the bidirectional reflectivity function must satisfy the relation

$$f(\vartheta_l, \varphi_l; \vartheta_e, \varphi_e) = f(\vartheta_e, \varphi_e; \vartheta_l, \varphi_l).$$

   This result can also be derived from the thermodynamic equilibrium of two surfaces illuminating each other (von Helmholtz).

2. *Isotropy:* We generally consider only isotropic surfaces, that is, those for which only differences $\varphi_e - \varphi_l$ in the azimuth angle are significant. Rotating isotropic surfaces around their normal has no effect on their radiance.

3. *Parallel illumination:* In this case, all of the irradiance is concentrated in a direction $\vec{l}$; this direction is the same for all illuminated points. Parallel illumination occurs, for example, in the case of very distant sources of light which are effectively point sources.

4. *Lambertian surfaces:* The radiance L of perfectly dull surfaces does not depend on the angle of emission. Equal amounts of light are reflected in every direction. The reflectivity function f is, then, a constant for all directions. A natural material whose surface reflection is very closely Lambertian is stucco.

5. *Mirror:* In the case of a perfect mirror, all light is reflected such that the angle of reflection equals the angle of incidence. f therefore is zero for all other pairs of directions ($\vartheta_e = \vartheta_l, \varphi_e = \varphi_l + \pi$).

2.1.3 Examples

Next we will examine several special cases of simple reflection with parallel illumination. Parallel illumination can occur when a point light source is at an infinite distance; the sun approximates these conditions. Since only a single reflection occurs, it is sufficient to consider two directions, namely that to the light source $\vec{l}$ and that to the observer's eye $\vec{e}$, the only direction of light reflection which is of interest in this case.

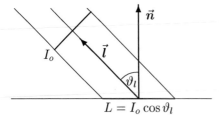

Figure 2.2
Illustration of Lambert's cosine law. For explanation see text.

$$L = I_o \cos \vartheta_l$$

Lambertian reflection

A dull surface, for example a plaster disk, is illuminated with parallel light. No matter from which direction such a surface is observed, its brightness does not change. On the other hand, the direction of the light source does affect the brightness of the surface; the brightness is greatest when the light falls vertically on the surface ($\vartheta_l = 0°$), and is reduced to zero when the direction of the source is parallel to the surface ($\vartheta_l = 90°$). This case describes an ideal diffuse or Lambert reflection.

A more precise description of the Lambert reflection comprises two steps. First, consider the incident light I_o passing through an aperture of unit area at right angles to the direction of the light. This light falls on a surface which is greater than that of the aperture by a factor of $1/\cos \vartheta_l$ (Fig. 2.2); the irradiance per unit area is therefore $E = I_o \cos \vartheta_l$. This formula explains the change in brightness when the light source is moved. The direction of incidence of the light plays no further role.

A part, c_d, of the incident light is reflected equally in all directions ("diffusely"). The surface therefore appears equally bright when observed from any direction. Taking all these effects into account, the following relationship results:

$$L = c_d I_o \cos \vartheta_l = c_d I_o (\vec{n} \cdot \vec{l}) \quad \text{for } (\vec{n} \cdot \vec{l}) \geq 0. \tag{2.5}$$

In the Lambertian case, the reflectivity function f of Eq. 2.4 is constant. If the dot product $(\vec{n} \cdot \vec{l}) < 0$, in other words, if $\cos \vartheta_l < 0$, the light source is behind the surface, and so the surface is not illuminated. In this case, L is 0. In computer graphics applications, it is always important to make sure that the normal to the surface points toward the observer. The part c_d of the light which is reflected is a property (called the albedo) of the material of which the surface is composed, and varies with wavelength, determining the brightness and color of the surface. If the light source includes multiple spectral components, Lambert's rule must be applied independently to each of them; c_d then becomes a function of the wavelength λ, that is to say, an absorption spectrum. If the incident light is white, then the color of the reflected light is that of the surface.

Real surfaces often conform to Lambert's rule only approximately, or not at all. In particular, surfaces which are metallic, polished, or wet appear to have different brightnesses when viewed from different directions. As an example, consider specular highlights changing their position on the surface as the observer moves. In computer graphics, Lambert reflection represents an especially simple case. Since the brightness of the surface does not depend on the position of the observer, brightness changes or shading can be "painted" onto the surface by the computer application.

Example: Dull spheres illuminated by parallel rays of light.
In a coordinate system whose origin is at the center of the sphere, let the surface of a sphere be described by the set of points $\vec{p}$. The observer's position is on the z axis. We assume that the radius of the sphere is unity. For the special case of a sphere, the surface normals $\vec{n}$ are equal to the radius vectors $\vec{p}$:

$$\vec{p} = \begin{pmatrix} x \\ y \\ \sqrt{1 - (x^2 + y^2)} \end{pmatrix} = \vec{n}.$$

The intensity of the parallel illumination is given by I_o. We calculate the intensity as a function of x and y, that is, we calculate the image of a shaded sphere under parallel (orthographic) projection (cf. below, Eq. 2.19).

a. Let $\vec{l} = (0,0,1)^\top$, that is, the illumination is frontal, from the direction of the observer. From Eq. 2.5 we obtain

$$L = I_o(\vec{l} \cdot \vec{n}) = I_0\sqrt{1 - (x^2 + y^2)}.$$

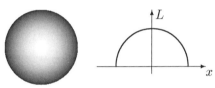

b. Let $\vec{l} = (1,0,0)^\top$, that is, the illumination is from the side. We obtain:

$$L = \begin{cases} I_o\, x & x \geq 0 \\ 0 & \text{otherwise} \end{cases}.$$

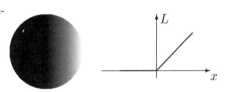

The image and the intensity distribution for both cases are shown in the illustrations at the right. In case **b.**, a self-shadowing boundary occurs at the mid-line of the image, where $(\vec{l} \cdot \vec{n}) = 0$ (see also Figure 7.1).

This calculation of the intensity profile of a sphere rests on the assumption that the surface is completely smooth. On rough surfaces, patches that are illuminated vertically will be found even in the vicinity of the self-shadowing boundary. This effect may explain the fact that the intensity distribution of the moon does not follow the function calculated above (Nayar & Oren 1995). In fact, rather than showing a smooth transition from bright to dark, the moon appears to have a roughly constant brightness all over its visible parts, with a sharp step edge at the inner outline of the crescent. This is in contradiction to the Lambert model for smooth surfaces, according to which the transition from bright to dark at the self-shadowing boundary should be gradual.

Mirrors

In a sense, mirrors are the complete opposite of Lambertian surfaces. While Lambertian surfaces reflect the same radiance to all directions, mirrors concentrate all of the radiance in one direction; we call this direction the vector of specularity, $\vec{s}$ (Figure 2.3a). The vector of specularity lies in a plane with $\vec{n}$ and $\vec{l}$, and the angle of incidence is equal to the angle of reflection. In vector notation, this can be expressed by requiring the projections of $\vec{l}$ and $\vec{s}$ on $\vec{n}$ to be equal. Therefore,

$$\vec{s} = 2(\vec{n} \cdot \vec{l})\, \vec{n} - \vec{l} \quad \text{or}$$
$$\vartheta_s = \vartheta_l; \quad \varphi_s = \varphi_l + \pi \tag{2.6}$$

and for the radiance emitted from the surface:

$$L(\vartheta_e, \varphi_e) = \begin{cases} I_o & \text{if } \vartheta_e = \vartheta_s, \varphi_e = \varphi_s; \ (\vec{e} = \vec{s}) \\ 0 & \text{else} \end{cases} \tag{2.7}$$

The brightness distribution of a mirror can not be "painted on," since it depends on the position of the observer. The reflected light has the color of the incident light.

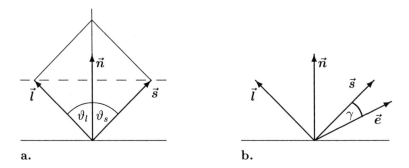

a.   b.

Figure 2.3
Reflection in a mirror (**a**) and from glossy surfaces (**b**). $\vec{n}$, normal to the surface. $\vec{l}$, unit vector to the light source. $\vec{s}$ mirror vector. $\vec{e}$, unit vector to the eye of the observer.

Glossy surfaces

Most real surfaces are neither purely diffuse nor purely specular. There are various models for glossy surfaces; that of Cook & Torrance (cf. Foley et al. 1995) is the most satisfactory one from a physical standpoint. It models surfaces statistically, that is, by means of many small mirror-like facets, and calculates the distribution of radiance from the distribution of orientations of the individual facets. For a thorough description of the physics of reflection at realistic surfaces, see Nayar et al. (1991).

A model which is sufficient for simple computer graphics applications is that of Phong, in which the incident light is reflected in a solid angle whose center is at $\vec{s}$. While all of the radiance from an ideal mirror is at $\vec{s}$, other directions $\vec{e}$ will also receive part of the radiance in the Phong model. The radiance emitted towards $\vec{e}$ is assumed to be proportional to some power of the cosine of the angle between $\vec{s}$ and $\vec{e}$, γ (Fig. 2.3b). This may be described as:

$$L = I_o \cos^n \gamma = I_o(\vec{s} \cdot \vec{e})^n. \tag{2.8}$$

Realistic highlights correspond to $10 \leq n \leq 100$; if $n = \infty$, then Eq. 2.8 degenerates into that for a mirror. However, $n = 1$ does *not* correspond to Lambert's rule, but rather to a physically unrealistic model of illumination.

The complete Phong model includes the term for specular reflection, as well as a term for diffuse (Lambert) reflection and one for ambient (nondirectional) background illumination:

$$L = \underbrace{I_a c_d}_{\text{ambient}} + I_p(\underbrace{c_d(\vec{n} \cdot \vec{l})}_{\text{diffuse}} + \underbrace{c_g(\vec{s} \cdot \vec{a})^n}_{\text{glossy}}). \tag{2.9}$$

In this equation, c_d represents the reflectivity (albedo) for the diffuse reflection. Reflectivity depends on the wavelength of the light, and so the Lambert term must be split up into a sum of terms for various spectral bands, if color is to be modeled. The factor c_g is the reflectivity of the specular term, which does not depend on the wavelength, since specular reflections have the same color as the incident light. I_a is the intensity of the nondirectional (ambient) illumination and I_p is the intensity of the parallel, directional illumination.

2.1.4 Distributed light sources and multiple reflections[*]

In the case of simple reflection, only two rays need be considered: those from the light source to the surface and from the surface to the observer. This simple description is insufficient, however, in the case of multiple reflections (indirect lighting) or of light sources of large angular extent. In the field of computer graphics, algorithms have been developed which permit a complete modeling of all inter-reflections, at least for Lambert surfaces. These algorithms are known as radiosity computations (Greenberg 1989, Foley et al., 1995).

In cases with distributed light sources or multiple reflections, irradiance is a nontrivial function of the direction (ϑ_l, φ_l). The irradiance from a solid angle $\Delta\omega = \sin\vartheta_l \Delta\vartheta_l \Delta\varphi_l$ is, then,

$$E(\vartheta_l, \varphi_l) \sin\vartheta_l \Delta\vartheta_l \Delta\varphi_l.$$

To compute the total irradiance E_{tot} at a point, each directional contribution must be weighted by $\cos\vartheta_l$, since the illuminated surface is foreshortened by this factor with respect to the light source. For each point on the surface, then,

$$E_{tot} = \int_{-\pi}^{\pi} \int_{0}^{\pi/2} E(\vartheta_l, \varphi_l) \sin\vartheta_l \cos\vartheta_l d\vartheta_l d\varphi_l. \tag{2.10}$$

---

[*]This section can be omitted when reading the book for the first time.

E_{tot} is the total irradiance at one point on the surface. When reflection is diffuse, the radiance emitted from this point is the same in all directions, and proportional to irradiance.

Let us assume that the surfaces in the scene are approximated by a set of n planar polygons, each of which emits a power of $\Phi_i, i = 1, ..., n$. This power comprises a reflection term Φ_i^R and, if the surface is a light source, a source term Φ_i^S. Φ_i^R is given by the integral of E_{tot} over all of the points of the surface. Since the reflected light flux is proportional to the illumination due to the Lambert characteristic,

$$\Phi_i^R = c_i \sum_j (\Phi_j^S + \Phi_j^R) F_{ij}. \tag{2.11}$$

Here, c_i is the reflectivity of the surface i and F_{ij} is a "form factor" which depends on the size and orientation of the surface elements i and j to one another; it represents the geometry of the imaged scene. Eq. 2.11 is a linear matrix equation; Φ_i^R results from the solution of this equation for a given distribution of light sources (Φ_i^S). Because of the Lambert characteristic, the radiance of a surface element in the direction of the observer is proportional to the total flux $\Phi_i = \Phi_i^R + \Phi_i^S$.

The radiosity technique allows realistic models of multiple reflections and inter-reflections. In addition, it has an advantage that makes it very suitable for animated walk-throughs of Lambertian scenes: since the light flux does not depend on the direction of the observer, Φ_i has to be determined only once. Once it has been determined, realistic gray levels or color values can be generated for any desired viewpoint. This advantage increases, in particular, the speed of calculation of shaded animations for flight simulators and similar computer applications.

2.2   Imaging systems

Having analyzed reflectivity, we can find the intensity values for individual points in an image. The spatial organization of the image follows from the ray optics of the imaging system, which is the topic of this section.

A basic issue underlies the problem of imaging: each point in a scene sends out light in many different directions (as described by its radiance distribution $L(\vartheta, \varphi)$), while, on the other hand, each point in an image should receive light from only one point in the outside world, or from one direction in space. Two approaches to imaging, both of which exist in nature, can realize this transformation (Fig. 2.4; cf. Land & Fernald 1992).

Collimators are bundles of tubes, each of which transmits light which falls within a certain solid angle determined by the diameters and lengths of the tubes. Depending on how the tubes are positioned, images are projected in different ways. The array shown in Fig. 2.4a produces parallel projection. The tubes could also be located on the surface of a sphere, so that all of their axes meet at a point. In this case, a central projection is generated. The image generated by a collimator is generally upright and in front of the point where the columns of light meet, if they do meet. The field of

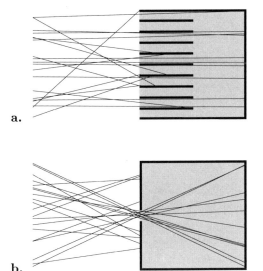

a.

b.

Figure 2.4
Imaging principles. **a.** Collimator. Only light rays which are approximately parallel can pass through a bundle of tubes. It follows that only light from a small solid angle falls on each point in the imaging plane. **b.** Pinhole camera. Unwanted rays are prevented from entering by the mask with its small aperture. Each point of the image plane receives light from a conical region which is defined by the size of the aperture. In the animal kingdom, the principle of the collimator is realized in the complex eyes of insects and crustaceans. Camera-like eyes are found in vertebrates, mollusks and arachnids.

view can be of any angular extent, even a full sphere. The complex eyes of insects and crustaceans provide examples of the collimator principle, though lenses, fiber optics and reflective surfaces improve the performance of these eyes over that of the device sketched in Fig. 2.4a.

In the pinhole camera, one aperture (i.e., the pinhole) acts as the common filtering device for all points in the image. The sharpness, that is, the width of the area in the image which receives light from one point, depends on the size of the aperture. Aside from this limitation, the image is sharp in any plane behind the aperture; in other words, the depth of field is infinite. Since all of the light rays must pass through the aperture, the image in the pinhole camera is a central projection; it is upside down. In the ideal case, the opening is a point. The point is then called the nodal point of the camera, which we designate with the letter N. The field of view is limited to the half-space in front of a plane through the aperture parallel to the image plane since light rays which come from the rear can not enter through the opening. A true pinhole camera eye exists in nature in, for example, the nautilus, a primitive cephalopod. Other animals including vertebrates, other mollusks and arachnids have more highly developed camera eyes with lenses. Goldsmith (1990) and Land & Fernald (1992) survey the structure of eyes in the animal kingdom.

2.2.1 Eyes with lenses

Thin lenses

Pinhole cameras generally produce very dim images, since light is collected only within a very small solid angle. Lenses make it possible to direct more light to a point in

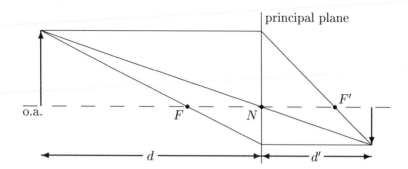

Figure 2.5
Ray diagram for a thin lens. o.a.: optical axis; F, F': front and rear focal points; N: nodal point (center of projection), d: distance to object, d': distance to image. $f = \overline{FN}$ is the focal length of the lens.

the image. For the purpose of ray tracing, a thin lens can be modeled by a *principal plane* at which transmitted rays are bent. The nodal point is then the intersection of the principal plane with the optical axis, that is, the axis of rotational symmetry of the lens surfaces.

The refractive power P of curved boundary surfaces between two media with different indices of refraction n is

$$P := \frac{\Delta n}{r}; \quad [P] = m^{-1} = \text{diopters}. \tag{2.12}$$

Here, r represents the radius of curvature of the refractive surfaces. In the case of a symmetrical thin lens, which has two refractive surfaces of equal refractive power,

$$\frac{1}{d} + \frac{1}{d'} = \frac{1}{f} = \frac{2(n - n_0)}{r} = P. \tag{2.13}$$

Here, d and d' are the distance to the object and to the image, f is the focal length and n_0 is the refractive index of the surrounding medium, $n_0 = 1$ for air. (cf. Fig. 2.5).

The brightness of the image is determined by the angular extent of the lens aperture. The increase in image brightness obtained by using a lens is accompanied by two disadvantages. One is that the location of the image plane (d' in Eq. 2.13), depends on the distance to the object, and so accommodation of the lens is necessary for objects at different distances. This results in a limited depth of field, which, however, can be increased by choosing smaller apertures if illumination is sufficient. The second problem results from aberrations of the lens, most significantly, distortions of the image and chromatic aberration. Chromatic aberration may be compensated by the use of lens systems composed of lenses with differing indices of refraction (achromats). Interestingly, the human eye is not achromatic, a deficit which is held responsible for certain perceptual effects such as color stereopsis.

The imaging characteristics of a thin lens are equivalent to those of a pinhole camera with its center of projection at N.

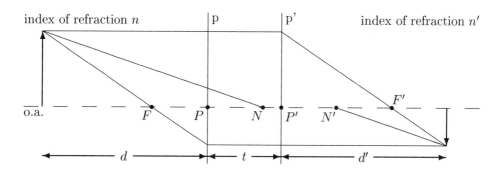

Figure 2.6
Ray tracing in a thick lens. p, p': principal planes, P, P': principal points, N, N': nodal points, F, F': focal points. The focal distances f, f' are the distances $\overline{FP}$ and $\overline{F'P'}$. t: interval (distance between P and P'), d: distance to object, d': image distance. If the refractive index is the same on the image and object sides of the lens, then N coincides with P and N' coincides with P'.

Thick lenses (lens systems)

Thin lenses have no effect on central rays (rays which pass through the nodal point N). Thick lenses do affect central rays. A ray whose angles as it approaches and leaves the lens are the same is displaced along the optical axis as it passes through the lens. The displacement is the "interval" t of the lens.

Ray tracing of a thick lens makes use of the following geometric reference points and planes (Fig. 2.6):

1. The principal plane is divided into two parallel planes, the image or rear principal plane, p' and the object or front principal plane, p. An incident ray from the object side and parallel to the optical axis is, for purposes of analysis, assumed to be refracted at the image principal plane, so that this ray passes through the focal point on the image side. The inverse is true of rays which pass through the focal point of the object side. The intersections of the principal planes with the optical axis are called principal points. The distance which separates them is the "interval" t.

2. The nodal point is also split up into two points, the image or rear nodal point, N' and the object or front nodal point, N. Rays which approach the lens from one of the nodal points, pass through the other nodal point as they move away from the lens. The distance $\overline{NN'}$ between the nodal points is equal to t.

The principal planes are formal construction aids that say nothing about the actual light path inside the lens. In particular, in some lens systems, the locations of the principal planes may be reversed ($t < 0$), or one or both principal planes may lie outside the lens. In the case of a thin lens, p, p' as well as N, N' coincide.

The principal points and nodal points of a lens differ from one another only when the indices of refraction of the media in front of and behind the lens, n and n' are different. If a ray reaches the principal point P at an angle γ to the optical axis, and leaves the principal point P' at an angle γ', then:

$$\frac{\gamma'}{\gamma} = \frac{n}{n'}. \tag{2.14}$$

Lens systems may suffer from an additional type of aberration which does not occur with thin lenses, namely, errors in the centering of the refractive surfaces to a common optical axis. For the purpose of analyzing the imaging properties, however, a thick lens can be modeled well by a pinhole camera with its center of projection at the object (frontal) nodal point N.

The vertebrate eye

Eyes with lenses evolved independently in mollusks and vertebrates. We will here briefly discuss ray tracing in the human eye (Fig. 2.7). In land animals, the largest

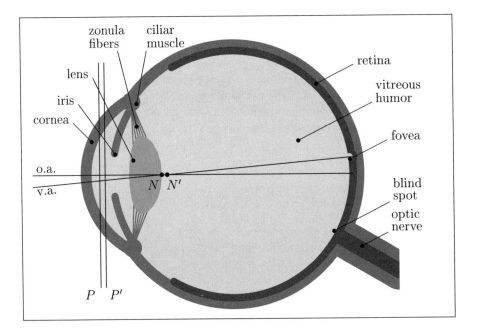

Figure 2.7
Simplified horizontal section through a right eye accommodated for distant vision. P, P': principal planes; N, N': nodal points. o.a.: optical axis. v.a.: visual axis (direction in which the fovea looks). Not labeled: anterior chamber (between the cornea and the iris) and posterior chamber (between the iris and the lens). These two chambers are filled with the aqueous humor.

	accommodation		
	far	any	near
index of refraction			
cornea		1.376	
aqueous humor		1.336	
lens		varying, 1.376 – 1.406	
vitreous humor		1.336	
radius of curvature in mm			
cornea: front side		7.7	
cornea: back side		6.8	
lens: front side	10.0		5.33
lens: back side	-6.0		-5.33
position in mm			
cornea: front side		0.0	
cornea: back side		0.5	
lens: front side	3.6		3.2
lens: back side		7.2	
object focal point F	-15.707		-12.397
image focal point F'	-24.387		21.016
object nodal point N	7.078		6.533
image nodal point N'	7.332		6.847
object principal point P	1.348		1.772
image principal point P'	1.602		2.086
fovea		24.0	
refractive power in diopters			
cornea		43.053	
lens	19.11		33.06
eye	58.636		70.57

Table 2.2
Some optical data on the human eye, after Gullstrand (1908), from Le Grand & El Hage (1980). The refractive index of the lens can not be described by a single quantity, since it varies within the lens.

part of the refractive power of the eye is at the front side of the cornea, and is due to the very different refractive indices of the media on either side of the cornea, air and the aqueous humor. The lens adds relatively little refractive power, but is important for accommodation. The lens is suspended by the zonula fibers, which do not themselves contract, but connect at their outer ends to the ring-shaped ciliar muscle. If the ciliar muscle is relaxed, the opening in the ring is large, and the elasticity of the eyeball stretches the lens into a flattened shape; the eye is accommodated for distance. If the muscle is contracted, the zonula fibers do not pull as strongly, and the elasticity of the lens itself makes it more nearly spherical; the eye is accommodated for near vision.

Some of the optical parameters of the eye are listed in Table 2.2 (cf. Le Grand & El Hage 1980). The refractive surfaces of the eye are centered on the optical axis with a precision of only about ±2 degrees; the fovea, the part of the retina where vision is sharpest, lies 5 degrees temporal of this axis. The axis through the fovea is called the visual axis.

The fibers of retinal ganglion cells which lead to the brain pass across the inner surface of the retina, and the receptor cells are deeper in the surface (cf. Figure 3.3). As a consequence, there can be no receptor cells at the location where the ganglion cell fibers leave the eyeball; at this location, the eye is blind. The blind spot is about 15 degrees away from the centerline of the eye, on the nasal side of the retina. It can easily be found (for example in the left eye) by closing the right eye and holding both arms outstretched with the thumbs held upwards. While looking at the right thumb and moving the left hand slowly away from the right hand horizontally, the left thumb may be made to disappear at a certain point. The retinal image of the left thumb is then on the blind spot.

As a model of the imaging properties of the vertebrate eye, we can again use the pinhole camera with a center of projection at the object nodal point N.

2.2.2   The general camera model

It has been shown in this section that imaging can always be modeled for our purposes in the way sketched out in Fig. 2.8. We will call the system of coordinates $\{\vec{x}, \vec{y}, \vec{z}\}$ with the origin N the camera coordinate system. The vectors $\vec{x}'$ and $\vec{y}'$, along with the intersection of the optical axis and the image plane, establish the coordinates for the image. In the next section, we will examine the mathematics of this model in

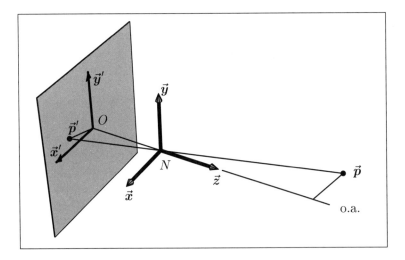

Figure 2.8
Generalized camera model. The image plane is at a right angle to the optical axis (o.a.). The projection center of the nodal point N lies at a distance $f = \overline{NO}$ in front of the image plane. In what follows, it is generally assumed that $f = 1$.

more detail, describing the projection as a mapping

$$\mathcal{P} : \vec{x} \in \mathbb{R}^3 \mapsto \vec{x}' \in \mathbb{R}^2 \tag{2.15}$$

In some cases, we will apply simpler models of projection, such as parallel projection.

In general, the camera model of Fig. 2.8 is defined by means of the following parameters:

1. External parameters of the camera

   (a) Position of the nodal point in space (three degrees of freedom)

   (b) Orientation of the camera coordinate system, as described by a 3×3 orthonormal matrix or three Euler angles (three degrees of freedom)

2. Internal parameters of the camera

   (a) Focal length f (one degree of freedom)

   (b) Position of the intersection of the optical axis with the image plane, in image plane coordinates, e.g., pixels (two degrees of freedom)

In all, then, nine numbers are necessary in order to define the imaging geometry. These numbers can be defined in different ways. For example, if the image plane and the nodal point are known, the optical axis has no independent significance, and can be defined simply as the one normal to the image plane which passes through the nodal point. The total of nine parameters, however, remains unchanged. Additional parameters may be necessary in the case of lens aberrations or of divergence between the normal to the camera target and the optical axis. Determining the camera parameters from images of gauge objects, or from supplemental measurements, is called "camera calibration". See for example Faugeras (1993) for a thorough discussion of the issues involved in this process.

2.3 Perspective projection

Before tackling the mathematics of perspective, note that the glossary at the end of this book explains a number of elementary mathematical concepts.

2.3.1 Projection of points in perspective

Building on the general camera model (Fig. 2.8), we now will examine the rules of perspective, that is, a function $\mathcal{P} : \vec{p} \in \mathbb{R}^3 \mapsto \vec{p}' \in \mathbb{R}^2$, which gives a point in the image $\vec{p}'$ for every point $\vec{p}$ in the outside world. To be precise, only points which are not in a plane which is parallel to the image plane and passes through the center of projection can be centrally projected: that is, points for which $p_3 \neq 0$. (In projective geometry, the projection of such points is, however, permitted. The image plane, extended to include the images of these points, which lie "at infinity," is then called

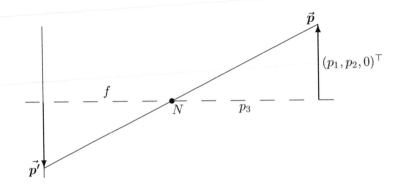

Figure 2.9
Derivation of the formula for central projection. The plane of the page in this figure
is the plane through $\vec{p'}$, O, and $\vec{p}$ in Fig. 2.8.

the *projective plane*.) The result of projection, $\vec{p'}$ is given in image coordinates, that
is, relative to the intersection of the optical axis with the image plane; $\vec{p'}$ has only two
components, p'_1 and p'_2. The construction follows from the parallel proportionality
theorem. For points $\vec{p}$ outside the optical axis, we consider the plane through $\vec{p}$ and
the optical axis (Fig. 2.9). Since $\vec{p}$ and N lie in this plane, the entire ray, and therefore
also the point $\vec{p'}$ of the image, also lie in this plane. The vector $\vec{p'}$ is therefore parallel
to the vector $(p_1, p_2, 0)^\top$, the normal of the optical axis connecting to $\vec{p}$. The length
of $\vec{p'}$ follows from the parallel proportionality theorem

$$\frac{\|\vec{p'}\|}{f} = \frac{\|\vec{p}\|}{p_3}. \tag{2.16}$$

The definition of projection in perspective (central projection) results:

$$\mathcal{P} : \{(p_1, p_2, p_3)^\top \in \mathbb{R}^3 \mid p_3 \neq 0\} \quad \mapsto \quad \mathbb{R}^2$$

$$\vec{p} = \begin{pmatrix} p_1 \\ p_2 \\ p_3 \end{pmatrix} \quad \mapsto \quad \begin{pmatrix} p'_1 \\ p'_2 \end{pmatrix} := -\frac{f}{p_3} \begin{pmatrix} p_1 \\ p_2 \end{pmatrix}. \tag{2.17}$$

Properties of central projection will be discussed in the following sections. We note
here some extensions and special cases of this rule.

1. *General viewing position and gaze direction:*
   If the coordinate systems for the outside world and for the camera are different,
   and, in particular, if the origin of the coordinate system for the outside world
   does not coincide with the center of projection of the camera, the following
   equation holds:

$$\vec{p'} = -\frac{f}{((\vec{p} - \vec{N}) \cdot \vec{z})} \left(\begin{array}{c} ((\vec{p} - \vec{N}) \cdot \vec{x}) \\ ((\vec{p} - \vec{N}) \cdot \vec{y}) \end{array} \right). \tag{2.18}$$

The coordinates of the nodal point and the three quantities which are required in the orthonormal coordinate system $(\vec{x}, \vec{y}, \vec{z})$ correspond to the six external parameters for calibration of a camera.

2. *Parallel projection*
   For many purposes, parallel (or orthographic) projection is satisfactory. In this projection, the $\vec{z}$-components may simply be ignored:

$$\left(\begin{array}{c} p_1 \\ p_2 \\ p_3 \end{array} \right) \mapsto \left(\begin{array}{c} p_1 \\ p_2 \end{array} \right). \tag{2.19}$$

Central projection degenerates into orthographic projection when p_3 goes to $+\infty$ and, at the same time, f goes to $-\infty$, that is, when the image is an enlarged one of a distant object (a telephoto view). The situation is plausible, since the differences in distance p_3 within an object can be neglected if the object is very distant. Another example of parallel projection is that of shadows cast in sunlight, which is parallel.

3. *"Paraperspective Projection"*
   Another approximation of perspective which has many applications is paraperspective (Aloimonos 1988). Around a fixed point $\vec{q}$,

$$\left(\begin{array}{c} p_1 \\ p_2 \\ p_3 \end{array} \right) \mapsto -\frac{f}{q_3} \left[\left(\begin{array}{c} p_1 \\ p_2 \end{array} \right) + \frac{q_3 - p_3}{q_3} \left(\begin{array}{c} q_1 \\ q_2 \end{array} \right) \right]. \tag{2.20}$$

Formally, this is simply a first order Taylor expansion of Eq. 2.17 around the point $\vec{q}$. It can be regarded as a parallel projection of the neighborhood of point $\vec{q}$ onto a frontoparallel plane containing $\vec{q}$ (a plane parallel to the image plane). The resulting image is then projected in central perspective onto the image plane. Since the reference plane was parallel to the image plane, the "central" projection proves only to be a scaling by the factor $-f/q_3$.

2.3.2 Perspective imaging of straight lines

Up to now, we have been examining only the imaging of individual points. We now will examine the imaging of simple geometric figures, starting with straight lines in three-dimensional space.

It is easy to understand that straight lines are generally imaged as straight lines. All light rays for a straight line between the points $\vec{a}$ and $\vec{b}$ which reach the image plane must be in the plane defined by $\vec{a}$, $\vec{b}$ and the nodal point N. Consequently, the

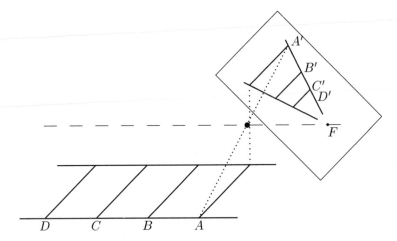

Figure 2.10
Construction of an image in perspective. The "railroad ties" which are parallel to the image plane are represented as parallel line segments, while the images of the "rails" meet at the vanishing point F. (Adapted from a drawing by Penna & Patterson 1986.)

intersection of this plane with the image plane holds the image of the straight lines, and this intersection is the straight line in the image between the points $\vec{a'}$ and $\vec{b'}$.

Let us consider a straight line l:

$$l : \vec{x} = \begin{pmatrix} s_1 \\ s_2 \\ s_3 \end{pmatrix} + \lambda \begin{pmatrix} l_1 \\ l_2 \\ l_3 \end{pmatrix}, \tag{2.21}$$

where $\vec{s}$ is an arbitrary starting point on the line and $\vec{l}$ the direction of the line. The points of l, $\vec{x}$, are projected onto an array of points in the image plane which satisfy the following equation:

$$\vec{x'} = \frac{-f}{s_3 + \lambda l_3} \begin{pmatrix} s_1 + \lambda l_1 \\ s_2 + \lambda l_2 \end{pmatrix}. \tag{2.22}$$

This looks somewhat like the equation for a straight line. However, we must distinguish three cases:

Case 1 : $l_3 = 0, s_3 \neq 0$. In this case, the straight line is parallel to the image plane, like the "railroad ties" in Fig. 2.10. From Eq. 2.22:

$$l' : \vec{x'} = -\frac{f}{s_3} \left[\begin{pmatrix} s_1 \\ s_2 \end{pmatrix} + \lambda \begin{pmatrix} l_1 \\ l_2 \end{pmatrix} \right]. \tag{2.23}$$

This is the full-length representation of a straight line in the image plane.

Case 2 : $\vec{s} = \lambda_0 \vec{l}, l_3 \neq 0$; This is a straight line through N which is not parallel to the image plane. Eq. 2.22 leads to:

$$g' : \vec{x'} = -\frac{f}{(\lambda + \lambda_0)l_3} \begin{pmatrix} (\lambda + \lambda_0)l_1 \\ (\lambda + \lambda_0)l_2 \end{pmatrix} = -\frac{f}{l_3} \begin{pmatrix} l_1 \\ l_2 \end{pmatrix}. \qquad (2.24)$$

In this case, the parameter λ cancels out of the equation. The image of a straight line through the origin is therefore only a single point; the line is viewed "end-on".

Case 3 : Normally, the image of a straight line is a "straight line with one end", that is, a ray. If we designate as $\vec{l}(\lambda) \in \mathbb{R}^3$ the point which is parameterized by λ, then the corresponding image point will move slower and slower as λ increases. In fact, $\vec{l'}(\lambda)$ converges to a *vanishing point**:

$$\lim_{\lambda \to \infty} l'(\lambda) = -\frac{f}{l_3} \begin{pmatrix} l_1 \\ l_2 \end{pmatrix}. \qquad (2.25)$$

The vanishing point does not depend on where the line starts; in other words, the images of all straight lines which are parallel to one another meet at a common vanishing point. In each such group of parallel lines, there is one line passing through the nodal point. This line will be imaged entirely at the vanishing point (case 2). Conversely, every point in the image plane (x', y') is the vanishing point of a set of straight lines, whose direction vector is $(-x', -y', f)^\top$.

Vanishing points have a special meaning in the geometric construction of images in perspective. In painting, constructions which use one, two or three vanishing points are called one-point, two-point and three-point perspective. These terms do not describe different rules of perspective; the difference, rather, is in the orientation of the object being represented relative to the image plane. If one face, and therefore eight edges, of a cube are parallel to the image plane, only one vanishing point is necessary for the construction of the remaining four edges. If only one direction of edges is parallel to the image plane, two vanishing points are necessary, etc.

Fig. 2.11 illustrates this geometric construction of the image of a three-dimensional cube. An additional example is given in Fig. 2.12, in which two groups of lines in a plane, meeting at right angles to each other are imaged. The vanishing points for all directions in a plane lie along a straight line in the image, the *horizon* of this plane. Clearly, parallel planes have the same horizon. If a stack of parallel planes is defined by the normal vector $\vec{n}_o$, then the common horizon of all planes in the stack is the intersection of the image plane with the plane defined by $(\vec{x} \cdot \vec{n}_o) = 0$.

---

*de l'Hospital's rule is used to calculate this limit: if $f(x)$ and $g(x)$ are two functions with $\lim_{x \to \infty} f(x) = \lim_{x \to \infty} g(x) = \infty$ and if limits exist for the derivatives f', g', then, for $\lim g'(x) \neq 0$:

$$\lim_{x \to \infty} \frac{f(x)}{g(x)} = \frac{\lim_{x \to \infty} f'(x)}{\lim_{x \to \infty} g'(x)}.$$

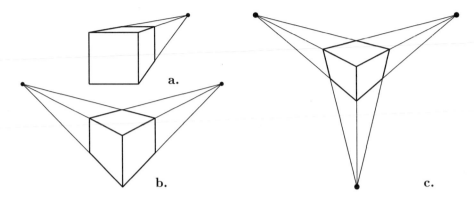

Figure 2.11
Images of a cube in perspective in different orientations to the image plane. **a.** Two of the three directions of edges are parallel to the image plane. Only a single vanishing point is required for construction (*one-point perspective*). **b.** Only one of the directions of edges is parallel to the image plane, and so two vanishing points are needed for the two remaining directions of edges (*two-point perspective*). **c.** None of the three directions of edges is parallel to the image plane; three vanishing points are necessary (*three-point perspective*).

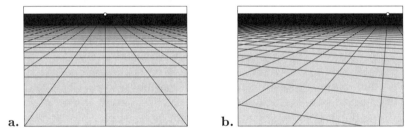

Figure 2.12
Image of a tiled plane **a.** in one-point perspective (one vanishing point in the middle of the image). **b.** in two-point perspective (two vanishing points, one of which is outside of the part of the image plane shown).

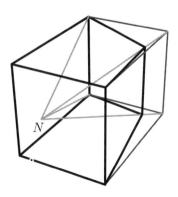

Figure 2.13
The geometric construction of the Ames room. If the polyhedron shown in black is viewed from the point N, it is indistinguishable from the rectangular parallelepiped shown in gray. The odd room with tilted floor and ceiling shown in black is therefore seen as a normal room with right-angled corners. Because of the resulting errors in judging distance, people appear to change size as they move from one side to the other of the back wall, which appears to be parallel to the image plane.

The dimensions of objects in Euclidean geometry are generally not preserved in perspective projection. This applies to length and the area of surfaces; also to angles, parallelism of lines, and other values. An important exception is the (*"cross ratio"*, see below). Topological and qualitative properties such as convexity and the coherence of objects, on the other hand, are maintained in the image.

Perspective imaging can not be reversed, since projection involves the mapping of an entire straight line onto a single point of the imaging plane. This fact is illustrated by a famous optical illusion, the Ames room (Fig. 2.13).

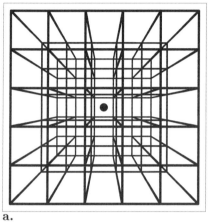

a.

Figure 2.14
Spherical perspective. **a.** Image of a three-dimensional grid in central perspective. The black dot marks the point of view. **b.** Image assembled from images in perspective when looking in different directions (once again indicated by black dots). In each part of the image, straight lines are imaged as straight lines. **c.** Increasing the number of directions of view results in an image in which straight lines are imaged as curves.

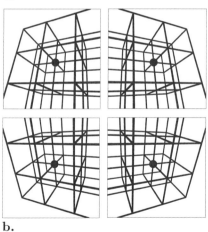

b.

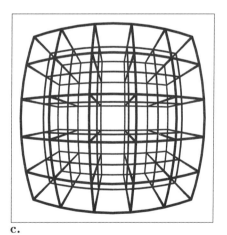

c.

2.3.3 Central projection onto a sphere

Up to now, we have assumed projection onto a plane surface, the image plane. In this type of projection, straight lines are always imaged as straight lines, rays or points, and never as curves. This seems to contradict the perception obtained when standing in a corridor with one's back to one wall and viewing the opposite wall. When asked to produce a perspective drawing of this situation, it is tempting to show the lines where the floor and ceiling intersect the opposite wall as curved lines whose tangents are parallel in the part nearest the point of view, but which converge towards both ends of the corridor. The described image, however, is not in agreement with the laws of perspective and, indeed, no curvature of the edges can be seen in the real world.

The reason for the imagined curvature is that, when the observer is looking toward either end of the corridor, both edge lines converge to a point. That they do is in full agreement with the theory of central perspective. When the observer is looking toward one end, the lines spread apart toward the other end, which is not visible. But if one part of the image is drawn at a time, with the direction of view always in the center of the currently drawn part, curvature actually does occur in the image assembled from these parts (Fig. 2.14). The piecewise construction of the image approximates a projection onto the surface of a sphere described in polar coordinates. It is necessary in this case to define not only the nodal point N but also the vertical axis $\vec{y}$. If r is the distance of a point, φ is its azimuth and ϑ is its elevation or height, then:

$$r = \sqrt{p_1^2 + p_2^2 + p_3^2} = \|\vec{p}\|$$
$$\varphi = \arctan\frac{p_1}{p_3}$$
$$\vartheta = \arctan\frac{p_2}{\sqrt{p_1^2 + p_3^2}}. \tag{2.26}$$

The projection results simply from omitting r. The images of straight lines which do not pass through the nodal point are halves of great circles on the surface of the sphere. The ends of these half-circles correspond to the vanishing points in a projection onto a plane; however, in spherical projection, vanishing points always occur in pairs. We will return to the subject of spherical perspective in Chapter 10 when we examine optical flow.

In Fig. 2.14c, the projection onto the surface of the sphere is stereographically projected onto the plane of the paper. In his well-known drawing "Up and Down," M. C. Escher used a similar geometric construction in which the projection was first onto a cylindrical shell, which was then unrolled into the plane of the paper. (Cf. Ernst, 1976, for a mathematical analysis of this and other drawings by Escher). A thorough treatment of spherical perspective may be found in Flocon & Barre (1987).

2.3.4   Quantitative characteristics

The general analysis of imaging in perspective leads to difficult mathematical problems. Textbooks which provide an introduction to the subject of projective geometry are those of Coxeter (1987) and Penna & Patterson (1986). In this chapter, only two aspects of analytic projective geometry will be discussed briefly.

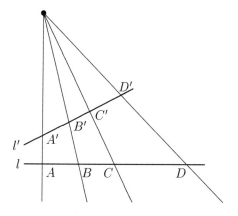

Figure 2.15
The cross ratio is a metrical quantity which is not changed by perspective projection.

The cross ratio

As already mentioned, the cross ratio is a quantity described in Euclidean geometry which is not altered by perspective transformations. If four points A, B, C, D on a straight line l are given, then the cross ratio c is given by the equation

$$c := \frac{\overline{AC}\ \overline{BD}}{\overline{AD}\ \overline{BC}}. \tag{2.27}$$

As is illustrated in Fig. 2.15, the straight line l is represented by the straight line l' after perspective transformation. The cross ratio defined in the same way on l' is unchanged.

Example. One consequence of the invariance of the cross ratio is that perspective along any given line is unambiguously defined by three points. If, for example, the two "rails" in Fig. 2.10, that is, the two straight lines which point away from the observer, and three of the "ties" have been defined, then the position of additional ties is determined by the cross ratio. Let $A, B, C, \ldots$ denote the "ties". If the spacing between the ties is taken to be constant, the cross ratio is then

$$c = \frac{\overline{AC}\ \overline{BD}}{\overline{AD}\ \overline{BC}} = \frac{2 \times 2}{3 \times 1} = \frac{4}{3}.$$

If the distances $\overline{A'B'} = 1$ and $\overline{B'C'} = 1/2$ in the image have been chosen, then $\overline{C'D'}$ results from the relationship

$$\frac{4}{3} = \frac{\overline{A'C'}\ \overline{B'D'}}{\overline{A'D'}\ \overline{B'C'}} = \frac{\frac{3}{2}(\overline{C'D'} + \frac{1}{2})}{(\overline{C'D'} + \frac{3}{2})\frac{1}{2}}$$

$$\overline{C'D'} = \frac{3}{10}.$$

By iteration, the image positions of further ties are determined as well.

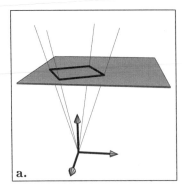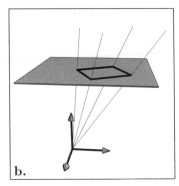

Figure 2.16
Homogeneous coordinates in two dimensions. The homogeneous coordinates of the
corners of a quadrilateral in a plane correspond to the rays from the origin through
these points. The change in position of the quadrilateral in Fig. **b.** corresponds to
a shearing transformation of the ray configuration. This is a linear operation in the
embedding three-dimensional space.

Homogeneous coordinates

Up to this point, we have assumed Cartesian coordinates in the scene and the image
plane. Besides some mathematical difficulties, this assumption has the disadvantage
that the perspective projection has a inconvenient, nonlinear form which is often
difficult to apply in practice. *Homogeneous coordinates* make it possible to simplify
the calculations considerably, especially when different imaging steps are combined.
Homogeneous coordinates are frequently used in computer vision and in robotics.

Homogeneous coordinates are not a transformation of coordinates in the usual
sense, but rather, they represent the embedding of the space being observed (image
plane or three-dimensional space) into a space with more dimensions. For coordinates
in a plane, this means that a point $\vec{x} = (x_1, x_2)^\top$ is identified with the straight
line $(\lambda x_1, \lambda x_2, \lambda)$ through the origin. The image plane is therefore considered to be
the plane $z = 1$ of a three-dimensional coordinate system, and the point (x_1, x_2)
is identified with the straight line through the origin which intersects the plane at
$(x_1, x_2, 1)$ (Fig. 2.16). This process can be applied formally in three-dimensional
space as well, resulting in the following relationships:

Let $\vec{x} = (x_1, x_2, x_3)^\top$ be a point in (projective) space. We designate the *homogeneous representation* of $\vec{x}$ as $\tilde{x}$:

$$
\tilde{x} = \begin{pmatrix} \lambda x_1 \\ \lambda x_2 \\ \lambda x_3 \\ \lambda \end{pmatrix} \quad \text{for } \lambda \in \mathbb{R} \backslash \{0\}. \tag{2.28}
$$

Clearly, the representation in homogeneous coordinates is redundant: for example, $[1, -4, 2, 5]$ and $[2, -8, 4, 10]$ describe the same point. If, conversely, a point $\tilde{y}$ is described in homogeneous coordinates, the Cartesian representation follows:

$$\vec{y} = \begin{pmatrix} y_1/y_4 \\ y_2/y_4 \\ y_3/y_4 \end{pmatrix}. \tag{2.29}$$

Points for which $y_4 = 0$ have no Cartesian representation, yet they are no less elements of projective space.

In the homogeneous representation, a number of transformations which are non-linear in Cartesian coordinates can be described by linear matrix multiplications. In particular, perspective itself and translations, as well as rotations, shear and mirroring, which are always linear, can be described in this way. An example in two dimensions is the conversion of a (nonlinear) translation into a (linear) shear transformation in Fig. 2.16.

In the three-dimensional case, projection onto the image plane $z = -f$ results in:

$$\tilde{x}' = \begin{pmatrix} 1 & 0 & 0 & 0 \\ 0 & 1 & 0 & 0 \\ 0 & 0 & 1 & 0 \\ 0 & 0 & -1/f & 0 \end{pmatrix} \begin{pmatrix} \lambda x_1 \\ \lambda x_2 \\ \lambda x_3 \\ \lambda \end{pmatrix} = \begin{pmatrix} \lambda x_1 \\ \lambda x_2 \\ \lambda x_3 \\ -\lambda x_3/f \end{pmatrix} \rightarrow -\frac{f}{x_3} \begin{pmatrix} x_1 \\ x_2 \\ x_3 \end{pmatrix}. \tag{2.30}$$

Translations, rotations etc. can be described in exactly the same way through appropriate entries in the fourth column of the matrix. The projection formula given here is therefore applicable to any center of projection through simple multiplication of the corresponding matrices. Generally, the term *collineation* is used to describe mappings which are linear in homogeneous coordinates.

2.4 Eye movements

2.4.1 Geometry

Anatomy

The eye is freely mobile in the eye socket (*orbita*) and is moved by the six external eye muscles. The four straight eye muscles (*Mm. recti*) attach to the eyeball above, below and at the nasal and temporal sides. These muscles all pull to the rear, where they form a common, fibrous ring that encircles the optic nerve. In addition, the two oblique eye muscles (*Mm. obliqui*) wrap around the eyeball from above and from below and enable rolling movements. The upper oblique eye muscle (*M. obliquus superior*) arises at the rear of the eye socket, but its direction changes where it passes over a bony hook, (*trochlea*) on the nasal side. The lower oblique muscle passes from the nasal wall of the eye socket directly to the underside of the eyeball. The effects of the various muscles are shown in Fig. 2.17 and Table 2.3. To a first approximation, it can be said that each muscle, with its attachment point, corresponds to a plane of

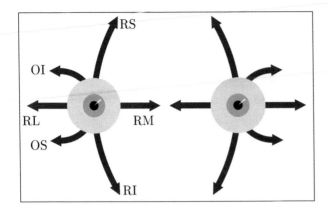

Figure 2.17
Effects of the external eye muscles. RS: *rectus superior*, RI: *rectus inferior*, OI: *obliquus inferior*, OS: *obliquus superior*, RL: *rectus lateralis*, RM: *rectus medialis* (after Hering cf. Kandel et al. 2000)

Table 2.3
The external eye muscles with their innervation and effects. Abduction: motion toward the outside (toward the temple). Adduction: toward the inside (toward the nose). The cerebral nerves which connect to the muscles are: III = *N. oculomotorius*, IV = *N. trochlearis* and VI = *N. abducens*

Muscle	Nerve	Effect
M. rectus superior	III	Raising (greatest when looking to the side); also adduction and rolling inwards.
M. obliquus inferior	III	Raising (greatest when looking across the centerline); also abduction and rolling outwards. Wraps around the bottom of the eyeball from the nasal side.
M. rectus inferior	III	Lowering (greatest when looking to the side); also adduction and rolling outwards.
M. obliquus superior	IV	Lowering (greatest when looking across the centerline); also abduction and rolling inwards. Passes over the *trochlea* where it changes direction.
M. rectus lateralis	VI	Abduction
M. rectus medialis	III	Adduction

rotation and, perpendicular to this, an axis of rotation around which the eyeball can rotate. In reality, the relationships are somewhat more complicated, since the effects of the muscles depend on the position of the eyeball (cf. Hallett 1986).

The eyeball occupies only a small part of the volume of the *orbita*. At the rear, it is supported by Tenon's capsule (the *vagina bulbi*), through which pass the optic nerve and the straight eye muscles. Together with a bed of fatty tissue, Tenon's capsule resists the rear-ward component of the forces exerted by the *Mm. recti*.

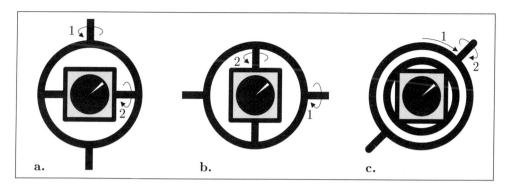

Figure 2.18
Degrees of freedom of rotation of camera systems and eyes. The square in the center with the pupil represents the camera. **a.** Fick system. The primary rotation is around the vertical axis, and the secondary is around a horizontal axis which rotates with the vertical one. **b.** Helmholtz system. The primary rotation is around the horizontal axis, and the secondary is around the vertical axis which rotates with the horizontal one. **c.** Listing system. The camera is suspended in a ring. The primary rotation affects only the external ring and establishes the axis of rotation. The secondary rotation pivots the entire system around the axis thus established. The third degree of freedom in all three systems, rolling around the axis of vision, is omitted.

Degrees of freedom

As a solid body, the eyeball theoretically has six degrees of freedom to move, three of which are translational and three rotational. Since the eyeball moves as if in a spherical socket within Tenon's capsule and cushioned by its bed of fat, the translational motion is small. A fairly well-defined center of rotation exists, though this can change by one to two millimeters as the eye rotates. The center of rotation lies between 13 and 15 mm behind the cornea and therefore about 5 mm behind the nodal point. Eye movements are therefore not pure rotations as defined for purposes of imaging geometry.

This fact can be proven by a simple experiment. When looking far to the right with the left eye, the right index finger is positioned so it just disappears behind the bridge of the nose. Then, when looking straight ahead without moving the finger, the finger will become visible in one's peripheral vision. It could not become visible if the center of rotation and the eye's nodal point were the same.

In what follows, we will ignore the minor translational movements and examine the rotational degrees of freedom. From first principles, rotations in space are defined by three angles, but different sets of angles may be used. Here, we will discuss three systems of coordinates that can be used to describe eye movements (Fig. 2.18). These systems of coordinates are also useful in the design of artificial camera systems (cf. Murray et al. 1992).

1. Fick coordinates. In Fick coordinates, the primary rotation is around a vertical axis, and the secondary is around a horizontal axis which is carried along
   with the vertical axis. The third rotation is rolling around the axis of vision
   established by the other two rotations. Rolling does not change the axis of
   vision.

2. Helmholtz coordinates. In this system, the order of the first two rotations is
   reversed. The primary rotation is around the horizontal axis, and the secondary
   is around the vertical axis, which rotates with the horizontal axis. The tertiary
   rotation is rolling around the axis of vision. Helmholtz coordinates have the
   advantage that the primary axis of rotation of both eyes is the same for binocular
   vision. In camera systems, this means that both cameras can be mounted on a
   common horizontal axis.

3. Listing-coordinates. The primary axis of rotation is fixed in the two systems
   already described, but in the Listing system, an axis of rotation is first adjusted
   so as to allow the direction of vision to be turned from the rest position to the
   desired direction in one step. The rotation therefore takes the shortest possible
   path: the pupil travels in a great circle. Here also, the tertiary rotation is rolling
   around the axis of vision. If $\vec{r}_o$ is the axis of vision in its rest position and $\vec{r}_1$
   is the desired axis, then the shortest path is rotation around the axis $\vec{d}$, which
   is at right angles to the two vectors, $(\vec{d} = \vec{r}_o \times \vec{r}_1)$. All of these vectors lie in
   a plane at right angles to $\vec{r}_o$. Since $\vec{r}_o$ points directly forward, this "Listing's
   plane" is orthogonal to the principal direction of gaze.

The rolling around the axis of vision which is the third step in all three systems
has no effect on the information available to the retina. Still, it is desirable that the
roll position of the eye at a given direction of vision does not depend on the way in
which this direction was reached. If this were not the case, the image for the same
direction of vision could be considerably different at different times. In fact, Donders'
Law in physiology states that the roll angle of the eye is always the same for a given
direction of vision, regardless of how this direction was reached. During fixation,
Donders' law is accurate to about ±6 minutes of arc of roll angle. In camera systems,
independence of the roll angle from the path is achieved simply enough by using the
Fick or Helmholtz system and omitting the third degree of freedom.

Though the Helmholtz system is most commonly used in the design of stereoscopic camera systems, the Listing system is the one which occurs in nature. This
is demonstrated by experiments which show that the roll angle of the eye is always
the same as if it had turned by the shortest possible path from the rest position to
any other position (Listing's law). This law holds even when the rotation does *not*
start from the rest position. The eye must, therefore, carry out compensatory rolling
movements. Listing's law does not follow from the geometry of the eye and of its
muscles, but is neuronally controlled.

Table 2.4

Types of eye movements

	abrupt (fast)	smooth (slow)
conjugate	saccades, fast phase of nystagmus	smooth pursuit, slow phase of optokinetic and vestibular nystagmus
disjunctive		convergence and divergence

2.4.2 Types of eye movements

Types of eye movements may be identified based on two criteria (cf. Hallett 1986). Fast (abrupt) and slow (smooth) movements are distinguished according to their speed. Same-direction (conjugate) eye movements or *versions* are distinguished from opposite-direction (disjunctive) movements or *vergence* movements. An overview of different types of eye movements is given in Table 2.4.

Saccades or jumps between directions of view are abrupt, conjugate eye movements, which can reach speeds of 20 – 600 degrees per second and which last between 20 and 100 milliseconds. Saccades are the only eye movements which can be carried out voluntarily and which can also be suppressed, though there are also involuntary saccades.

Smooth pursuit movements occur when a small object's motion is being followed, and can reach approximately 20 to 30 degrees per second. If the object moves more rapidly, saccades are interspersed in order not to lose the object. Smooth pursuit movements can not be carried out voluntarily. If an attempt is made to carry out such a movement with the eyes, what occurs is not a smooth pursuit movement but a number of small saccades. This fact can be demonstrated easily by closing the eyes and placing the tips of the index and middle fingers lightly on the eyelids. The intermittent motion of the eyes can be felt through the eyelids. If one eye is then opened and a real object is followed, for example one's own finger, the smooth motion of the other eye can be felt through the eyelid.

Other smooth, conjugate eye movements are compensatory eye movements which hold the direction of vision constant in spite of movements of the head and body. A distinction is made between *vestibular* movements which arise in response to stimuli from the semicircular canals in the inner ears, and *optokinetic* movements, which arise in response to large visual stimuli. If the stimulus continues for a long time (for example, when rotating in a swivel chair or looking out the window of a railroad car), the smooth compensatory movement is periodically interrupted by abrupt movements in the opposite direction. The combination of smooth pursuit movements and abrupt restoring movements is called nystagmus.

Vergence movements   are smooth eye movements in opposite directions, and can reach speeds of approximately 10 degrees per second. There are no abrupt eye movements in opposite directions, though the distances of saccades in the two eyes can be slightly different, so that they include a vergence component (Collewijn et al. 1997, Enright 1998). Vergence movements are closely related to stereoscopic depth vision and will be discussed in connection with that topic. They also are closely linked to accommodation in that the axes of vision intersect in a distance range in which imaging is sharpest.

Residual movements during fixation.   If a point is fixated, the axes of vision of the two eyes are directed at this point, which is imaged in the fovea, the part of the retina with the highest resolution (cf. Chapter 3). Fixation is not held exactly, but rather is broken up slightly by residual movements in each eye. The *microtremor* is a rapid, trembling movement whose amplitude is approximately half a minute of arc, at a frequency of 30 to 100 Hz. This amplitude corresponds approximately to the spacing of receptors in the fovea. *Microsaccades* with amplitudes of about 5 minutes of arc (extreme values of 2 to 28 minutes of arc) occur about once or twice per second. Finally, the eyes drift during fixation, at a rate of approximately 4 minutes of arc per second. The drift is compensated about once or twice per second by the microsaccades. Binocular residual movements are not fully conjugate.

Part II

Contrast, Form, and Color

Vision and image processing are processes which start with images and recover various types of data from them. In this part of the book, we will consider intensity data, which is present for each pixel. The product of image processing is itself a kind of image, and generally differs from the original image in that certain aspects are emphasized and others are suppressed. In contrast, depth perception primarily generates maps of depth values, and motion perception primarily generates maps of motion vectors. Neither of these representations is itself image-like.

Image processing is closely related to the concept of neighborhood operations; that is, to the calculation of neighboring intensity values. Two examples of this type of processing are local averaging (low-pass filtering) to reduce noise, and local differentiation to increase contrast. These concepts originated with the Austrian physicist Ernst Mach (1838 – 1916), who applied them to the study of perceptual effects such as lateral inhibition. In neurobiology, the corresponding concept is that of the receptive field (Kuffler 1953). Generalization to more complex patterns of lateral interactions (not just lateral inhibition) leads to the concept of the extraction of features: each neuron, through its receptive field, is regarded as establishing whether a specific image feature is present (Lettvin et al. 1959). The early development of the discipline of image processing was decisively influenced by these concepts.

Chapter 3 describes some of the fundamental processes of image processing, as well as the most important issues and experimental results concerning image resolution. The optical resolution limit of the eye is not as central to this discussion as is the question of the fineness of resolution at which a particular image processing operation is best performed; or to put it another way, how large the scope of the neighborhood operations should be. Obviously the limit of resolution is set by the optical characteristics of the imaging device. Coarser resolution may, however, be of advantage for some types of processing. Human vision makes use of this approach.

Edge detection is part of image processing, but is discussed in a chapter of its own (Chapter 4) because of its great practical importance. Edge detection will be used as an example of how filters for image processing are constructed.

In computer processing of images, color still plays a relatively minor role. But in the human visual system, the perception of relative brightness can not meaningfully be distinguished from that of color. Since, in addition, color vision is one of the most striking capabilities of the sense of vision, it deserves thorough examination. Mathematical approaches have a long tradition in the study of color vision. In Chapter 5 we will discuss the application of linear algebra in the trichromatic theory of color vision. Another theoretical issue that can be clearly illustrated in color vision is population coding, an approach which has many applications in perceptual psychology and which has far-reaching consequences for information processing in general.

Chapter 3

Representation and processing of images

Images are two-dimensional arrays of brightness and color values (Fig. 1.2). This very general definition can be made more concrete in various ways using different branches of mathematics, each leading to different possibilities for manipulating images—that is, for image processing. This chapter will explore some of the basic issues relative to this topic; for reference, see Ballard & Brown (1982), Rosenfeld & Kak (1982), and Pratt (1991). In later chapters, we will return frequently to the topics of representation and processing of images as we examine more concrete problems. At the end of this chapter, we will examine the topic of resolution, which is closely related to those of representation and processing.

Table 3.1
Different models of images (representations) allow different mathematical and computing techniques to be applied.

image model	applicable mathematical tools
analog intensity functions	analysis and functional analysis
temporal and spatial sampling (pixels)	linear algebra
quantization of the gray values	numerical techniques
point sets	set theory; mathematical morphology
random fields	stochastics
lists of image features	logic and artificial intelligence

3.1   Examples

Table 3.1 lists a variety of possibilities used in image representation together with the applicable mathematics. Some examples include:

Intensity functions: The intensity of an image can be represented as an analog function of location in the image (and also of time; cf. Fig. 9.1). If the spectral composition of the light which illuminates each point of the image is also considered, then in the most general sense, an entire spectrum—that is, another function—must be considered at every point in the image. Since human color vision as well as standard color cameras and monitors employ three spectral channels, a representation as a vector with three components is, however, sufficient. The components represent the activity in three classes of receptors sensitive, for example, to red, green and blue light. Clearly, intensity values are not negative; we will always assume that they fall within the range $[0, 1]$. Images are therefore functions from a two-dimensional space, or from three-dimensional space-time into the set of intensities or color vectors:

$$\mathbb{R}_x \times \mathbb{R}_y \times \mathbb{R}_t \mapsto \left\{ \begin{array}{ll} [0, 1] & \text{gray value image} \\ [0, 1]^3 & \text{color image} \end{array} \right. \tag{3.1}$$

Here, the indices x, y and t represent the appropriate variable names.

Sampling in time and space: In the process of image capture, spatially sampled representations of the analog gray value function are acquired both in biological and most man-made systems (e.g., CCD cameras). Sampling always occurs at discrete points or in "sampling windows." The points in the image are called *pixels* (abbreviated from picture element). In artificial systems, the time axis is usually also sampled, for example at the video frame rate of 30 Hertz. The representation of time in biological systems is theoretically continuous; nonetheless, the release of action potentials at the output of the retina occurs at discrete times, but with no fixed rate and no synchronization among nerve fibers.

Quantization of gray value and color: Intensity, as well, can generally not vary continuously; rather, it takes on discrete values. In computer vision systems, 8 bits are commonly available, making it possible to represent a $2^8 = 256$ step gray scale or $2^{3 \times 8} = 16,777,216$ colors.

Point sets: Quantization with only one bit per pixel results in binary (0/1) images: black and white images without gray scale steps. Such images can be represented as point sets, for example, as the set of all black pixels. This representation makes it possible to apply the technique of mathematical morphology to image processing (cf. section 3.3.2).

Random fields: The intensity value of each pixel may be regarded as a random variable; means and correlations are then examined. One especially important technique based on this approach is the Karhunen-Loève-transform, which uses principal component analysis to identify repeated patterns in the image (cf. Rosenfeld & Kak 1982, Mardia et al. 1979). Another application of stochastics is the examination of the image as a Markov random field. In this case, the concept of the Markov chain is expanded to two dimensions; each pixel is examined as a random variable in a random field, and dependencies are restricted to the immediate neighborhood of that pixel. Stochastic descriptions are used most commonly in noise reduction, image compression, image segmentation (Geman & Geman 1984, Blake & Zisserman 1987) and pattern recognition.

Sketches and symbolic descriptions: Sketches are lists of primitives or features and their locations in the image. Edge elements and intersections of contours are types of features which are frequently used. Sketches in the usual sense of the word include only such features, but are often easier to recognize than the original image. More complex elements lead to more general symbolic descriptions. Such symbolic descriptions of an image may be regarded on the one hand as results, or on the other hand as input data for further information processing. If, for example, a particular object—for example, the letter "G"—is found in the image, then the "representation" ("the image is of a capital 'G' ") is the result of the image processing. In general, it is not possible to distinguish clearly between representations and processing steps.

Physical nature: If image processing is carried out in hardware, the type of image processing must reflect the physical nature of the image signal. Examples are analog electronics for video signals, optical image processing using coherent light (Feitelson 1988) and the processing of visual information in the nervous system.

The following definitions are generally applicable: a representation is data about an image in an appropriate form for the type of information processing which is to be performed. Information processing can then be regarded as the calculation of specific, better representations. Marr (1982) calls this the "making explicit" of information. One danger of this approach is that the construction of representations, that is, the description of the environment, is seen itself as a goal of information processing. In a behavior-oriented approach, on the other hand, representations are subjugated to the requirement that they be useful for the generation and control of behavior.

3.2 Sampling

3.2.1 Uniform sampling grids

Images are always quantized spatially, in natural vision as well as in computer vision: that is, images are represented as grids of pixels. The pixels are considered to be either small patches of a plane (rectangles, hexagons) or the center or corner points of such patches. Since image processing operations always are based on comparison between neighboring pixels, the pixel grids and the proximities which they define are of great importance.

Cartesian grids. The simplest and therefore almost universally applied grid is the Cartesian grid, Fig. 3.1a. Often, the pixels are not square, and so the horizontal and vertical resolutions differ.

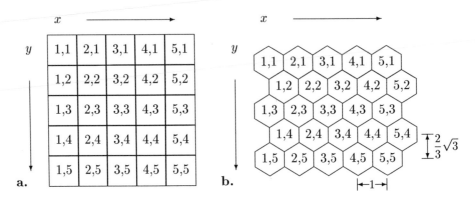

Figure 3.1
Equally-spaced sampling grids **a.** Cartesian **b.** Hexagonal

There are two possible ways to define adjacency in the Cartesian grid. Two pixels may be designated as neighbors if they have an edge in common. In this case, each pixel (except those along the margins of the image) has four immediate neighbors:

$$\mathcal{N}_4(x_o, y_o) := \{(x, y)|\ |x_0 - x| + |y_0 - y| = 1\}. \tag{3.2}$$

If pixels which only have a corner in common are also considered adjacent, then each pixel has eight neighbors:

$$\mathcal{N}_8(x_o, y_o) := \{(x, y)|\ \max(|x_0 - x|, |y_0 - y|) = 1\}. \tag{3.3}$$

Neither of these definitions is fully satisfactory in the context of actual patterns in images. A checkerboard pattern, for example, leads to the following paradox: if we regard only pixels with a common edge as adjacent, then neither the white nor the black squares are seen as forming connected patterns. If we use 8 pixel neighborhoods, then both the black and white squares are seen as forming connected patterns.

Hexagonal grid.   In this case, there is only one type of adjacency, in which two pixels have an edge in common; for this reason, there are no conceptual difficulties like those with rectangular pixels. A grid of rectangular pixels in a pattern like a brick wall, with each row offset from the next by a half pixel, is topologically equivalent to a hexagonal grid.

If the pixels are numbered with the suffixes i, j then the positions of the pixels of the hexagonal grid in (Fig. 3.1b) are given by:

$$x_{i,j} = \begin{cases} ai & \text{if } j \text{ is even} \\ a(i + \frac{1}{2}) & \text{if } j \text{ is odd} \end{cases},$$

$$y_{i,j} = \frac{a}{2}\sqrt{3}j. \tag{3.4}$$

Here, a is the distance between the centers of two neighboring pixels.

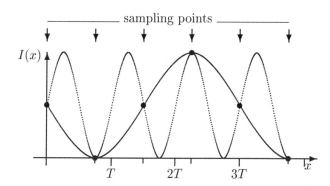

Figure 3.2
Sampling of a periodic pattern using a sampling frequency which is too low. An alias results, with a frequency which was not originally present in the image. High frequency pattern: signal. Low-frequency pattern: alias.

Sampling theorem. It is easy to see that image structures which are finer than the sampling grid can be reproduced only imperfectly if at all. The exact relationship between the sampling grid and the image content is described by the sampling theorem. Here, we examine a one-dimensional example (Fig. 3.2). Details can be found in image processing textbooks, e.g., Rosenfeld & Kak (1982).

Consider a striped pattern, as defined by the periodic intensity function $I(x) = (1 + \sin(\omega x))/2$ with a frequency of $\omega = \frac{2\pi}{T}$. T is the wavelength. We now sample this pattern at discrete values of x with a uniform separation $\Delta x = \frac{3}{4}T$. The distance between these points is called the sampling rate. The intensity values at the points $i\Delta x$ form a pattern which is significantly different from the original pattern; the name *alias* is given to the new pattern. As Fig. 3.2 shows, this is once again a periodic pattern, but with a frequency of $\omega_a = \frac{2\pi}{3T}$. It is easy to see that the highest frequency which can be correctly represented is $\frac{2\pi}{2\Delta x}$ or in other words, that two sampling points per period are necessary (the Nyquist limit).

Undersampling not only fails to represent some of an image's content, but even more disturbingly results in the generation of false patterns (aliases). Generation of such false patterns must be forestalled before sampling, for example by low-pass filtering. In the case illustrated in Fig. 3.2, such filtering would result in no detectable remaining signal to sample. So-called Moiré-patterns, which can be seen in draperies, are related to alias patterns. If one layer of cloth lies on top of another, then one layer serves more or less as the sampling filter for the other. Low-frequency patterns result, and these change markedly when the fabric moves only slightly.

3.2.2   Space-variant sampling

The retina

The vertebrate retina consists of several layers of cells which play different roles in the sampling and preprocessing of the image. Here, we will describe only the most important types of cells and their roles in imaging. A detailed description of the retinal neurons and their connections can be found in Wässle & Boycott (1991).

Receptor cells. Transformation of light into a neuronal signal occurs in the receptor cells. In humans and most mammals, there are two types. The *cones* function at relatively high levels of lighting (photopic vision). Their selective response to different wavelengths makes color vision possible. The *rods* function at low levels of lighting, for example, on moonless nights (scotopic vision) and are color blind. In an intermediate luminance range from about 10^{-3} to 10^2 candela per square meter, both the cone and the rod vision are active. In this case, vision is said to be mesopic.

The resolution of the image is limited by the density of receptors. Primates have a particularly specialized area of the retina, the optical pit or *fovea centralis* (Fig. 2.7), in which the density of receptors is especially high. In a central area approximately 1/3 degree across (*foveola*), there are only cones, in a nearly perfect hexagonal array. Their separation is about 30 seconds of arc, the same as the optical limit of resolution of the eye. There are no rods at the center of the fovea; rods reach their highest density approximately 20 degrees away from the fovea(cf. Fig. 3.3b). The total number of cones in the human eye is approximately 6 million, and that of the rods is approximately 120 million.

Connecting neurons. Between the receptive layer and the "output layer" of the retina, there is a layer of three types of neurons, the *bipolar, horizontal* and *amacrine-cells*. The bipolar cells pass through the retina, connecting the receptor cells to the

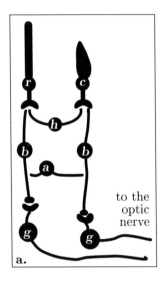 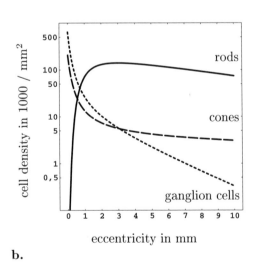

Figure 3.3
a. the most important types of cells in the retina and their connections. **a** Amacrine cell; **b** Bipolar cell; **g** Ganglion cell; **h** Horizontal cell; **r** Rod; **c** Cone. **b.** Density of cones, rods and ganglion cells in the retina of the rhesus monkey *Maccaca mulatta* as a function of distance from the fovea. After Wässle & Boycott 1991.

ganglion cells. Both other types of cells connect mostly laterally. The horizontal cells connect primarily between receptor cells and between the distal ends of bipolar cells; the amacrine cells connect between ganglion cells and between the proximal ends of bipolar cells. Complex spatial and temporal interactions between the levels of stimuli to the individual receptors take place in this network. Nerve conduction in this network is as analog signals; action potentials are not released until the signals reach the ganglion cells.

Ganglion cells. The nerve fibers which lead from the retina to the brain are the axons of the *ganglion cells*, which are connected to the receptor cells directly through the bipolar cells, and indirectly through the entire network. Three types of ganglion cells can be distinguished according to their morphological and physiological characteristics. These are called α (large cells, fast reaction time, physiologically "Y"), β (smaller cells, slower reaction time, physiologically "X") and γ (small cells with a sparse though extensive dendrite tree, weak action potentials, physiologically "W"). There are no ganglion cells in the fovea itself; those which serve the fovea are located outside the fovea in order to improve optical imaging. In the rhesus monkey, the density of ganglion cells reaches 50,000 per mm^2 at the margins of the fovea and falls to about 100 per mm^2 at 40 degrees away from the fovea. The fall in the density of ganglion cells is intermediate between that of the cones and rods. In the cat, the total number of retinal ganglion cells is approximately 150,000; in primates, 1.5 million. This is the number of fibers in the optic nerve and the number of image points which reach the brain. While the resolution may seem rather low as compared with that achieved in artificial systems, it must be noted that the signal in each individual fiber has been preprocessed and therefore holds more information than an individual camera pixel usually does.

Visual cortex

In the visual cortex, information from the different parts of the retina is systematically ordered, resulting in what is called a retinotopic map or image. This image can be charted by recording from cortical neurons using an electrical probe and then determining which location on the retina delivers peak stimulation to each cortical location. The cortex of primates has a large number (> 20) of areas each one of which contains a more or less retinotopic image of the retina.

If it is assumed that each retinal ganglion cell corresponds to the same amount of space in the cortex, then the spatial distribution of the ganglion cells results in a distortion of the cortical image such that the retinal areas with a lower density of ganglion cells are represented by smaller amounts of cortical tissue. If $\varrho(x,y)$ represents the density of ganglion cells and $\mathcal{R}$ represents the imaging function described by the retinotopic map, then the hypothetical equal representation of all ganglion cells can be formulated as follows:

$$\varrho(x,y) = const.|\det J_{\mathcal{R}}(x,y)|. \tag{3.5}$$

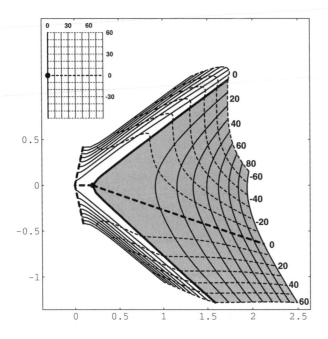

Figure 3.4
Retinotopic imaging of the right visual field onto the left visual cortex of the cat. Inset: coordinates in the visual field. Gray shading: the primary visual cortex (area V1), and to its left, the crescent-shaped area V2. The drawing shows an analytical model of the mapping (Mallot 1985), based on measurements by Tusa et al. (1979).

Here, $|\det J_{\mathcal{R}}|$ is the cortical magnification factor (for an explanation of the mathematics, cf. Section 8.3.2).

Equation 3.5 is fairly accurate for actual cortical retinotopic maps: the cortical magnification factor corresponds to the ganglion cell density in the retina (cf. Wässle et al. 1990). However, there is generally not a unique solution of Equation 3.5 for $\mathcal{R}$. For some interesting specific cases, cf. Mallot & Giannakopoulos (1996).

Fig. 3.4 gives an analytical approximation of the retinotopic maps of areas V1 and V2 in the cat. In area V1 of primates, there are more pronounced distortions, which can be modeled as a transformation into logarithmic polar coordinates (Fischer 1973, Schwartz 1980). If Cartesian coordinates are chosen for the mapping of the retina and the cortex, this transformation may be expressed as:

$$\mathcal{P}(x,y) = \begin{pmatrix} \frac{1}{2}\log(x^2 + y^2) \\ \arctan \frac{y}{x} \end{pmatrix}. \tag{3.6}$$

If retinal and cortical locations are described in complex coordinates, $z = x + iy$, then $\mathcal{P}$ turns out to be the complex logarithmic function. The magnification factor decreases, then, as the inverse square of distance from the fovea.

Space-variance in computer vision systems

Sensors with nonuniform characteristics are appropriate when the image, or the image structure of interest, has systematic spatial variations. If, for example, the observer moves on a ground plane, there is a fixed relationship between the height of a point in the image and the distance of the object. In this case, spatial variation in the sampling rate can, for example, make the resolution of the ground plane constant. An application of this idea to obstacle avoidance is described in Section 6.3.4.

For cameras and eyes in motion, the most important source of systematic spatial variation is the motion itself. If, for example, an object is being tracked, the image of the object remains centered, while large motions occur in the peripheral parts of the image. Saccadic eye movements make it possible for only the fovea to have a high density of receptors, and to deploy this high density as needed. In active camera heads, spatially nonuniform sensors are often used, and for this same reason. Such sensors are especially useful when the spatial variance is realized in hardware design of the camera target (Tistarelli & Sandini 1992). As a rule, the complex logarithmic function, Equation 3.6, is used in determining the non-uniformity.

3.3 Image processing

Once an image exists as a sampled array of gray levels, various image processing operations may be performed on it in order, for example, to detect particular objects or to make them more distinct. Image processing is a broad discipline which can not be fully described here. Textbooks are Rosenfeld & Kak (1982), Pratt (1991) or Duda & Hart (1973).

3.3.1 Convolution

Discrete convolution

The most common image processing operation is *discrete convolution*. Consider, as a simple example, an image sampled in a Cartesian grid, which may be described as an array of gray levels, $\{g_{ij}\}$. If it is desired to "smooth" the image, that is, to make it less sharp and so to reduce noise, a new image $\{h_{ij}\}$ may be generated by processing each pixel (i, j) with relation to its immediate neighbors; for example,

$$h_{i,j} := \frac{1}{5}(g_{i,j} + g_{i-1,j} + g_{i+1,j} + g_{i,j-1} + g_{i,j+1}). \tag{3.7}$$

The contrast between pixels may be increased by subtracting from each pixel the average gray value of its neighbors: for example

$$h_{i,j} := g_{i,j} - \frac{1}{4}(g_{i-1,j} + g_{i+1,j} + g_{i,j-1} + g_{i,j+1}). \tag{3.8}$$

The formula must be modified for pixels at the edge of the image. As a rule, the gray values for pixels outside the image are simply set to zero.

In these examples, the influence of a pixel g_{ij} on a pixel h_{kl} in the new image depends only on the difference in their coordinates $(k - i, l - j) = (m, n)$; in other words, the same operation is performed at every location in the image. Operations of this type are called "space-invariant" or "translation-invariant." This type of operation may be described most generally by assigning a "weight" c_{nm} to each difference in coordinates (m, n). The weight describes how the pixel being considered affects another. The matrix $\{c_{nm}\}$ may be called a *template* or *mask*, or the *kernel* of the convolution. Discrete convolution can then be notated as:

$$h = g * c,$$

$$h_{kl} = \sum_{m=-M}^{M} \sum_{n=-N}^{N} c_{m,n} g_{k-m,l-n}. \tag{3.9}$$

The two examples already given, (Equation 3.7 and 3.8) therefore may be described by the masks:*

$$c_{nm} = \begin{array}{|c|c|c|} \hline 0 & 1/5 & 0 \\ \hline 1/5 & 1/5 & 1/5 \\ \hline 0 & 1/5 & 0 \\ \hline \end{array} \text{ and } c_{nm} = \begin{array}{|c|c|c|} \hline 0 & -1/4 & 0 \\ \hline -1/4 & 1 & -1/4 \\ \hline 0 & -1/4 & 0 \\ \hline \end{array}. \tag{3.10}$$

The operation described in equation 3.9 is called *discrete convolution* or *discrete filtering*. As a rule, the mask is much smaller than the image which is being processed. However, if its array indexing is chosen appropriately, the mask may itself also be regarded as an "image". In fact, the intensity of the output image h is maximized when the original image g and the mask are locally identical (cf. the Cauchy-Schwarz inequality in linear algebra). A mask used in this way to find a pattern in the original image is called a *matched filter*.

Mathematically, the set of all gray values tables $\{g_{i,j}\}$, $1 \leq i \leq I, 1 \leq j \leq J$ (i.e. sampled images) constitutes a vector space of $I \times J$ dimensions; discrete convolution defines a linear mapping of this space into itself. Without giving proofs, we will note some of the important characteristics of discrete convolution.

1. *Commutativity:* by choosing the indices appropriately, it may be shown that the image and the mask in Equation 3.9 can be substituted for one another,

$$g * c = c * g. \tag{3.11}$$

2. *Linearity:* If convolution is considered as a mapping in an image space, then the operation is linear. As usual, an operation is said to be linear if the following relations hold:

$$(f + g) * c = f * c + g * c; \quad (\lambda f) * c = \lambda(f * c). \tag{3.12}$$

Here, $\lambda \in \mathbb{R}$ is a real number, f and g are images and c is a convolution mask. Addition of images and multiplication by λ are on a pixel-by-pixel basis.

3. *Associativity:* If g is an image and c, d are two masks, then

$$(g * c) * d = g * (c * d). \tag{3.13}$$

---

*We write masks as "tables" rather than matrices to make clear that they are not matrices in the sense of linear algebra, cf. Table 3.2.

Table 3.2
Convolution operations and linear algebra

linear algebra	image processing
vector	image, mask; the vector space has $I \cdot J$ dimensions
linear mapping a) "Toeplitz" matrix: $m_{ij} = m_{pq}$ if $i - j = p - q$. A single row of this matrix corresponds to the convolution mask, extended by zeroes at the margins.	convolution with a mask (space-invariant)
b) Orthonormal (unitary) matrix (coordinate transformation)	integral transform (e.g. Fourier transform)
c) any matrix	any linear mapping, may be space-variant.
dot product	correlation

This type of image processing is, then, largely an application of linear algebra. Each pixel corresponds, however, to one vector component, and so the "matrix" representation of images and masks must not be confused with the matrices of linear algebra. If the convolution of an image by means of a mask is formulated algebraically, the image is described as a vector with $I \cdot J$-dimensions, and the convolution results in an $(I \cdot J \times I \cdot J)$-matrix. As a result of translational invariance, the matrix is highly redundant, since each row has the same coefficients, only displaced by one column (this is sometimes called a Toeplitz matrix). A summary of these issues may be found in Table 3.2.

Convolution of continuous functions

The equivalent of discrete convolution for images described as continuous two-dimensional gray value functions is an analog, continuous operation. As the size of pixels goes to zero, Equation 3.9 approaches:

$$h(x, y) = \int \int c(x', y') g(x - x', y - y') dx' dy'. \tag{3.14}$$

The range of the integration is the entire plane; however, the image and mask values are set to zero outside a finite region. A continuous expression may serve as an approximation for images with large number of pixels, and is mathematically more tractable than the discrete case, since functional analysis may be applied. Readers who are not interested in the mathematical details may skip the rest of this section.

Neutral element (δ impulse).   When the image and mask are discrete, it is easy to describe a mask which leaves the image unchanged; this is the one-location mask

d, which has only one nonzero element, $d_{oo} = 1$. Convolution with this mask is the "neutral element" of discrete convolution. If the image and mask are continuous, the mask of the neutral element can be approximated, for example, in the form

$$d_n(x,y) := \begin{cases} n & x^2 + y^2 < \frac{1}{n\pi} \\ 0 & otherwise \end{cases}.$$ (3.15)

In this case, $\int d_n(\vec{x})d\vec{x} = 1$ for all $n \in \mathbb{N}$. Convolution with d_n transforms each point of the image into a local average taken over a disk with an area of $1/n$. As n goes to infinity, the disk becomes a point, and

$$\lim_{n \to \infty} \int d_n(\vec{x}')g(\vec{x} - \vec{x}')d\vec{x}' = g(\vec{x}).$$ (3.16)

The limit operation can not, however, simply be brought inside the integral, since the series d_n at $\vec{x} = (0,0)$ does not converge. In other words, the neutral element in continuous convolution is not a function in the usual sense. It is called the Dirac or δ impulse, $\delta(\vec{x})$. Intuitively however, it is nonetheless a type of limit of the series d_n, which is to say that $d(\vec{x}) = 0$ holds for all $\vec{x} \neq (0,0)$ and

$$\int \delta(\vec{x})g(\vec{x})d\vec{x} = g(0,0).$$ (3.17)

The δ-impulse belongs to a class of objects called "distributions" or "generalized functions" in functional analysis. They occur if linear functionals, i.e. mappings from a function space to the space of real numbers are represented as integral equations. In the example given in Equation 3.16, the functional maps the function g to its value at the coordinate origin, $g(0,0)$.

The eigenfunctions of convolution.   In describing linear mappings, use is often made of eigenfunctions; that is, functions which remain unchanged by the mapping except for a multiplicative factor (the eigenvalue). When processed by continuous convolution, the sine and cosine functions have a characteristic of this type: namely, if two sine waves of the same frequency but of differing phase and amplitude are added together, the result is a sine wave at the same frequency. This characteristic is maintained for convolution, which after all is nothing but an additive process. No matter with what mask a sinusoidal function is convolved, then, the result is still a sinusoidal function with the same frequency, although generally with a different amplitude and phase. In order to treat amplitude and phase jointly as one eigenvalue, we use the complex representation of sinusoids given by Euler's formula,

$$e^{i\varphi} = \cos\varphi + i\sin\varphi.$$ (3.18)

Here $i = \sqrt{-1}$ is the imaginary unit. If the complex exponential function $\exp\{i\omega x\}$ is inserted into the convolution equation, then in the one-dimensional case,

$$\int c(x')\exp\{i\omega(x - x')\}dx' = \exp\{i\omega x\} \underbrace{\int c(x')\exp\{i\omega x'\}dx'}_{\tilde{c}(\omega)}.$$ (3.19)

The eigenvalue associated with the eigenfunction $exp\{i\omega x\}$ is, then, $\tilde{c}(\omega)$.

The same ideas apply to the two-dimensional case. The eigenfunctions of two-dimensional convolution are sinusoidal grids or plane waves with arbitrary frequency, orientation and phase (see below, Equation 3.23).

The Fourier transform. The eigenvalue $\tilde{c}(\omega)$ in Equation 3.19 is a complex number which depends on the frequency of the input pattern. If the number is determined for all frequencies $\omega \in \mathbb{R}$, the result is a complex function of one real variable, which is called the Fourier transform of c. Since sinusoidal functions are orthogonal,

$$\int \exp\{i\omega_1 x\} \exp\{i\omega_2 x\} dx = \delta(\omega_1 - \omega_2), \tag{3.20}$$

two results can be proven, which are fundamental to the significance of the Fourier transform for the theory of convolution operators:

1. Every (sufficiently) continuous function can be unambiguously and reversibly represented by its Fourier transform:

$$\text{forward:} \quad \tilde{g}(\omega) := \int g(x) \exp\{i\omega x\} dx, \tag{3.21}$$

$$\text{backward:} \quad g(x) := \frac{1}{2\pi} \int \tilde{g}(\omega) \exp\{-i\omega x\} dx.$$

    The real and imaginary part of $\tilde{g}$ are also called the Fourier cosine and Fourier sine transforms. Intuitively, Equation 3.21 says that every continuous function can be represented as the sum of sine and cosine functions.

2. (Convolution theorem.) If the original function is replaced by its Fourier transform, then convolution is replaced by multiplication:

$$(g * h)^\sim(\omega) = \tilde{g}(\omega) \, \tilde{h}(\omega). \tag{3.22}$$

    The commutativity and associativity of convolution, already noted above, follow directly from this theorem.

In order to extend the Fourier transform to two or to n dimensions, it should first be noted that the exponential function in this case takes on the form of a plane wave,

$$\exp\{i(\omega_1 x_1 + ... + \omega_n x_n)\} = \exp\{i(\vec{\omega} \cdot \vec{x})\}. \tag{3.23}$$

The term ωx in the exponent of Equation 3.21 is in this case simply replaced by the inner product $(\vec{\omega} \cdot \vec{x})$. The Fourier transform is in this case a complex function of n real variables.

From the convolution theorem and the Fourier representation of the image function, it follows that convolution may be interpreted as *filtering*. If the Fourier transform of a mask goes to zero, let us say, outside some interval, then all of the spatial frequencies outside of that interval are filtered out, while the others are retained. Smoothing masks are in this sense low-pass filters, since they allow only low spatial frequencies to pass. Differentiating masks, on the other hand, are highpass or bandpass filters.

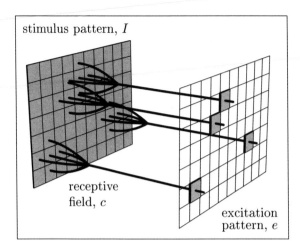

stimulus pattern, I

receptive
field, c

excitation
pattern, e

Figure 3.5
Convolution and receptive fields in neural networks. Each point of the output layer receives inputs from the locations in the mask c which are weighted by the factors c_{ij} (Eqn. 3.24). The mask therefore corresponds to the weightings in a feed-forward network. If the weightings for all cells are the same except for the position on the mask, the result is a convolution.

Receptive fields

Convolution also underlies the theory of the *receptive field* in neurobiology. Put most simply, the receptive field is a protocol for measuring the excitation of a neuron. Most generally, all stimuli which excite a neuron comprise its receptive field. In the stages of the visual system close to the input, receptive fields can be defined according to the location on the retina or in the visual field at which a stimulus must occur in order to lead to an excitation. To each location is assigned a weighting factor which represents the strength of the resulting excitation, or, if negative, the strength of inhibition. The receptive field is, then, a function which assigns this weighting factor to the points of the visual field. If the cell sums its inputs linearly, then:

$$e = \int \int c(x,y) I(x,y) dx dy. \tag{3.24}$$

Here, e is the excitation of the cell, $c(x,y)$ is the weighting function, and $I(x,y)$ is the function which describes the image. In reality, receptive fields are always also time-dependent.

If it is assumed that a neuronal structure (for example, an area of the visual cortex) contains many neurons whose receptive fields are displaced relative to one another, then Equation 3.24 is transformed into a convolution. This model is, however, only neurophysiologically accurate to a first approximation. In reality, the nonuniform magnification of the retinotopic image (cf. Fig. 3.4) and also different specializations of the internal connectivity make the receptive fields of neighboring cells different from one another. The image processing is, therefore, spatially nonuniform (cf. Mallot et al. 1990).

Fig. 3.5 illustrates the analogy between masking operations and receptive fields. The connections between the input and output layers do not, however, correspond exactly to the actual neuronal networks, but rather only indicate the signal flow

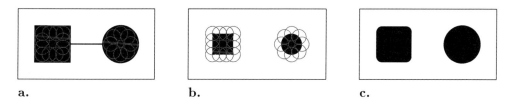

a. **b.** **c.**

Figure 3.6
Diagrammatic representation of morphological operations on images. **a.** The input image composed of a square, a circle and a line. The circular mask B is shown at some positions which are entirely inside the pattern. **b.** Erosion of the input image by the mask B. The small circles show positions of B whose point of reference is inside the pattern. **c.** The area enclosed by the small circles of b constitutes the opening of the input pattern by the circular mask The line has been lost through erosion, and the square is smoothed.

schematically. The actual networks can have multiple stages with feedback, and so the receptive fields can have complicated spatial and temporal characteristics.

3.3.2 Morphological filters

The last section examined image processing operations in which the output was a weighted sum of the intensity values of a region of an image with a continuous gray scale. An alternative approach to image processing proceeds from the representation of "0/1 images" as sets of points. This approach underlies *mathematical morphology*, a field which is closely related to set theory and to algebra (cf. Serra 1982, Haralick & Shapiro 1992, Heijmans 1995).

We will consider here only a few simple examples. If an image is defined by a set X such that X is the set of all black pixels, it follows that:

$$\begin{aligned} X &:= \{\vec{\mathbf{x}} = (x_i, y_j) | I(\vec{\pmb{x}}) = 0\}, \\ X^c &= \{\vec{\mathbf{x}} = (x_i, y_j) | I(\vec{\pmb{x}}) = 1\}. \end{aligned} \tag{3.25}$$

We designate the fundamental set of all pixels as Ω. Then $\Omega = X \cup X^c$. We also need another set, B, which has a role similar to that of the mask in convolution. As before, we want to displace the mask across the image so that all locations in the image are processed in the same way. The displacement of a set is here regarded as the displacement of all of its elements. Furthermore, with relation to B, we define the reflected set $\check{B} := \{\vec{\mathbf{x}} | -\vec{\mathbf{x}} \in B\}$. In this light, let us consider the following operations:

Erosion. Here, the input image X is transformed into a filtered image $X \ominus B$ which includes only the points in X for which the mask B lies entirely inside X:

$$X \ominus B := \{\vec{\pmb{x}} \in \Omega | \vec{\pmb{x}} + \vec{\pmb{b}} \in X \text{ for all } \vec{\pmb{b}} \in B\}. \tag{3.26}$$

Instead of positioning the mask B at every point and determining whether it is entirely inside X, it is possible to speed up calculation by displacing X by all vectors that are inside B and then finding the intersection of these displaced versions.

Dilation.   Erosion of the set X extends the "background" X^c of that set. Analogously, the extension of X by B to $X \oplus B$ is defined as the set of all points for which one point of the input image coincides with one point of the mask.

$$X \oplus B := \{\vec{y} \in \Omega | \vec{y} = \vec{x} + \vec{b} \text{ for any } \vec{x} \in X \text{ and } \vec{b} \in B\}. \tag{3.27}$$

As with erosion, dilatation may be calculated efficiently by first displacing the image X by all vectors in B and then constructing the union of all of these sets. Erosion and dilatation may, then, be calculated efficiently from the same data by calculating the intersection and the union of the displaced sets.

As already mentioned, the erosion of an image is related to the dilatation of its complement. For symmetric masks, i.e. masks satisfying $B = \check{B}$, the two operations are equivalent.

$$
\begin{aligned}
(X \ominus B)^c &= X^c \oplus \check{B}, \\
(X \oplus B)^c &= X^c \ominus \check{B}.
\end{aligned}
\tag{3.28}
$$

Here, $\check{B}$ is the reflected set as defined above.

Opening and closing.   Dilation is not the reverse of erosion; if a set B (for example a circle) is used in erosion and the result is dilated with the same circle, the result is not X but a set with a smoothed outline. This smoothing of the outline is different from the smoothing of the intensity landscape as is done by the convolution operations discussed in Section 3.3.1. Of course, smoothing the gray values will also affect the outlines—that is, individual contour lines—but the outcomes of both types of smoothing may be quite different.

The sequence of erosion and dilatation is called *opening*:

$$X \circ B := (X \ominus B) \oplus B. \tag{3.29}$$

The closing is defined analogously,

$$X \bullet B := (X \oplus B) \ominus B. \tag{3.30}$$

The algebraic structure of dilatation and erosion is studied in mathematical morphology. For example, $(X \circ B)^c = X^c \bullet \check{B}$. Fig. 3.6 illustrates an example of morphological filtering.

The "skeleton" of a figure.   The "skeleton" is sometimes used to describe a figure X (cf. Fig. 3.7). Let us first consider the opening of a figure with a small disk. As shown in Fig. 3.6c, this process, so to speak, "sands off" the corners. If the corners

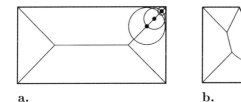

a.   b.

Figure 3.7
The skeleton used to describe a shape. **a.** The centers of maximal disks (that is, those that are not entirely inside any other disk inside X) comprise the skeleton of a figure X. **b.** Small changes in the figure can have a great influence on the skeleton. The derivation of the skeleton should therefore always be performed in conjunction with morphological smoothing operations at various levels of resolution.

sanded off using masks of different sizes are joined together, the result is the skeleton or the "median axis" of the figure. A different way to define the skeleton applies the concept of maximal disks. A maximal disk is a disk completely inside the figure which is not inside any other disk which is itself completely inside the figure. It can be shown that the centers of maximal disks constitute the median axis (Fig. 3.7)a. Another, especially intuitive explanation is given by Duda & Hart (1973): Think of the outline of a figure as a line in a prairie which is set afire at the same time all along its length. The lines along which the expanding burned areas merge and the fire goes out also define the skeleton. We do not attempt to give a formal definition of the medial axis in this introductory text; for various versions of formal definitions, see Serra (1982), Haralick & Shapiro (1992) and Rosenfeld & Kak (1982). For a more recent algorithm for the computation of skeletons, see Deseilligny et al. (1998).

3.4 Resolution

3.4.1 Psychophysics

Resolution and acuity of vision depend in the first instance on the optical characteristics of the imaging system, but are influenced further by the sampling in the retina or camera target, as well as by later image processing operations. The optical resolution limit can be described by the width of the image of a single point of light ("point spread image"); this depends on the diameter of the pupil and the wavelength of the light. In the human eye, this is on the order of 30 seconds of arc, and corresponds approximately to the spacing of receptor cells in the fovea.

A number of different test patterns may be used for psychophysical measurement of the resolution limit. Some of these are illustrated in Fig. 3.8.

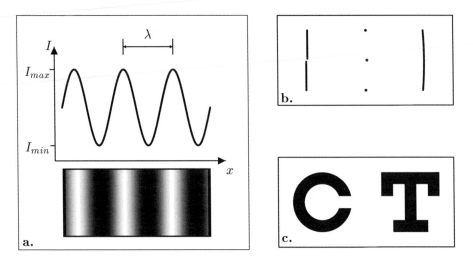

Figure 3.8
Various types of test patterns for measurement of the acuity of vision. **a.** Sinusoidal grating. **b.** Test patterns for hyperacuity: left, vernier, middle, row of dots, right, arc. **c.** Test pattern for form perception. Left: Landolt ring, right: Snellen letter.

Sensitivity to contrast

Modulation transfer function.   Let us consider a sinusoidal intensity pattern such as that shown in Fig. 3.8a. Resolution is measured by determining the contrast at which a sinusoidal pattern with a period λ is visible. Here, λ is the wavelength of the sinusoidal pattern, not of the light. The inverse of λ is the spatial frequency of the pattern; this is measured in cycles per degree. The contrast is defined as the quotient of the sum and difference of the extremes of intensity:

$$\text{contrast} := \frac{I_{max} - I_{min}}{I_{max} + I_{min}}. \tag{3.31}$$

This dimensionless quantity is more accurately called the two-point or Michelson contrast. Its value can be between 0 and 1. If the illumination of an image changes, the contrast remains the same, since the illumination affects the intensities multiplicatively and cancels out of the quotient in Equation 3.31. The name *sensitivity* is given to the inverse of the threshold contrast, defined as the contrast at which the pattern is correctly recognized in 75% of trials. Fig. 3.9 diagrammatically shows the results of such a test, and also gives a simple demonstration of the frequency dependence of contrast sensitivity.

Contrast sensitivity reaches its peak in the range of approximately 2 through 10 cycles per degree and falls off rapidly at higher spatial frequencies. Sinusoidal patterns with spatial frequencies of 60 periods per degree are never resolved. The outline curve in Fig. 3.9a is called the modulation transfer function. In linear systems, it corresponds to the Fourier transform of the input masks.

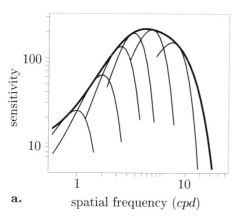

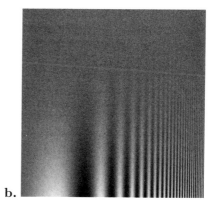

a.   spatial frequency (*cpd*)   **b.**

Figure 3.9
a. Outline: Contrast sensitivity of the human eye as a function of spatial frequency (*cpd: cycles per degree*). A sensitivity of 100 indicates that contrast at the threshold of perception is 1/100. Family of curves under the outline: modulation transfer functions of individual spatial frequency channels (combined, after DeValois & DeValois 1988, and Wilson et al., 1983). **b.** Illustration of contrast sensitivity. The illustration shows a stimulus with spatial frequency increasing from left to right and contrast decreasing from bottom to top. At intermediate spatial frequencies, sinusoidal modulation is visible even at relatively low contrasts; the limit at which the modulation becomes visible traces the outline in **a.** (After Cornsweet 1970).

Resolution channels.   The contrast sensitivity illustrated in Fig. 3.9 is not generated by one single mechanism. Rather, the image is captured through distinct, parallel "channels" which are specialized as to spatial location, spatial frequency, and temporal frequency. Responses of spatial frequency channels are shown in the curves under the outline in Fig. 3.9a. Evidence for the existence of these channels is provided mostly by adaptation experiments. If the visual system is adapted by long observation of a striped pattern, the sensitivity to this pattern decreases. If contrast sensitivity were mediated by only one channel, it would be expected that sensitivity to all other spatial frequencies would also decrease, since a single channel could not distinguish among the different spatial frequencies. In fact, however, local adaptation occurs: sensitivity decreases for spatial frequencies near the frequency of adaptation, but sensitivity remains unchanged at frequencies that differ more greatly (Blakemore & Campbell 1969).

Harmon & Julesz (1973) have devised a stimulus showing different images when viewed at different resolutions. In their example, the face of Abraham Lincoln is shown with just 15 by 20 pixels. When viewed at low resolution, the face is clearly visible. At high resolution, however, the raster of the pixel boundaries masks the perception of the face.* Clearly, the image of the face is still present in the low spatial frequency

---

*The Spanish painter Salvador Dalí (1904 – 1989) has created a version of this picture showing

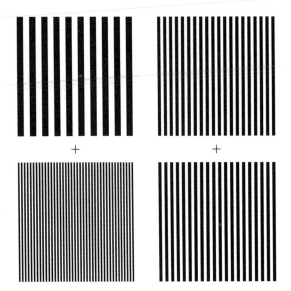

Figure 3.10
Demonstration of the shift in perceived spatial frequency after adaptation. After closing one eye and looking at the small cross at the left for at least one minute, then looking at the cross on the right, the two striped patterns at the right appear to have different spatial frequencies. (After Olzak & Thomas 1986).

band, but interactions between the channels prevent its perception. Interestingly, the interaction is "fine-to-coarse", in contrast to the various "coarse-to-fine" schemes to be discussed later.

An additional experiment is shown in Fig. 3.10. Adaptation changes not only the sensitivity to a pattern, but also the perception of spatial frequency. This observation, which at first seems astonishing, is also explained by the existence of parallel perceptual channels whose spatial sensitivity response differs (Fig. 3.11). The proof of parallel channels for spatial frequency in human perception has led to the development of similar strategies in image processing (pyramids, resolution space), which will be discussed further in what follows.

With the encoding of contrast information in parallel channels which have overlapping sensitivity curves, we encounter for the first time an important principle in neuronal information processing, namely that of population coding. Some fundamental issues relative to population coding, and additional examples, will be discussed in Section 5.1.5.

Hyperacuity

Fig. 3.8b shows some patterns which also may be used to measure resolution. The versions of the patterns shown, or their mirror images, are shown to the test subject. Then the subject is asked whether the upper line is to the left or the right of the lower one (example at the left); whether the middle of the three points is to the left or the right of the line connecting the two other points (middle example) or in which direction the arc is bent (example at right). All of these experiments reveal

---

Lincoln's face in the low spatial frequency band and the painter's wife Gala in the high spatial frequency band.

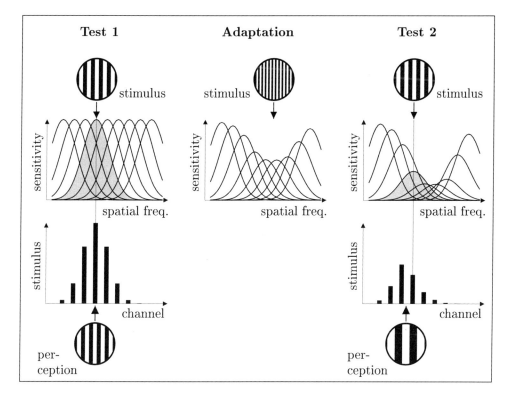

Figure 3.11
Population coding in the perception of spatial frequencies. In the first test, the channels are excited in proportion to their sensitivity. The perceived frequency, here established as the center of gravity of the distribution of excitation among the channels, is the same as the frequency of the stimulus. In the adaptation phase, a high-frequency stimulus is presented which selectively reduces the sensitivity of the channels. Next, the original pattern is presented again (test 2). This time, the pattern of excitation in the channels is shifted towards the left, conveying the impression of a lower spatial frequency. The channel shaded in gray is the one which "corresponds" to the stimulus. After adaptation, the channel's sensitivity to this stimulus is, however, less than that of the neighboring channel, which codes for a lower frequency. (After Braddick et al. 1978)

perceptual thresholds on the order of 10 seconds of arc or less. This phenomenon is called hyperacuity, since this level of acuity should seemingly not be possible with a minimal receptor spacing of 30 seconds of arc (cf. McKee et al. 1990). The explanation for this phenomenon is that many receptors take part in the imaging of the pattern. By examining the relationship between the stimuli to two neighboring receptors with bell-shaped, overlapping input characteristics, it is in fact possible to attain resolutions smaller than that of the pixel grid (Fahle & Poggio 1981). Hyperacuity is another example of population coding.

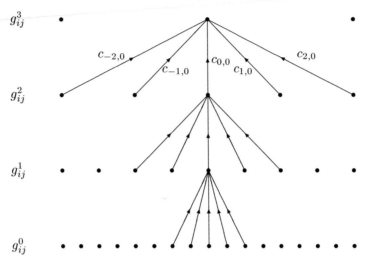

Figure 3.12
Data flow diagram for the calculation of a resolution pyramid as in Equation 3.32, after Burt & Adelson (1983). Each row of points represents pixels in one level of the pyramid. The pixels in the lowest level are the gray values of the image. In each level, five pixels are weighted and averaged, and construct a point in the next higher level. The pixel spacing increases from level to level by a factor of two, while the kernel of the smoothing mask remains the same at every level.

3.4.2   Resolution pyramids

The concept of parallel channels states that each point in the image is processed in different channels with different resolution, localization and time dependence. In computer processing of images, the corresponding concept is that of *pyramids* in which the same mask (for example, undersampling subsequent to the original sampling) is applied repeatedly.

Let $\{g_{ij}\} = \{g_{ij}^0\}$ be the original image and $\{c_{mn}\}$ be a mask. We then designate as the **reduction** of g^l onto g^{l+1} the sequence of undersampling and convolution (cf. Burt & Adelson 1983, Jähne 1997, Lindeberg 1994):

$$g_{ij}^{l+1} = \sum_{m=-M}^{M} \sum_{n=-N}^{N} c_{m,n} g_{2i-m,2j-n}^l. \tag{3.32}$$

In an image with $2^L \times 2^L$ pixels, this operation may be performed a maximum of $L+1$ times. Fig. 3.12 illustrates this process.

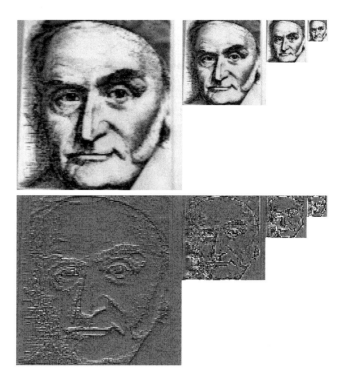

Figure 3.13
Four levels of the Gauss and Laplace pyramid. The upper row shows the low-pass filtered and undersampled images $g^{0,0}$ through $g^{3,0}$. Each level of the Laplace pyramids (lower row) is the difference between the corresponding level of the Gauss pyramid and the next higher level, which has been expanded once, $g^{0,0} - g^{1,1}$ through $g^{3,0} - g^{4,1}$ (after Gillner et al. 1993; the picture of C. F. Gauß is taken from the German 10 mark bill).

Let c be a sampling of the two-dimensional Gaussian function

$$G_\sigma(x,y) = \frac{1}{2\pi\sigma^2}\exp\{-\frac{1}{2\sigma^2}(x^2+y^2)\}. \tag{3.33}$$

The Gaussian function has the useful characteristic that convolution with itself generates another Gaussian function: $G_\sigma * G_\sigma = G_{\sqrt{2}\sigma}$. The pyramid may therefore be generated without iterations, by direct convolution with $G_{\sqrt{2^l}\sigma}$ and subsequent l-times undersampling. Clearly, however, this procedure would be computationally less efficient.*

In order to reconstruct the original image, the steps of the pyramid must be correctly interpolated. We will designate the appropriate mask as d. Since this "expansion" is not the exact inversion of the reduction, we will denote the result of the k-times expansion of g^l as $g^{l,k}$. Note that $g^l = g^{l,0}$.

$$g_{ij}^{l,k+1} = \sum_{m=-M}^{M}\sum_{n=-N}^{N} d_{m,n}g_{(i-m)/2,(j-n)/2}^{l,k}. \tag{3.34}$$

---

*The *central limit theorem* of probability theory guarantees that the limit case of repeated convolutions with a non-negative mask is a convolution with a Gaussian. If another low-pass filter is chosen, then the higher levels of the pyramid generated in this way will approximate the Gaussian pyramid more and more closely.

Here, we consider only those terms for which $(i-m)/2$ and $(j-n)/2$ are integers. The images $g^{l,l}$ are simply blurred versions of the original g. The level of undersampling is proportional to the unsharpness or blur at each level $g^{l,0}$.

Laplace pyramids are generated from Gaussian pyramids by storing only the difference $g^{l,0} - g^{l+1,1}$ at each level l (Fig. 3.13). Starting at the coarsest level, each step, then, holds only the additional information which corresponds to better image resolution. The same image as for this step is obtained through convolution by the difference of two Gaussian functions of appropriate widths (DoG-filter; cf. Gl. 4.18). This result follows from the distributivity of convolution. The name "Laplace-pyramid" reflects the similarity between the DoG-operator and the Laplacian of a Gausian, LoG (see Section 4.3).

In the case of continuous functions, the methods of functional analysis may be used to generate more elaborate expansion and reduction functions. The totality of the expansion and reduction functions defines a set of basis functions through which the original image may be described by means of a series of coefficients. As in the case of the Fourier expansion, it can be required that the set of basis functions be complete and orthogonal. This requirement leads to what is called the *wavelet* expansion (cf. Mallat 1989). Basis functions in wavelet expansions are self-similar families of Gabor functions which may be of the form

$$\psi_{\omega,b}(x) = \frac{1}{\sqrt{\omega}} \exp\{-\frac{1}{2} \left(\frac{x-b}{\omega} \right)^2\} \exp\{-i\omega x\}. \qquad (3.35)$$

Because of the completeness of the function system, perfect reconstructions are possible when using wavelets.

The (continuous) totality of all of the low-pass filtered versions of an image g is called the *scale space* of the image; this will be discussed in connection with edge detection in Chapter 4.

Chapter 4

Edge detection

4.1 The significance of edges

4.1.1 Examples

Edges are locations in an image where intensities change abruptly or at least "rapidly". For reasons which will be discussed in the following sections, edges play an important role in the early stages of image processing. This chapter will describe not only edge detection itself but will also give examples of how to construct image processing masks appropriate for specific tasks.

Information content. The highest spatial density of information in images occurs where the intensity changes rapidly, that is, at edges (Srinivasan et al. 1982). The best estimate of the gray level of a pixel from its surroundings is a weighted average of the gray levels of neighboring pixels. At edges and lines, the actual gray level of the pixel differs from that average. These locations are of special interest. For a discussion of the choice of image features for optimal encoding and of reproduction of images using statistical techniques, cf. Olshausen & Field (1996).

Neurophysiology. Most visual neurons in the primary areas of the visual cortex in mammals react to intensity jumps or edges which have a particular orientation, and especially so when these edges move across the image at right angles to their orientation ("orientation selectivity" Hubel & Wiesel 1962). Orientation-selective edge detection is probably the one neurophysiological result applied most widely in image processing, and has become the basis for many computer vision architectures. An overview of the neurophysiology of edge detection is to be found in DeValois & DeValois (1988). Mathematical models of orientation selectivity are based on the theory of lateral inhibition, first advanced by Ernst Mach (1922; cf. also Ratliff 1965). Isotropic lateral inhibition is usually modeled with Gaussian functions (e.g., von Seelen 1970) while

Gabor functions are used to model oriented receptive fields (e.g., Pollen & Ronner 1983).

Primal sketch. It is sometimes useful to describe an image by means of a list of features, so the image can be processed as symbolic information. Edge elements are suitable features for this type of processing, as are points where edges cross or branch, the ends of lines (terminators), dots etc. Marr (1976) defines the *primal sketch* as a list of declarations, each of which describes such an image feature. An entry in this list consists more or less of the following elements: type of feature, position, contrast, sharpness and orientation. Some types of features may have additional characteristics, for example the curvature of a line or the possible spatial interpretations of a T junction of two edge elements (e.g, concealment of the edge that ends by the one that is continuous). Features are robust against noise and of changes of illumination.

Image segmentation. Abrupt intensity changes tend to occur at the boundaries of objects. Together with discontinuities in other local characteristics (motion, depth, color etc.), these edges may be used to divide the image into segments, which may be assumed to correspond to representations of separate objects. Another assumption which contributes to this interpretation is that the environment consists of objects of more or less constant reflectivity, whose images are bounded by edges. Here, also, the robustness of edges in spite of changes in illumination is important.

One complicating factor in the relationship between edge detection and image segmentation is that not all intensity jumps correspond to boundaries of objects. Difficulties are presented by cast shadows, textures and "surface" patterns. The camouflage patterns of many animals provide especially illustrative examples, and are often stronger visually than the animals' actual outlines, causing the shape of an animal to "dissolve" into the background (e.g. Metzger 1975, Fig. 109).

Interpretation of image intensities. As already discussed, the relationship "image intensity = illumination × reflectivity" does not allow the illumination and reflectivity to be determined without further analysis. Generally, however, the following heuristic analysis is helpful:

Intensity change		Interpretation
very gradual	→	variation in illumination
more abrupt, but still continuous	→	curvature (shading), highlights
very abrupt, discontinuous	→	boundaries of objects

Edges can, therefore, be used to separate the influences of reflectivity and illumination on intensities in the image. A process which accomplishes this is discussed in Chapter 5 ("retinex theory").

Psychophysics. Neighborhood effects play an important role in the perception of brightness. Generally, intensity jumps are enhanced, while minor and, especially,

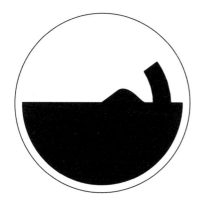

Figure 4.1
Following a suggestion by Helmholtz, any desired one-dimensional gray scale function $I(r)$ can be generated using rotating black and white disks. At every radius r on a white disk, a black arc of length $\varphi(r) = 2\pi(1 - I(r))$ is drawn. If the disk is rotated rapidly enough that no flickering is visible, the desired gray scale function appears across the disk's diameter. The illustration shows a disk with a blurred step-edge and a sharp-edged line.

Image	Intensity profile $I(x)$	Observed brightness

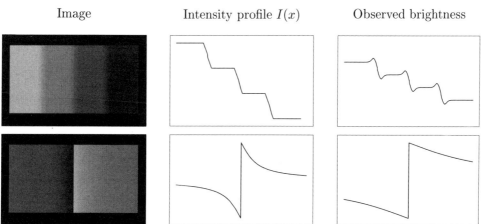

Figure 4.2
Lateral interactions in contrast perception. **Top:** Mach bands. The intensity jumps are perceived as intensified. **Bottom:** Craik-O'Brien-Cornsweet illusion. Brightness in each half of the image appears more even than it is.

gradual intensity variations are more usually suppressed. A simple device for the generation of one-dimensional intensity functions without any need for calibration is shown in Fig. 4.1. Two classic brightness effects are illustrated in Fig. 4.2.

1. Mach bands: Adjacent to intensity jumps of moderate steepness, bright and dark bands are perceived which increase the contrast of the edges. These bands can be explained by lateral inhibition, that is, by convolution of the intensity function with filtering functions (such as the difference between two Gaussian functions) which subtract the local average from the central intensity value (see below, Equation 4.18 on page 90). This mechanism, which was suggested already by Mach (1922), does not, however, explain why the Mach bands are weaker with very sharp edges than with blurrier ones.

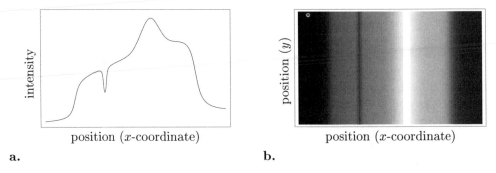

position (x-coordinate)   position (x-coordinate)

a.   **b.**

Figure 4.3
Gray value function with various types of edges: (step-edge, line, highlight, step-edge)
and a superimposed illumination gradient (brighter toward the right). **a.** Intensity
function. **b.** Image.

2. Craik-O'Brien-Cornsweet illusion: Given the same level of contrast, steep intensity changes are more visible than gradual ones. In the extreme case, the
   intensity function shown in Fig. 4.2 (bottom) appears to be an abrupt step edge
   between two surfaces of constant brightness. More readily visible is the darker
   appearance of the left end of the gray value function in comparison with the
   right end. It goes away if the middle of the figure is covered by a sheet of paper.
   The Craik-O'Brien-Cornsweet illusion as well can be at least partially explained
   by lateral inhibition.

Pessoa (1996) gives an overview of the extensive literature on Mach bands and related phenomena. Detailed theories of the perception of brightness postulate several
levels of processing which carry out other, non-linear operations in addition to lateral
inhibition (cf. Neumann 1996).

An additional psychophysical argument for the importance of edges in perception
is provided by the subjective contours which were described briefly in Chapter 1.
These demonstrate that not all edges are locations where intensity changes abruptly;
edges can also be generated in the process of perceptual organization, in which image
elements are grouped together. Edges therefore are not only a cause, but sometimes,
rather, a result of image segmentation.

4.1.2   Formal analysis of the problem

Intensity steps are representations of borders of objects, or of reflectivity changes, in
the external world, corrupted to a greater or lesser degree by noise. The reconstruction of boundaries between objects is therefore a problem of "inverse optics" which,
in general, is not completely open to solution. The biggest problem in the reversal of
the optical imaging in edge detection is random noise superimposed on the intensity
profile. Differentiation is therefore not entirely satisfactory as a means of edge detection. We will now first consider only one-dimensional gray value functions. Various

types of edges of this type are shown in Fig. 4.3.

A good edge detector should satisfy the following conditions (Canny 1986):

- Quality of detection: small probability of detection errors or of edges that are not identified. This is equivalent to the requirement for a high signal-to-noise ratio at the output of the detector.

- Localization: The maximum detector output should appear at the position of the edge.

- Unique output: There should be only one result per actual edge. This requirement follows in part from that of the quality of detection.

An additional requirement might be that the edge elements, detected in two dimensions, can be assembled into continuous lines. An edge detector does not normally assemble them; rather, the problem is addressed in a separate stage of image processing called image segmentation.

The stated requirements can in general not be perfectly fulfilled: there is more than one way to define edges in any given image. It is possible either to ignore this problem (and retain all potential edges) or to force unique solutions through "regularizations," which are formulations of plausible additional conditions which exclude some solutions. Approaches to edge detection may be categorized as follows:

1. *Differentiation:* If a one-dimensional intensity function is differentiated spatially, step-like edges correspond to sharp minima or maxima of the first derivative or to zero crossings of the second derivative (points of inflection). Lines correspond to extremes of the imaging function or of its second derivative. In the case of two-dimensional functions, more complicated combinations of the partial derivatives I_x and I_y, including nonlinear combinations, are used. These will be discussed in Section 4.3.

2. *Regularization through noise reduction:* Noise reduction preprocessing can lead to unique edge detection solutions in noisy images. The preprocessing is followed by differentiation as already described. The resulting operators are somewhat different from those for differentiation alone (cf. Marr & Hildreth 1980, Torre & Poggio 1986).

3. *Regularization through error minimization:* Canny (1986) formalizes the requirements already described into a cost function which can be minimized for given edge functions by varying the filter mask. The resulting operators (numerical results) are similar to those derived from noise reduction but allow some image-specific adjustments.

We will consider here only the first two of these approaches.

4.2   Edge detection in one dimension

4.2.1   Differentiation

Fig. 4.4 shows the relationship between edges and zero crossings of the second derivative for a one-dimensional intensity function as can be derived from elementary analysis of curves. Step-like edges are points of inflection of the intensity function, i.e, points at which the curvature of the intensity function changes between leftwards and rightwards, and where the function changes between convex and concave. Such points of inflection are characterized by zero crossings of the second derivative where the third derivative is not zero. This last condition ($I''' \neq 0$) is important: as can be seen in Fig. 4.4, there are places where the second derivative is zero but which do not correspond to edges. These correspond to points of inflection at which the second derivative changes only very slowly and the third derivative therefore is near zero.

A line behaves like a pair of edges close to one another with opposite polarities of the intensity step, and is characterized by the first derivative's going to zero and a large value of the second derivative.

Numerical differentiation

We want now to construct linear operators (masks) to approximate the differentiation of the sampled image. The technique applied is that of numerical differentiation,

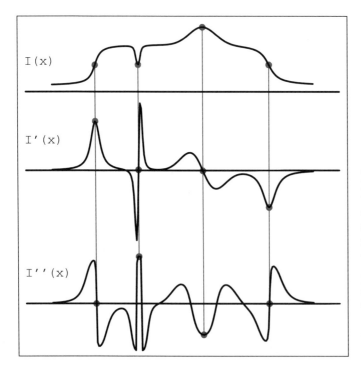

Figure 4.4
Intensity   function
$I(x)$ and   first   and
second   derivative   (as
in Fig. 4.3 but with
uniform   lighting).
Step-like edges can be
localized at the point
of inflection of the step
($I'' = 0$); lines generate
two zero crossings of
the second derivative.

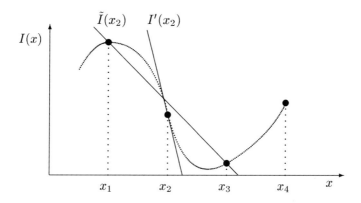

Figure 4.5
Determining the derivative of sampled functions. The "real" tangent at point x_2, $I'(x_2)$ can not be determined from the sample points alone. A possible estimate is $\tilde{I}(x_2)$, which corresponds to the secant through $(x_1, I(x_1))$ and $(x_2, I(x_2))$. Note that this estimate does not depend in any way on the value of the function at the point x_2.

which is thoroughly described in textbooks on numerical analysis (e.g., Press et al. 1986, Stoer & Bulirsch 1992).

We define the one-dimensional derivative of the imaging function $I(x)$ in the usual way, as:

$$I'(x) = \lim_{h \to 0} \frac{I(x+h) - I(x-h)}{2h}. \tag{4.1}$$

The transition to the limit for $h \to 0$ can, however, not be calculated, since I for the sampled image is known only at discrete points. We set the pixel spacing to 1 and also assume that x is an integer. An obvious approximation to $I'(x)$ is achieved when $h = 1$:

$$\tilde{I}(x) = \frac{1}{2}(I(x+1) - I(x-1)). \tag{4.2}$$

Fig. 4.5 shows an example of the derivative I' of a function and an approximation $\tilde{I}$. Clearly, there are many differentiable functions I, which pass through the same two sample points, but which have different derivatives at x_2. The approximation $\tilde{I}(x_2)$ is, however, the same for all such curves. If it is assumed that I is sufficiently smooth (e.g., continuously differentiable at least once), better approximations can be constructed by taking more distant sample points into account.

Polynomial interpolation

A better estimate for I can be attained by constructing a smooth curve through a number of sample points. The interpolation curve is then analytically known and can be differentiated exactly.

We choose polynomial functions as our interpolation functions, and we note an important analytical result: The interpolation of $n + 1$ paired sample points using an nth order polynomial (i.e. a function of the form $p(x) = \sum_{i=0}^{n} a_i x^i$) is unique, i.e. there is only one polynomial whose highest power is x^n and which passes through all of the sample points. We prove this assertion in two steps:

a. *If two polynomials p, q are everywhere the same ($p(x) \equiv q(x)$), then they are of the same order, and all of their coefficients are equal.* To see this, let

$$p(x) := \sum_{i=0}^{n} a_i x^i, \quad q(x) = \sum_{i=0}^{m} b_i x^i \qquad (4.3)$$

be two polynomials of degree n and m (i.e. $a_n \neq 0$, $b_m \neq 0$). Since their values are everywhere the same, then all of their derivatives must also be the same, $p^{(j)} \equiv q^{(j)}$ for all $j \in \mathbb{N}_o$. We calculate the jth derivative of p at $x = 0$:

$$p^{(j)}(x) = \sum_{i=j}^{n} a_i \frac{i!}{(i-j)!} x^{i-j} \quad \text{and} \quad p^{(j)}(0) = j! a_j. \qquad (4.4)$$

If, analogously, we calculate the jth derivative of q, it follows immediately from the equality of the derivatives at $x = 0$ that $j! a_j = j! b_j$, and furthermore, $a_j = b_j$ for all $j \geq 0$. The first part of the assertion has therefore been proven.

b. *If two polynomials whose highest degree is n have the same values at $n+1$ points, they are identical.*
In this case, the difference polynomial $r(x) := p(x) - q(x)$ has at least $n + 1$ zero crossings. Now, the degree of r as well can be no higher than n, i.e. r can contain no higher powers of x than p or q. According to the fundamental theorem of algebra, a polynomial of the nth degree with $n + 1$ zero crossings is zero everywhere; therefore, $r = p - q \equiv 0$, and therefore, as asserted, $p \equiv q$. Since we have already shown in (a) that identical polynomials must have the same coefficients, the uniqueness of the solution has now been proven.

In general, the coefficients of an interpolation polynomial with $n + 1$ sample points $(x_0, I(x_0)), ..., (x_n, I(x_n))$ may be obtained using Lagrange's formula,

$$p_n(x) = \sum_{i=0}^{n} I(x_i) \frac{(x - x_0) \ldots (x - x_{i-1})(x - x_{i+1}) \ldots (x - x_n)}{(x_i - x_0) \ldots (x_i - x_{i-1})(x_i - x_{i+1}) \ldots (x_i - x_n)}. \qquad (4.5)$$

This polynomial can not be of a higher degree than n. We will, however, not use this formula. Instead, we will undertake a step-by-step solution of the conditional equations for a simple example.

Example

Let us consider the image function I at five equidistant sample points $(-2, -1, 0, 1, 2)$, aligning the coordinate system so $I(0) = 0$. We want to find a fourth degree polynomial

$$p(x) = ax + bx^2 + cx^3 + dx^4.$$

through the sample points. Because of our choice of coordinate system, $p(0) = 0$, and only four coefficients need be determined. If the polynomial p is known, then the coefficient a is the derivative to be evaluated:

$$p'(x) = a + 2bx + 3cx^2 + 4dx^3$$
$$p'(0) = a.$$

We consider two cases:

1. Interpolation between three sample points by a parabola ($c = d = 0$)
2. Interpolation between five sample points by a fourth degree polynomial.

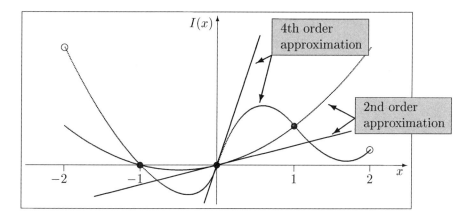

Figure 4.6
An approximate evaluation of derivatives of sampled functions. If three sample points are used ($\bullet$), the result is a second degree function (parabola) and a less steep tangent. If five sample points are used ($\bullet$ and $\circ$), the result is a fourth degree function, and a steeper tangent in the case illustrated.

Case 1: We set $c = d = 0$, and we examine only the sample points $I(1), I(0)$ and $I(-1)$. By substitution into the equation $p(x) = ax + bx^2$, we obtain the conditional equations

$$\left. \begin{array}{rcl} I(-1) & = & p(-1) & = & -a + b \\ I(1) & = & p(1) & = & a + b \end{array} \right\} \Rightarrow a = \frac{1}{2}(I(1) - I(-1)). \qquad (4.6)$$

This is the heuristic approximation from equation 4.2. The corresponding mask for discrete convolution is of the form $\boxed{-\frac{1}{2} \mid 0 \mid \frac{1}{2}}$.

Case 2: In this case, we must solve a system of four equations for a. We start with the sample points $x = \pm 1$:

$$\left.\begin{array}{rclcrcrcrcr} I(-1) & = & p(-1) & = & -a & + & b & - & c & + & d \\ I(1) & = & p(1) & = & a & + & b & + & c & + & d \end{array}\right\} \quad (4.7)$$

$$\Rightarrow \quad I(1) - I(-1) = 2a + 2c.$$

We can also eliminate the unknowns b and d from the equations for $x = \pm 2$:

$$\left.\begin{array}{rclcrcrcrcr} I(-2) & = & p(-2) & = & -2a & + & 4b & - & 8c & + & 16d \\ I(2) & = & p(2) & = & 2a & + & 4b & + & 8c & + & 16d \end{array}\right\} \quad (4.8)$$

$$\Rightarrow \quad I(2) - I(-2) = 4a + 16c.$$

We now eliminate c from the intermediate results (Equations 4.7, 4.8), and obtain

$$(I(2) - I(-2)) - 8(I(1) - I(-1)) = 4a - 16a = -12a$$

$$a = \frac{2}{3}(I(1) - I(-1)) - \frac{1}{12}(I(2) - I(-2)).$$

In this case, then, we obtain the five-location mask $\boxed{\begin{array}{c|c|c|c|c} \frac{1}{12} & -\frac{2}{3} & 0 & \frac{2}{3} & -\frac{1}{12} \end{array}}$.

Summary

Numerical approximations of derivatives depend linearly on the values of the image function at the neighboring image points. The exact numbers in the mask depend on assumptions about the "real" function between the sample points. Possible interpolations are:

1. Segments of nth degree polynomials, which pass through $\frac{n}{2}$ points on either side of the point at which the derivative is to be determined, as in the example given above. Interpolations using polynomials of degree higher than four should be avoided, since the interpolations between the sample points tend to oscillate strongly. This tendency is immediately apparent when interpolating a function that has the same value at all sample points.

2. Segments of third-degree polynomials which pass through two sample points and which are continuously twice differentiable, i.e. have the same first and second derivatives where they meet. These *cubic splines* minimize the curvature $\int (f''(x))^2 dx$ of the interpolation function. Large masks (theoretically, masks of infinite width) must be used in calculating these interpolations, since the requirement for smoothness can make changes at one sample point propagate through the entire interpolation.

3. Smoothing splines. These are not interpolations in the usual sense, since they do not necessarily pass through the sample points, but rather only approximate

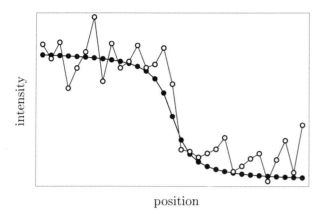

intensity

position

Figure 4.7
Intensity function showing a step-like edge. Black dots: without noise; White dots: with additive random noise. The noise changes the estimated height and position of the edge, and has a greater effect on the derivative than on the original image function.

them. If all sample points are equally reliable, the smoothing spline minimizes the functional

$$E_\lambda(f) = \lambda \sum_i (I(x_i) - f(x_i))^2 + (1 - \lambda) \int (f''(x))^2 dx.$$

The parameter $\lambda \in [0, 1]$ adjusts the relationship between reliability of data and smoothness.

4. Finally, it should be noted that other functions as well, e.g., trigonometric functions, may be chosen as the basis of an interpolation.

In all of these cases, the enhancement and detection of edges can be achieved by means of linear convolution. However, with spline interpolation, the slope at any point depends on the values at all other points, and so the mask must extend throughout the entire image. In some cases, recursive filters can avoid this problem.

4.2.2   Edge detection in noisy images

Let us consider a one-dimensional gray value function I_x which is sampled at the equidistant points x. Random noise n_x is superimposed additively at each point. We assume that the distribution of the noise at all sample points is independent, and that its average value is zero (cf. Fig. 4.7). The relationship between the average image intensity and the standard deviation of the noise process is called the signal to noise ratio.

If the image is differentiated, the average value of the resulting signal (that is, the derivative of the imaging function) will approximately go to zero. For all masks c, the expected value of the filtered image function is the expected value of the original image, multiplied by $\sum_i c_i$, which is 0 in the case of our derivative mask in the above example. On the other hand, the noise occurs independently at neighboring pixels and is therefore just as likely to be intensified as reduced by the subtraction. It can be shown that the variance of the noise when convolved with a mask c is multiplied by the factor $\sum_i c_i^2$. All in all, the signal-to-noise ratio is changed by the factor

$$\frac{\sum_i c_i}{\sqrt{\sum_i c_i^2}} \tag{4.9}$$

when filtered using the mask c.

Differentiation therefore worsens the signal to noise ratio. The same mathematical reasoning can show that local averaging, for example by masks all of whose coefficients are positive and less than 1, improves the signal to noise ratio.

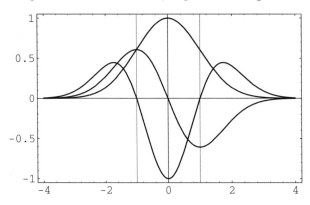

Figure 4.8
One-dimensional profile of the Gaussian curve $f(x) := \exp\{-x^2/2\}$ and its first and second derivatives. The second derivative can be approximated by the difference between two Gaussians of different width.

Differentiation with smoothing

This problem of increasing noise through image differentiation may be avoided by noise reduction preceding the calculation of the derivative. The noise reduction could be achieved by means of smoothing splines, though these do lead to infinitely wide masks, as has already been mentioned. Another possibility is local averaging (low-pass filtering) of the image: as also already mentioned, local averaging reduces noise while altering the signal I only slightly. As with the Gaussian pyramid, the mask used is a (sampled version of the) Gaussian curve

$$G_\sigma(x, y) := \frac{1}{2\pi\sigma^2} \exp\left\{ -\frac{1}{2\sigma^2}(x^2 + y^2) \right\}. \tag{4.10}$$

The averaging is therefore in a window weighted as G_σ.

Convolution and differentiation are linear, translation-invariant operations, in which associativity and commutativity hold. Smoothing and differentiation can therefore be performed in a single step. We will illustrate this for the one-dimensional case. We want to obtain the derivative of the convolution product

$$(I * G_\sigma)'(x) = \frac{d}{dx} \int I(x') G_\sigma(x - x') dx'. \tag{4.11}$$

If the integral exists, we can bring the differentiation inside it, obtaining:

$$(I * G_\sigma)'(x) = \int I(x') G_\sigma'(x - x') dx' = (I * G_\sigma')(x). \qquad (4.12)$$

The result, shown diagrammatically, is as follows:

$$\underbrace{\text{noisy image} * \text{Gaussian}}_{\text{smoothed image}} * \text{differentiation} =$$
$$\text{noisy image} * \underbrace{\text{Gaussian} * \text{differentiation}}_{\text{derivative of the Gaussian}}.$$

This process can be carried on through several differentiations, generating a new class of masks based on Gaussian curves and their derivatives (Fig. 4.8).

Scale space

The assumption that low-pass filtering reduces noise and leaves the actual image unchanged is of course only approximately true. The greater the range of integration, i.e. the greater the value of σ, the more the image is altered. The function

$$I(\vec{\mathbf{x}}; \sigma) := (G_\sigma * I)(\vec{\mathbf{x}}) \qquad (4.13)$$

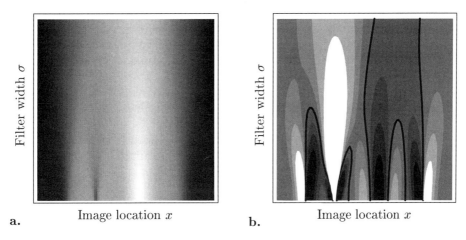

a.   Image location x b.   Image location x

Figure 4.9
Scale space. **a.** Gray value image of the edge function in Fig. 4.3 after low-pass filtering with different filter widths σ. The very bottom of the image shows the original function without low-pass filtering. **b.** Contour lines and values of the second derivative of the gray value function. Darker regions correspond to a negative second derivative and lighter regions, to a positive one. The thick contour lines indicate locations where the second derivative passes through zero ("zero crossings"). There are eight zero crossings at the highest resolution (bottom of the image; cf. also Fig. 4.4), but fewer and fewer zero crossings remain as the smoothing is increased.

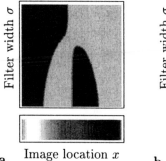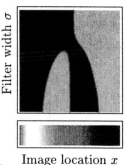

a. Image location x b. Image location x

Figure 4.10
Behavior of the zero crossings in scale space. At the bottom in both examples, the gray value function $I(x) = x^5/20 \pm x^4/240 - x^3/6$ is shown. In **a.**, the $\pm$ sign is assumed to be positive. The three zero crossings at $\sigma = 0$ blend into one as smoothing increases. Which of the original zero crossings becomes the single remaining one depends on very small differences in the gray value, and therefore on noise.

is called the *"scale-space"* of the image I; the variable σ represents the "scale". The concept of scale space is closely related to that of the Gaussian pyramid (Section 3.4.2), but differs in that resolution σ is a continuous function, and in that no under-sampling takes place when making the transition to a lower level of resolution.

The zero crossings of the derivatives of the intensity function are computed by convolution with the corresponding derivatives of the Gaussian. If the zero crossings of $G''_\sigma * I$ are plotted in scale space, they form lines which show how errors in localization and the blending of edge elements develop as the level of resolution changes (cf. Yuille & Poggio 1986). Fig. 4.9b shows an example of this. The blending of the zero crossing lines as smoothing increases is not simple: the high-contrast edges do not always persist and the weaker ones do not always disappear. Fig. 4.10 shows a "bifurcation", in which a very small change in the gray value function affects the relationship of the zero crossing lines in scale space. If scale space is used in a coarse-to-fine strategy as shown here, the results are very sensitive to noise. For more about the theory of scale space cf. Lindeberg (1994).

4.2.3   Lines and steps: "Edge energy"

Up to this point, we have discussed how to evaluate derivatives of the gray value map in sampled, noisy gray scale images. It has already been shown in connection with Fig. 4.4 how these derivatives are related to edges. One problem with this approach is the difference between the behavior of lines—for example, of black lines on a white background—and of step-like edges, i.e. boundaries between bright and dark areas of an image. Lines are, in a certain sense, the derivatives of steps, and for this reason, the two types of edges appear in derivatives of different orders. If an edge detector which uses the slope maxima (zero crossings of the second derivatives) is applied to

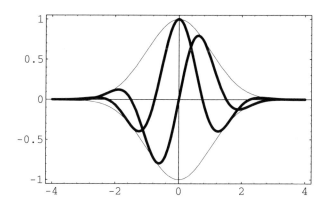

Figure 4.11
One-dimensional Gabor functions with $\omega = 1/3$ and $\sigma = 1$. The even (mirror symmetrical) function is the cosinusioidal Gabor function, and the odd (point symmetrical) function is the sinusoidal Gabor function. The thin lines show the enveloping Gaussian curves.

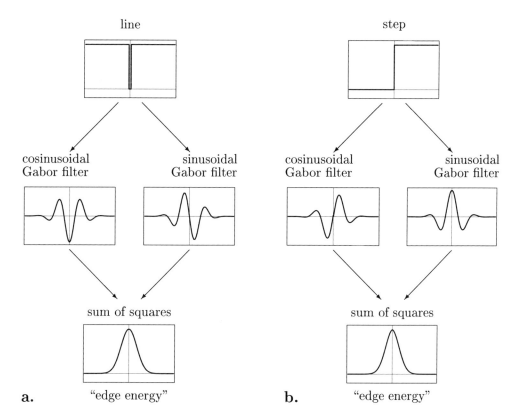

Figure 4.12
Diagram showing the detection of steps and line edges with quadrature filters. Top: image functions. Middle and bottom: Filter response as a function of the location in the images. Further discussion in the text.

line edges, it will detect two edges for each line, corresponding to the two sides of the line in the image.

This problem can be resolved by using two filters, one only for step-like edges and the other for line edges. An example is given in Fig. 4.8: The second derivative of the Gaussian function is suitable for the detection of line edges, while the first derivative may be used for step-like edges. However, the Gabor functions are more widely applied. These are sinusoidal and cosinusoidal functions multiplied by the Gaussian function:

$$g_c(x) \quad := \quad \cos(2\pi\omega x)\exp\left\{-\frac{x^2}{2\sigma^2}\right\} \qquad (4.14)$$

$$g_s(x) \quad := \quad \sin(2\pi\omega x)\exp\left\{-\frac{x^2}{2\sigma^2}\right\}. \qquad (4.15)$$

The cosinusoidal Gabor function is "even", i.e., it fulfills the condition that $g_c(x) \equiv g_c(-x)$; the sinusoidal Gabor function is odd, $g_s(x) \equiv -g_s(-x)$ (cf. Fig. 4.11).

Fig. 4.12 shows how the Gabor functions can be applied. The line edge (Fig. 4.12a) is evaluated correctly by the even, cosinusoidal Gabor filter; the odd, sinusoidal Gabor function generates two peaks, which correspond to the sides of the line. The situation with the step-like edge (Fig. 4.12a) is exactly the opposite. If the output of each filter is squared and these results are added, the result in both cases is unambiguous with the maximum at the position of the step or line edge. Results similar to those shown in Fig. 4.12 are obtained using a large number of filtering functions, of which one must be even and the other odd. Such filters are called quadrature pairs.* The output of a quadrature filter is often called "energy", and in the case of edges, "edge energy". An energy approach to the detection of motion will be described in Section 9.4.

The parameters of the Gabor functions to be applied, the window width σ and the spatial frequency ω, determine the resolution of the edge detection. Resolution pyramids (cf. Section 3.4.2) based on Gabor functions are described in Mallat (1989).

4.3   Edge detection in two dimensions

4.3.1   Kernels of continuous filters

There is more than one way to define derivatives of the Gaussian curve in two dimensions (Fig. 4.13). Oriented filters corresponding to the first derivative in one dimension are generated by directional differentiation of the two-dimensional Gaussian curve,

$$G'_{\sigma,\varphi}(x,y) = -\frac{1}{2\pi\sigma^4}(x\sin\varphi + y\cos\varphi)\exp\{-\frac{1}{2\sigma^2}(x^2+y^2)\} \qquad (4.16)$$

(Fig. 4.13a,b). Clearly, the filtering which results is different for every direction φ.

---

*Not every pairing of an odd and even function is a quadrature pair. If the even filter is designated as f_e and the odd one as f_o, then also, $f_e + if_o$ ($i = \sqrt{-1}$) must be an analytical (differentiable in the complex plane) function. Or, to state this another way, the Hilbert transform must convert the even function into the odd and vice versa. (cf. Papoulis 1968).

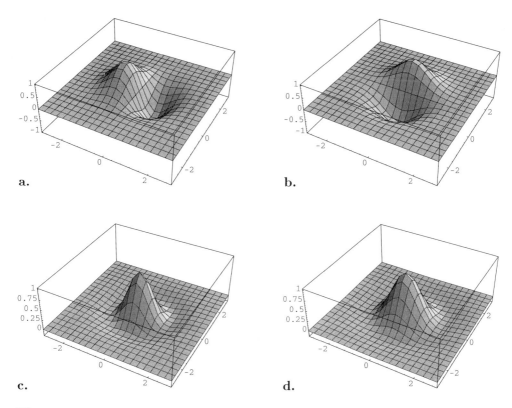

Figure 4.13
Continuous two-dimensional filtering functions. **a.,b.** Directional derivatives of the Gaussian function (Equation 4.16) for two angles φ. **c.** Laplace operator applied to the Gaussian function (Equation 4.17). **d.** Difference between two Gaussian functions of differing width (Equation 4.18).

By analogy to Equation 4.16, it is possible to define directional second derivatives and to use them as well for edge detection. An isotropic—that is, rotationally symmetrical—mask is obtained if the second partial derivatives are added ("Laplace operator").

$$\left(\frac{\partial^2}{\partial x^2} + \frac{\partial^2}{\partial y^2}\right) G_\sigma(x, y) = \frac{1}{\pi\sigma^4}\left(\frac{x^2 + y^2}{2\sigma^2} - 1\right)\exp\{-\frac{1}{2\sigma^2}(x^2 + y^2)\}. \qquad (4.17)$$

In mathematical physics, the Laplace operator is symbolized by Δ (Delta) oder ∇^2 (nabla squared). In image processing, the abbreviation *LoG* (for "Laplacian of a Gaussian") is commonly used. Models of brightness perception based on the Laplace operator ware first proposed by Mach (1922).

The difference between two Gaussian curves of different width provides a good approximation of the *LoG* operator. The symbol representing this curve is *DoG*, which stands for "difference of Gaussians":

$$DoG(x,y) := \frac{1}{2\pi\sigma_e^2}\exp\left\{-\frac{x^2+y^2}{2\sigma_e^2}\right\} - \frac{1}{2\pi\sigma_i^2}\exp\left\{-\frac{x^2+y^2}{2\sigma_i^2}\right\}. \qquad (4.18)$$

The approximation is good when $\sigma_i/\sigma_e = 1.6$ (Marr & Hildreth 1980). The DoG function is a straightforward formalization of the concept of lateral inhibition (Ratliff 1965): The average intensity (σ_i) of a large area surrounding each point is subtracted from the intensity in the immediate neighborhood (σ_e) of the point.

Gabor functions always conform to the orientation of the underlying sinusoidal and cosinusoidal waveforms; isotropic variants are not used. If the orientation is φ, then Equation 4.14 leads to

$$g_{c,\varphi}(x,y) := \cos(2\pi\omega(x\sin\varphi + y\cos\varphi))\exp\{-\frac{1}{2\sigma^2}(x^2+y^2)\}. \qquad (4.19)$$

An analogous equation results from Equation 4.15.

4.3.2   Discrete masks for straight edge elements

The approaches set forth in the previous sections can easily be applied to two dimensions if edge elements are (approximately) straight. In this case, the directional derivatives are at a right angle to the orientation of the edge. The zero crossing of the second derivative in this direction then represents the point of the greatest slope, which is to be identified as the edge location. Examples may be obtained by sampling the functions $G'_{\sigma\varphi}$ in Equation 4.16 (cf. Fig. 4.13a,b):

$$v = \begin{array}{|c|c|c|}\hline -1 & 0 & 1 \\\hline -1 & 0 & 1 \\\hline -1 & 0 & 1 \\\hline\end{array} \quad h = \begin{array}{|c|c|c|}\hline 1 & 1 & 1 \\\hline 0 & 0 & 0 \\\hline -1 & -1 & -1 \\\hline\end{array} \quad d = \begin{array}{|c|c|c|}\hline 0 & 2 & 1 \\\hline -2 & 0 & 2 \\\hline -1 & -2 & 0 \\\hline\end{array}.$$

Application of v results in an enhancement of vertical edges, h enhances horizontal edges and d diagonal edges. Masks approximating the second directional derivatives are obtained by taking the absolute values in the above masks and replacing the value 0 by -1. In practice, if the sinusoidal Gabor function is sampled instead of G', masks with very similar coefficients will result. In order to take advantage of the mathematical advantages of the Gabor functions, larger masks with a finer sampling interval are required.

Two more isotropic filters are the following:

1. **Lateral inhibition:** Rotationally symmetrical or isotropic filters evaluate edges identically regardless of their orientation. Examples are the Laplace filtered Gaussian curves LoG (Equation 4.17) and the difference between two Gaussian curves DoG (Equation 4.18; Fig. 4.13c,d). The result of sampling such an

isotropic operator is a mask such as

−1	−4	−1
−4	20	−4
−1	−4	−1

2. **Slope in the direction of the gradient:** The steepest slope in the gray value map is in the direction of the gradient $\mathrm{grad}I(x,y) = (I_x(x,y), I_y(x,y))$. The slope in this direction is exactly the magnitude of the gradient:

$$s(x,y) := \|I_g(x,y)\| = \left(\left(\frac{\partial I}{\partial x}(x,y) \right)^2 + \left(\frac{\partial I}{\partial y}(x,y) \right)^2 \right)^{\frac{1}{2}}. \qquad (4.20)$$

Here, I_g is the directional derivative I in the direction of the gradient. If the 3×3 masks h and v shown above are used to determine the partial derivatives, this edge detector is called the Sobel operator. It is nonlinear.

4.3.3 Curved edges

In the one-dimensional case, the locations where steepness is greatest correspond to the zero crossings of the second derivative of the image function. In the two-dimensional case, we have used the Laplace operator to define similar points. This is, however, only an approximation, and it leads to systematic localization errors when edges or lines are curved. It would be mathematically correct to determine the second directional derivative of I in the direction of the intensity gradient, by taking the derivative of I_g in Equation 4.20 again. Once again, we designate the direction of the gradient at a point (x,y) as g, $g = \mathrm{grad}I(x,y)/\|\mathrm{grad}I(x,y)\|$, and obtain:

$$I_{gg}(x,y) = \frac{I_x^2 I_{xx} + 2I_x I_y I_{xy} + I_y^2 I_{yy}}{I_x^2 + I_y^2}. \qquad (4.21)$$

The numerator of the fraction on the right side of this equation can be written as a quadratic form,

$$(I_x, I_y) \begin{pmatrix} I_{xx} & I_{xy} \\ I_{xy} & I_{yy} \end{pmatrix} \begin{pmatrix} I_x \\ I_y \end{pmatrix}; \qquad (4.22)$$

the matrix of the second partial derivatives is called the Hesse matrix H_I of the image function.

In this formulation, the Laplace operator is the trace of the Hesse matrix, i.e. the sum of the diagonal entries. Its going to zero is in general not equivalent to the going to zero of the entire quadratic form in Equation 4.21. Fig. 4.14 shows that the zero crossings of the *LoG*-filtered image where edges are curved (Fig. 4.14e) differ considerably from the locations of greatest slope (Fig. 4.14c).

The Gaussian curvature of the gray value map may serve as a criterion for the applicability of the Laplace operator. Where edges are straight, the Gaussian curvature

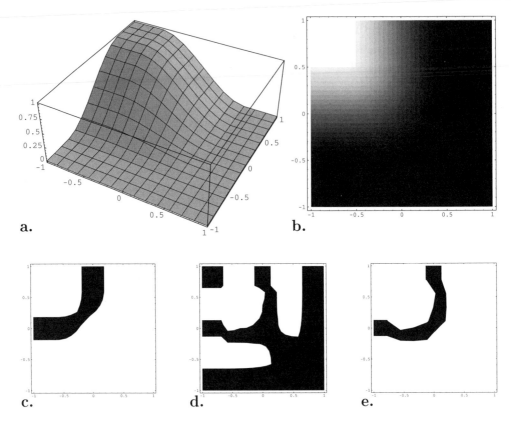

Figure 4.14
Localization of curved edges **a.** Intensity profile **b.** corresponding image. **c.** The
points where the steepness in (a) is greatest are identified by the Sobel operator. **d.**
Regions in which the Laplace operator returns values near zero. **e.** As in (d), except
that locations are omitted at which the sum of the first partial derivatives becomes
small, i.e. regions in which value of the Laplace operator is near zero for the trivial
reason that the gray value is constant. The Laplace operator does not localize the
edge exactly at the steepest point in the intensity profile shown in (c).

goes to zero. A curvature operator which differs from the Gaussian curvature only by
a normalization can be obtained from the determinant of the Hesse matrix (cf. Barth
et al. 1993):

$$\det H_I(x,y) = I_{xx}(x,y)I_{yy}(x,y) - (I_{xy}(x,y))^2. \qquad (4.23)$$

As can easily be confirmed, it follows that when the determinant of H_I and the Laplace
operator both go to zero, the entire Hesse matrix and therefore also the quadratic
from in Equation 4.21 also go to zero. If edges are straight, then, the Laplace operator
gives correct results. Conversely, the operator of Equation 4.23 may be used to locate
highly curved segments of edges.

4.3.4 Further questions

This chapter has examined only the localization of edge elements. For the extraction of a sketch and an edge-based segmentation of the image (separation into more or less homogeneous regions, which correspond accurately to surfaces in the scene being imaged), connection of edge elements into coherent contours is also of great importance. Some of the problems which must be solved in order to achieve this result have already been discussed:

- Uniqueness: A line edge is sometimes represented by two parallel edge elements.

- Intersections and junctions as well as ends of lines often lead to failures in the detection of edge elements. Intersections and junctions can, however, be detected directly as separate classes of features.

- It is often not possible to group edge elements into closed figures unambiguously, and so it may be necessary to make use of other, derived image information. For example, one might search for images of particular objects described by parametric models; cf. Brooks (1981), Biederman (1990). Locally consistent but globally inconsistent interpretations of line images are illustrated, for example, in the "impossible" drawings of M. C. Escher.

Examples of interesting neurobiologically and psychophysically motivated approaches to the perception of lines are found in the models of Grossberg & Mingolla (1985), Watt (1990) and Heitger et al. (1992).

Chapter 5

Color and color constancy

In the preceding chapters, and also in those to follow, intensity I, also called "gray value", is regarded as a scalar quantity. In reality, the irradiance which impinges on a point in the image plane is composed of light of different wavelengths, and consequently is perceived as having a particular color. There are three fundamental but different concepts of color:

Lights and spectra comprise the physical basis of color vision. The expression $I(\lambda)$ represents the spectral composition of light.

Pigments, paint and dye can change the spectral composition of light in the process of reflection. The change is described by means of an absorption spectrum which, when multiplied by the input spectrum, results in the output spectrum.

Color is a perception which results from a complex physiological process.

The (perceived) color does not correspond in a simple way to the spectrum of the light which reaches the eye; rather, color depends differently on the spectra of the illuminating light and of surfaces. In particular, surfaces which have the same absorption spectra usually appear to have the same color despite differences in illumination. This characteristic of vision, called "color constancy", relies not only on the spectral composition of individual points in the image, but also on the spatial distribution of spectra. From the point of view of information processing, the central problem of color perception is that of separating the contribution of illumination (the light source) from that of reflectivity (the surface).

The first section of this chapter concerns itself with space independent characteristics of color perception, while the second section examines local interactions within spatial distributions of colors and gray values.

5.1   The color of isolated points of light

Three concepts of color space are of importance in the theory of color vision:

- *Physics:* Spectra of light are studied as physical phenomena. The set of all spectra is a function space (in the sense of functional analysis) with an infinite number of dimensions, since intensities at all wavelengths are in theory independent of one another. However, the space is not a complete vector space, since there can be no negative intensities.

- *Physiology:* The possible excitation patterns of receptors are studied as physiological phenomena ("receptor space", see below). Since there are three types of receptors, this space is three-dimensional. With the exception that it may include only non-negative intensities and excitations, this space is a linear subspace of spectral space.

- *Psychophysics:* Psychophysical measurements of color use the proportions of primary colors in a mixture matching the color of some test light. These proportions constitute the perceptual color space. Different values of coordinates result from different choices of primary colors; nonetheless, all of the resulting color spaces are equivalent to each other and to the receptor space.

The trichromatic theory of color vision is based on the work of Thomas Young (1773 – 1829) and Hermann von Helmholtz (1821 – 1894) and, thanks to its formal elegance, has played a major role in the study of visual information processing. Modern descriptions are given by Wyszecki & Stiles (1982) and Pokorny & Smith (1986). Trichromatic color vision provides a classic example of population coding, i.e. the coding of a quantity by the relative excitations of channels which have different but overlapping sensitivity curves.

5.1.1   Color mixtures and metamerism

All color perceptions can be generated by the additive mixing of three primary colors. The term "additive color mixture" refers to the super-imposition of light of the corresponding individual colors; that is, in a physical sense, the point-wise addition of spectral intensities at each wavelength. Additive color mixing occurs, for example, when images from several projectors which throw different colors of light are super-imposed. Another example is Maxwell's spinning top, the multiple colors of whose paper surface are mixed over time due to the rapid rotation. By changing the size of the sectors of different colors, it is easily possible to create any desired color mixture (cf. von Campenhausen 1993). Of great practical importance is additive color mixing by the blending of small image elements, for example in color video displays, in offset printing, in weaving and in pointillistic painting. Additive color mixing is to be distinguished from the so-called subtractive color mixing, in which pigments are combined so that their absorption spectra multiply. Examples are the mixing of

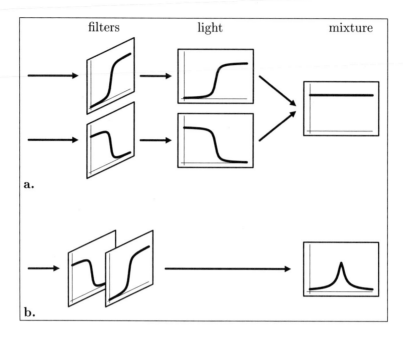

Figure 5.1
Diagrammatic representation of additive and subtractive color mixing. All curves shown are functions of wavelength, λ. The filter curves, shown in perspective, are absorption spectra; the other curves are spectra of light. **a.** Additive color mixing: White light falls on two filters which absorb shorter wavelengths (top) and longer wavelengths (bottom). Yellow light passes through one filter, and blue light through the other. If the light that passed through each of the two filters is superimposed, the result is a flat spectral curve, i.e. white light: blue "plus" yellow = white. **b.** So-called subtractive color mixing: the white light passes through the yellow and blue filters one after the other. The result is a multiplication of the two absorption spectra; the spectrum of the remaining light has a peak in the green spectral range: yellow "minus" blue = green.

pigments in painting and the super-imposition of colored filter sheets in one projector (Fig. 5.1).

The mixing of three primary colors is sufficient to produce (almost) all visible colors. It follows that light with very different spectral compositions can produce the same perception of color. An example of this is the generation of white light from a spectrum with three narrow peaks in the red, green and blue. This line spectrum leads to exactly the same perception of "white", as a flat spectral curve, in which components at all wavelengths are present. Intensity spectra which result in the same perception of color despite differing spectra are called *metamers*. Different light sources with the same spectrum, on the other hand, are called isomers.

The physiological basis for the generation of all colors from three primary colors, and so for metamerism, is the existence of three types of retinal cone cells whose spectral sensitivity is greatest at shorter, intermediate and longer wavelengths of light. Only the excitation of the three types of cones is decisive in color perception. Spectral differences which do not affect the excitation are of little significance, with the one exception of effects due to the chromatic aberration of the dioptric system. Recall that in bright light (daytime), vision is mediated exclusively by the cone system (photopic vision). Night vision (scotopic vision), which works at low levels of illumination by means of the rod receptors, is color blind, since intensity and wavelength can not be distinguished by only one type of receptor.

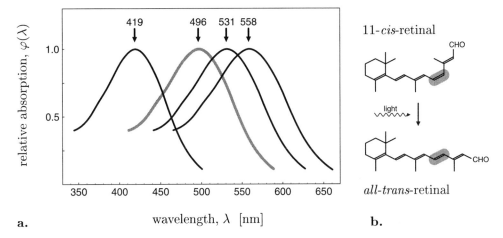

a.   wavelength, λ [nm]   b.

Figure 5.2
a. Absorption spectra of the three types of cones (dark lines) and of the rods (shaded curve) after data of Dartnall et al. (1983). The curves would be identical if absorption were plotted against the fourth root of wavelength. **b.** In all four cases, the absorbing molecule is the same, 11-cis-retinal. The differences between the spectra result from the *opsins*, i.e. the protein components of rhodopsin, which are involved. Cf. Sharpe et al. (1999).

The absorption spectra of the pigments of the human retina are shown in Fig. 5.2a. The curves in this illustration are derived from individual receptor cells, whose output was determined by means of very narrow beams of light under a microscope. The numbers of the individual types of receptors, which naturally are of great importance in perception, do not affect these measurements. The psychophysical sensitivity to shorter wavelengths (blue light) is less than that for red or green light by a factor of approximately 4.5. This factor, however, depends on the spatial extent and duration of the test stimulus. The peak sensitivities of the three types of cones are in violet (shorter), green (intermediate) and yellow (longer) wavelengths of light. There is no actual red receptor. This is surprising, considering the alerting function and striking quality of the color red. The sensory basis for the perception of red is, however, not a receptor specific to red, but rather the proportion of excitation of the medium and long wave receptors.

It is interesting that eyes throughout the animal kingdom, as well as all of the different types of receptors, use the same molecule, retinal (Fig. 5.2b), for the reception of light. The different absorption spectra depend on the protein component, or *opsin* of the receptors. The universality of the retinal molecule points to a common origin of the organ of sight, in spite of all of the variations in its structure. Recently, this common origin has been proven through the identification of a universal gene which initiates the development of eyes (Halder et al. 1995; see also footnote on page 7). A comparative overview of color vision in mammals is given by Jacobs (1993). It has been theorized that the evolution of receptors for intermediate and longer wavelengths in primates was closely bound up with life in the evergreen rain forest. Perception of yellows and reds could have made it possible to identify edible fruits and to evaluate their degree of ripeness (e.g. Osorio & Vorobyev 1996). For a modern introduction to the physiological and psychophysical foundations of color vision, see Gegenfurtner & Sharpe (1999).

5.1.2   Receptor space

If $\varphi_i(\lambda), i \in \{k, m, l\}$ represent the sensitivities of the three receptors (Fig. 5.2a) and $I(\lambda)$ represents the spectral content of a stimulus, then the excitation of the receptor can be calculated as the summation of the spectral components weighted by the sensitivity. Let us call the excitations of the cones with absorption maxima in the shorter, intermediate and longer wavelength ranges e_s, e_m and e_l:

$$
\begin{aligned}
e_s &= \int \varphi_s(\lambda) I(\lambda) d\lambda \\
e_m &= \int \varphi_m(\lambda) I(\lambda) d\lambda \\
e_l &= \int \varphi_l(\lambda) I(\lambda) d\lambda.
\end{aligned}
\tag{5.1}
$$

It is assumed here that the contributions of different spectral ranges are summed linearly. Equation 5.1 describes the projection of the spectral distribution of the light onto the absorption spectrum of the receptors by means of a dot product. The assumption of linearity is of course only approximately correct, since the receptor cells have a sensitivity threshold and a saturation level; these in turn depend on adaptation to the average light level. The quantities e_i as defined in Equation 5.1 are therefore more accurately called *photon catch*. Excitation is a monotonic function of photon catch.

Since the intensity at each wavelength can vary independently, the set of all possible spectra $I(\lambda)$ is a space with an infinite number of dimensions. Since there are no negative intensities, this space is, however, not a complete vector space as described in linear algebra. A coordinate system which represents this space well is defined by the spectral colors $I_{\lambda_o}(\lambda) = \delta(\lambda - \lambda_o)$, where δ is the Dirac impulse, cf. glossary.

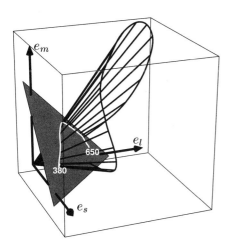 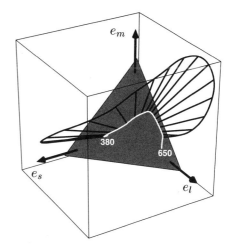

Figure 5.3
The space of receptor excitations as seen from different directions. The three-dimensional curve represents the excitations elicited by the spectral (monochromatic) colors, $(\varphi_s(\lambda), \varphi_m(\lambda), \varphi_l(\lambda))^\top$ for wavelengths from 380 to 650 nm. It corresponds to light of constant irradiance (physical power). Along the rays which connect the origin with this curve, only brightness varies, while the proportions in which the individual receptors are excited remains the same. The points at which these rays intersect the gray triangle represent colors with a constant sum of receptor excitations.

$I_{\lambda_o}(\lambda)$ is therefore a line spectrum with a single line at the wavelength λ_o. The space of all spectra, with an infinite number of dimensions, is projected onto the three-dimensional space of receptor excitations $\vec{e} = (e_s, e_m, e_l)^\top$ by means of equation 5.1. The loss of information which results from the reduction in the number of dimensions is responsible for the metamerism which has already been discussed.

If it is assumed that each type of cone can have an excitation in the interval $[0, 1]$, then the excitation of the receptors may be represented by the volume within the cube $[0, 1]^3$. In fact, however, the large overlaps between the absorption curves make some $\vec{e}$ vectors within the cube impossible: for example, there is no possibility that one type of receptor will be excited alone; the excitation patterns of the type $\vec{e} = (1, 0, 0)^\top$ can not occur. The shape of the receptor space, i.e. the set of all possible $\vec{e}$ vectors, can be inferred from the following considerations. First, it is obvious that those excitation vectors generated by pure spectral lines are within the space. For a fixed irradiance, the curve which describes these vectors is $(\varphi_s(\lambda), \varphi_m(\lambda), \varphi_l(\lambda))$ (Fig. 5.3). Secondly, $\vec{e} = (0, 0, 0)$ is an element of the excitation space. Finally, all other colors are linear combinations of the vectors which have been described, with positive coefficients. The resulting receptor space may therefore be formally described as the convex hull* of

---

*The convex hull of a set M is the smallest set $\hat{M}$ which includes M and which also includes all points x for which $x = \mu a + (1 - \mu)b$ for any two elements $a, b \in M$ and $\mu \in [0, 1]$. Stated more

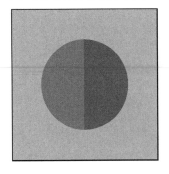

Figure 5.4
Color matching experiment. A two-colored field is presented against a uniform background. One half of the field holds the test color. In the other half, the primary colors can be mixed additively in any desired proportion. The task of the human observer is to match the test color as closely as possible.

the rays from $(0,0,0)$ through the curve of spectral colors, as long as these lie within the cube $[0,1]^3$.

The space of realizable receptor excitations therefore has a more or less conical shape. We note two important characteristics.

1. A coordinate system with orthogonal axes and the origin $(0,0,0)$ can not exist in this space, since the apex angle of the cone is too small. This condition results from the overlap of the absorption functions.

2. In cross-section, the cone is more or less triangular (Fig. 5.3); two sides of the cross-section are determined by the spectral color surface. The third side results from the construction of the convex hull of this surface; its intersection with the triangle in Fig. 5.3 is called the purple line (see below).

5.1.3   Psychophysical color space (Tristimulus space)

Color matching

The field of colorimetry is not concerned with the receptor space, but rather with the coordinate system of a psychophysical color space defined by three primary colors. Against a colorless background, a two-part field is displayed, one half of which is a test color. In the other half, the test color can be duplicated by additive mixing of three primary colors (Fig. 5.4). A crucial requirement is that none of the primary colors can be matched using the other two; in other words, the vectors of receptor excitation generated by the primary colors must be linearly independent.

Initially, let us choose three primary colors whose spectra are $b_j(\lambda)$, $j \in \{1,2,3\}$, which correspond e.g. to the colors red, green and blue. By means of additive mixing, all spectra of the form $\sum_j a_j b_j(\lambda)$ for $0 \le a_j \le 1$ can be generated. If the observer identifies a mixture with the components a_j as indistinguishable from a given spectrum $I(\lambda)$, then the receptor excitations of both of these stimuli must be equal; it

---

simply, this means that the lines connecting two points of M lie entirely within $\hat{M}$. $\hat{M}$ therefore has no concavities.

follows from Equation 5.1 that the following relationship holds:

$$\int \varphi_i(\lambda) \underbrace{I(\lambda)}_{\text{test}} d\lambda = \int \varphi_i(\lambda) \underbrace{\left(\sum_{j=1}^{3} a_j b_j(\lambda) \right)}_{\text{match}} d\lambda \quad \text{with } i \in \{s, m, l\}. \qquad (5.2)$$

The coefficients a_i are called the *tristimulus values* of the test light $I(\lambda)$. In Equation 5.2, it is formally possible for the components a_i to take on negative values. In the experiment, this means that the color is being added not to the comparison field, but rather to the test field itself. This adjustment can be described on the left side of Equation 5.2 with a positive sign. Describing it with a negative sign on the right side is mathematically equivalent.

Spectral tristimulus values

A large role in colorimetry is played by the *spectral tristimulus values*, $\bar{b}_i$. These are the tristimulus values with which pure spectral colors can be matched using three primary colors*. Once again, we designate the spectra of three primary colors as $(b_1(\lambda), b_2(\lambda), b_3(\lambda))$. The excitation of the i-th receptor type when observing a pure spectral color of the wavelength λ_o is clearly $\varphi_i(\lambda_o)$. Let a matching color produced by mixing the three primary colors be $\sum_i \bar{b}_i(\lambda_o) b_i(\lambda)$. Then, since the excitations of the receptors for the pure spectral colors and the matching color must be the same, it follows, as in Equation 5.2, that:

$$\int \varphi_i(\lambda) \left(\sum_{j=1}^{3} \bar{b}_j(\lambda_o) b_j(\lambda) \right) d\lambda = \varphi_i(\lambda_o). \qquad (5.3)$$

The functions $\bar{b}_j(\lambda_o)$ are the spectral tristimulus values; they take the place of the tristimulus values a_j of a general color in Equation 5.2.

It is important to understand that the tristimulus values of any light, including light sources with combined spectra, can be predicted if the spectral tristimulus values are known. It is easy to see this if one thinks of an arbitrary spectrum as being first decomposed into its individual spectral lines. Each individual line corresponds, then, to a spectral color, and this color can be matched using spectral tristimulus values. If, in turn, all of these matched colors, which are mixtures of the same three primary colors, are mixed together, the result is the original, combined spectrum.

This relationship can be described formally in the following way: we consider a light with an arbitrary spectrum $I(\lambda)$. The resulting excitations of the receptors are, as usual, (Equation 5.1),

$$e_i = \int \varphi_i(\lambda) I(\lambda) d\lambda. \qquad (5.4)$$

---

*Matching a spectral color fom three primaries will generally lead to negative tristimulus values as discussed in the preceding paragraph. This is due to the fact that a real mixture, i.e. a mixture with positive values, will always be less saturated than the spectral color.

We now substitute the left side of Equation 5.3 for $\varphi_i(\lambda)$, abandoning the subscript o and renaming the integration variable from Equation 5.3 as λ':

$$e_i = \int \int \varphi_i(\lambda') \left(\sum_j \bar{b}_j(\lambda) b_j(\lambda') \right) d\lambda' \, I(\lambda) d\lambda. \tag{5.5}$$

It is then possible to move the term $I(\lambda)$ into the inner integral and on into the sum, and to reverse the order of integration (Fubini's theorem). Thus, all terms depending on λ are grouped together:

$$e_i = \int \varphi_i(\lambda') \left(\sum_j b_j(\lambda') \int I(\lambda) \bar{b}_j(\lambda) d\lambda \right) d\lambda'. \tag{5.6}$$

The inner expression $\int I(\lambda) \bar{b}_j(\lambda) d\lambda$ turns out to be the projection of I on the spectral value function $\bar{b}_j$. Because the complete expression is equal to the right side of Equation 5.4, it follows that the color value a_j generated by mixing I is given exactly by the projection of I onto the spectral value functions $\bar{b}_j$,

$$a_j = \int I(\lambda) \bar{b}_j(\lambda) d\lambda. \tag{5.7}$$

The basis of color space

We have examined the spectra of the primary colors $\{b_i(\lambda)\}$ and the spectral value functions $\{\bar{b}_j(\lambda)\}$: two groups of three functions each, which exhibit certain characteristics of a basis or of a coordinate system. The coordinates of a color are the tristimulus values a_i. The primary colors constitute a "constructive" basis which makes it possible to determine the spectrum which corresponds to the tristimulus values, by means of the equation $I(\lambda) = \sum_i a_i b_i(\lambda)$. The spectral value functions constitute a "descriptive" basis which allows to determine the tristimulus values of a given spectrum: $a_i = \int I(\lambda) \bar{b}_i(\lambda) d\lambda$.

Primary colors and spectral tristimulus values are therefore related to each other as covariant and contravariant coordinates in affine geometry (Fig. 5.5). If we consider the tristimulus values of the primary colors, then we immediately obtain*

$$\int b_i(\lambda) \bar{b}_j(\lambda) d\lambda = \begin{cases} 0 & \text{if} \quad i \neq j \\ 1 & \text{if} \quad i = j \end{cases}. \tag{5.8}$$

Intuitively, this means that the matching of one of the primary colors consists only of that primary color itself. Equation 5.8 can be interpreted mathematically to show that b_i is orthogonal to all $\bar{b}_j$ with $j \neq i$. Consequently, not all b_i and $\bar{b}_i$ will fit

---

*Equation 5.8 follows also from the relationship $a_j = \int \bar{b}_j(\lambda) \sum_i a_i b_i(\lambda) d\lambda$, which must hold for every j and every tristimulus vector $(a_1, a_2, a_3)^\top$.

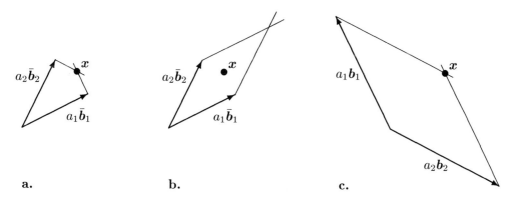

a.   **b.**   **c.**

Figure 5.5
The meaning of coordinate values in affine coordinate systems. **a.** The "descriptive" coordinates of a vector x can be defined by projections at right angles onto the axes $\bar{b}_1$ and $\bar{b}_2$. This process generates the coefficients a_1, a_2. **b.** If the same basis vectors are added together, using a_1 and a_2 as weights, the result will differ from vector x: $x \neq a_1\bar{b}_1 + a_2\bar{b}_2$. **c.** By solving the equations $(\bar{b}_i \cdot \sum_j a_j b_j) = a_i$, two vectors b_1, b_2 can be calculated, by means of which the reconstruction of x is possible. In n-dimensional space, b_i lies at a right angle to all $\bar{b}_j$ with $j \neq i$. The spectral tristimulus value functions correspond to the basis vectors $\bar{b}_i$, the spectra of the primary colors correspond to b_i, and the tristimulus values correspond to a_i.

simultaneously into the space of possible spectra, which can have only non-negative values between 0 and 1. To put it another way: when starting with realizable primary colors, the corresponding spectral tristimulus values will always exhibit negative values. If the coordinate system is transformed so as to make the spectral tristimulus values always positive, then there are no real primary colors for use in color mixture. The specific colorimetric systems to be described below (RGB and XYZ) use either realizable primary colors (RGB) or realizable spectral value functions (XYZ).

Primary colors may be chosen freely within the color space, as long as none of them can be matched by a mixture of the other two. Depending on the primary colors which have been chosen, the tristimulus values for a given color are different. It can be shown that the tristimulus values for different primaries are related to each other through a linear transformation whose 3×3 matrix consists of the tristimulus values of the new primary colors measured with respect to the old ones. Since this transformation is in general not orthonormal, distances and angles are not preserved when going from one system of primary colors to another. Since there is no reason to prefer one or the other system of primary colors, it is not possible to define distances and angles meaningfully in color space. This is to say that color space is an affine space.

Let us summarize once more the most important objects in color space.

1. The spectra of the primary colors $b_i(\lambda)$ establish the coordinate system in the

color matching experiment.

2. The tristimulus values a_i are the actual coordinates of a color. If the primary colors are mixed in the proportion given by the tristimulus values a_i, a metamer of the original spectrum is generated.

3. Spectral values $\bar{b}_i(\lambda)$ are the tristimulus values of pure, monochromatic colors. They can be used to calculate the tristimulus values of any color. They therefore correspond to the sensitivity distributions of real or theoretical receptors by means of which the tristimulus values can be measured directly. Since the primary colors can not be orthogonal to each other, spectral tristimulus value functions are not identical to the spectra of the primary colors (Fig. 5.5).

4. All systems of primary colors satisfying the requirement that no primary can be remixed by the other two (linear independence of the associated receptor excitations) are equivalent. Since angles and distances are not preserved when converting between different systems of primary colors, the angles and distances in color space can not be defined in any meaningful way.

The chromaticity diagram

Tristimulus space incorporates not only different colors but also variations in brightness. Since brightness is often not of interest, the normalized *chromaticities* are often considered, rather than the tristimulus values a_1, a_2, a_3.

$$c_1 = \frac{a_1}{a_1 + a_2 + a_3}; \quad c_2 = \frac{a_2}{a_1 + a_2 + a_3}. \tag{5.9}$$

Each color, then, is defined by two numbers; a quantity $c_3 = 1 - c_1 - c_2$ is no longer necessary. The conversion from the tristimulus values to the chromaticities corresponds to the central projection of the color space onto the triangle $a_1 + a_2 + a_3 = 1$ of Fig. 5.3. This triangle is called the chromaticity diagram.

The basic characteristics of the chromaticity diagram have already been shown in Fig. 5.3. The loci of the spectral colors trace an open curve. All real colors can be mixed from two spectral colors; that is, they lie on a line between two points on the spectral color path. The totality of these lines is the convex hull of the spectral color curve, which has already been mentioned. This region of real colors is shaded in the standard color triangle in Fig. 5.6; it is bounded at the bottom by the purple line. Due to the overlap among the receptor curves, colors outside this region are unrealizable.

The choice of the three primary colors establishes the coordinate system of the color space. In theory, all systems are equally valid; their color triangles can be converted into one another by linear transformations. In practice, two systems are commonly used:

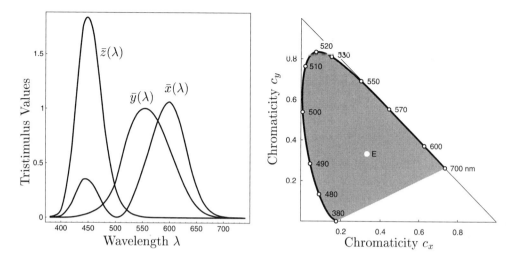

Figure 5.6
Left: Spectral tristimulus value functions for the "CIE 1931 standard observer"(XYZ system). **right:** CIE chromaticity diagram showing the spectral color loci, the white point E and the purple line (lower boundary of the color space).

The RGB system uses as its primary colors the spectral colors of wavelengths

$$\lambda_R = 700 \text{ nm}; \quad \lambda_G = 546.1 \text{ nm}; \quad \lambda_B = 435.8 \text{ nm}.$$

The spectral tristimulus values of this system (and any primary-based system) take on negative values. For example, the pure spectral color with $\lambda = 500$ nm can not be matched, but rather only a mixture including some red R (700 nm). In the chromaticity diagram, mixtures of the blue and green primary will fall on the straight line connecting the loci of these two primaries and will always be somewhat less saturated than the spectral color at $\lambda = 500$ nm. The loci of the colors resulting from mixtures of primaries with positive tristimulus values form a triangle connecting the loci of these primaries. No such triangle can occupy the entire area of realizable colors in the chromaticity diagram.

The XYZ system is the standard system of colorimetry, as defined by the *"Commission Internationale de l'Eclairage"* (CIE) in 1931. This system is based on measurements using the same primary colors as the RGB system; however, a transformation of coordinates is added. This lends certain simple characteristics to the spectral tristimulus values and the chromaticity diagram. The spectral tristimulus values of the XYZ system are everywhere non-negative, and so can be realized using filters, while the primary colors are unreal (Fig. 5.6). The spectral tristimulus values $\bar{y}(\lambda)$ are identical with the curve of brightness sensitivity for photopic (cone receptor) vision. The axes c_x and c_y of the standard chromaticity diagram are orthogonal to one another, so that the perceived brightness in the c_x direction is constant. In the XYZ chromaticity diagram, white light is represented by the point $(c_x, c_y) = (\frac{1}{3}, \frac{1}{3})$ (white dot E in Fig. 5.6).

To summarize the most important characteristics of the chromaticity diagram:

1. *White, or colorless, point:* When the tristimulus values are equal, $a_x = a_y = a_z$, the "color" is white. In the standard chromaticity diagram, its coordinates are $c_x = c_y = \frac{1}{3}$. Colors near the white point are described as "unsaturated".

2. *Real and unreal (imaginary) colors:* Not all coordinates c_x, c_y correspond to real colors. Because of the overlap of the spectral tristimulus functions there can, for example, be no physical spectrum which generates the tristimulus values $(1, 0, 0)$. The apices of the color triangle, and an area in the vicinity of each of them, are therefore unoccupied.

3. *Spectral color loci:* The upper boundary of the occupied region is the curve formed by the spectral colors. Along with the purple line, this represents the most highly saturated colors.

4. *Purple line:* The lower boundary of the occupied region is a straight line connecting the two ends of the spectral color curve.

5. *Color mixing:* All additive mixtures of two colors lie on the line connecting the locations of those two primary colors. All mixtures of n colors lie within the polygon defined by these colors (the convex hull of the loci of the primary colors). A color monitor screen with three phosphors can therefore never represent all colors, but rather only those in the triangle defined by the three primary colors which are generated by the monitor's phosphors.

6. *Complementary colors:* Spectral colors with loci on opposite sides of the white point in the chromaticity diagram can be additively mixed to white. Such colors are called "complementary". Green does not have a complementary color in the spectrum. Complementary colors must not be confused with opponent colors discussed below.

The HSB system

Representation of colors by means of vectorial coordinate systems in color space is very appropriate for the generation of colors through additive color mixing. Representation in terms of variables for hue, saturation and brightness is, however, more intuitive. Brightness is the length of the vector which is abandoned when making the transition from color space to the chromaticity diagram; hue and saturation are, more or less, the angle and radius in a representation in polar coordinates with white at the center. For example, in the DIN 6164 color chart, the lines of constant hue are straight lines from the white point to the spectral color path. The lines of constant saturation are not circles, but rather, are shapes which are elongated parallel to the purple line (cf.

Richter 1981, Wyszecki & Stiles 1982, p. 512). The psychophysical limit of resolution in the HSB system is shown in Table 5.1.

Attempts have been made in connection with the HSB system and similar systems to determine perceptually equal gradations of color. Such systems can not be based simply on the color matching experiment, which asks only whether two colors are the same or different. The question, for example, whether the visible difference is of hue or saturation, or whether the perceptual distance between two colors is the same as between two other colors leads to what is sometimes called "higher order colorimetry".

Table 5.1
HSB coordinates in color space

Dimension	Interpretation	Number of perceivable steps
Hue	Quality of color perception (red, green, yellow, blue), wavelengths of the spectral colors	ca. 200
Saturation	How highly colored. How much white is mixed in?	ca. 20
Brightness	Intensity of light, weighted by the spectral sensitivity curve (candela/m^2)	ca. 500
Total		> 1.000.000

5.1.4 Opponent colors

Neighboring colors in the color triangle blend continuously with one another. It is therefore not difficult to imagine a yellowish red or a bluish green. There are, however, pairs of colors between which a continuous transition which does not pass through white or a third color is unimaginable: there can be no greenish red or yellowish blue. According to Ewald Hering (1834 – 1918), there are three such pairs of opponents:

$$\text{red} \iff \text{green}$$
$$\text{yellow} \iff \text{blue}$$
$$\text{bright} \iff \text{dark.}$$

Opponent colors do not contradict the trichromatic theory, but rather, are indicative of a higher level of processing which can be confirmed to exist on as low a level as the retinal ganglion cells (Fig. 5.7). At this stage of processing, the differences between signals from the different types of cone receptors are evaluated.

Opponent color channels transmit differences (or sometimes also sums) of receptor excitations. The usefulness of opponent color coding is in its decorrelating the

excitations of the three types of cones (Buchsbaum & Gottschalk 1983). If the three
color opponent channels are represented by a, p, q and their excitations, correspondingly, by f_a, f_p, f_q, then the forward signal transmission path from the receptors to
the opponent color channels can be represented by a weighting matrix W:

$$\begin{pmatrix} f_a \\ f_p \\ f_q \end{pmatrix} = \begin{pmatrix} w_{as} & w_{am} & w_{al} \\ w_{ps} & w_{pm} & w_{pl} \\ w_{qs} & w_{qm} & w_{ql} \end{pmatrix} \begin{pmatrix} e_s \\ e_m \\ e_l \end{pmatrix}. \tag{5.10}$$

Here, w_{as} (and similarly for the other receptors) is the weighting with which a S cone
(short wavelength) excites or inhibits the opponent color mechanism a. Due to the
great overlap of the spectral sensitivities of the receptors, Fig. 5.2a, the excitations
e_s, e_m, and e_l are highly correlated. In its details, the correlation depends on the
spectral distribution of light in the scene being observed. By applying the methods
of multivariate statistics (principle component analysis, cf. Mardia et al. 1979), a
matrix W can be calculated which decorrelates the excitations of the opponent color
channels, i.e, the maximum possible information is transmitted. As Buchsbaum &
Gottschalk (1983) show, decorrelation results in an achromatic channel a in which all
of the receptor channels contribute with a positive sign, a difference channel p of the
M and L cones ("yellow minus green") as well as an additional difference channel q
in which the combined excitation of the M and L cones is subtracted from that or
the S cones ("blue minus yellow"). The largest amount of information is carried by
the achromatic (bright/dark) channel (97.2 % of the variance); the red/green channel
carries another 2.78 %, while the blue/yellow channel carries only another 0.02 %
of the signal variance. These channels, predicted through analysis using information
theory, have sensitivity curves which correspond well to those of the psychophysically
confirmed opponent colors.

Opponent colors do not lie exactly opposite each other in the chromaticity diagram. Nonetheless, it is possible to arrange the most highly saturated colors in a
circle in which the opponent colors are in fact opposite one another. This circle is
closed between red and blue by the perceived color "purple". The concept of the
"color circle" underlies the HSB system of colorimetry.

The physiological basis for opponent colors is the network of cones and ganglion
cells in the retina. In good agreement with psychophysical measurements and the
theoretical analysis presented above, ganglion cell types for all three opponent color
channels have been identified. The combining of input signals does not, however,
occur simply at each retinal location, as was assumed for the sake of simplicity in
the theory of Gottschalk & Buchsbaum (1983). Strictly speaking, this assumption
is not possibly correct, since cones of different types are never at exactly the same
place in the image. In reality, the processing pattern is that of lateral inhibition,
in which, for example, central longer-wavelength inputs are subtracted from lateral
medium-wavelength inputs ("green-on-center, red-off-surround"). Since no negative
excitations of the ganglion cells are possible, a total of four different types of ganglion
cells are necessary in the red-green channel. The achromatic channel and the yellow-
blue channel each have only two types of ganglion cells. (Fig. 5.7).

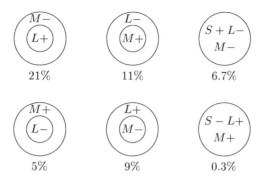

Figure 5.7

Receptive fields of retinal ganglion cells with opponent color characteristics. Upper row: on-center neurons. Lower row: off-center neurons. S, M, L: Types of cones from which the cell receives signals. $+, -$: Sign of the influence of this signal (excitatory, inhibitory). The percentages indicate the frequency of these cells in the rhesus monkey retina; the remaining 47% were not color-specific. After Zrenner 1983; cf. also Dacey 1996

The color-specific ganglion cells of the retina are of what is called the *parvocellular* type (cf. page 55: β-cells). This type is distinct from the achromatic *magnocellular* type (α- cells), which is characterized by greater temporal resolution. The separation of the two types of cells is maintained in the lateral geniculate nucleus (LGN) of the diencephalon, the first relay station for the ganglion cell axons, and in the visual cortex. Consequently, separate processing of color information and motion information in the visual system has been postulated ("color blind motion sensing system"). Recent research has shown, however, that there is interaction between the two systems and that motion sensing is not completely color blind (cf. Gegenfurtner & Hawken 1996).

5.1.5 Population coding

It might seem that the decorrelation of the color channels by opponent colors is simply a "remedial measure" which would not be necessary if the receptor sensitivity curves did not overlap. But it must also be understood clearly that this overlap allows a fundamentally more efficient coding than would be possible if the sensitivities did not overlap. Codes with overlapping sensitivities are called population codes, since each signal (here, each wavelength) is coded in a distributed excitation pattern which involves all channels. In contrast to this is interval coding, in which the sensitivities of the channels do not overlap.

The greater efficiency of population coding is clear if we consider that the largest amount of information is transmitted through a given number of channels when each of them is excited or not excited equally often (optimal coding as described in infor-

Table 5.2

Examples of population coding in visual perception

Encoded quantity	Channels with overlapping selectivity
Color	Spectral sensitivity of the receptors (Fig. 5.2)
Retinal position (hyperacuity in vernier resolution)	Receptive fields as the spatial distribution of sensitivity (Section 3.4.1)
Contrast and spatial frequency	Spatial-frequency channels (Fig. 3.11)
Stereopsis	Disparity tuning of binocular neurons (Fig. 6.17)
Egomotion	Matched filter for specific patterns of optical flow (Fig. 10.12)
Observer position in a large environment	Hippocampal place fields in rats (Section 11.4)

mation theory; cf. Cover & Thomas 1991). In interval coding, however, each channel is excited only when a signal falls into the exact interval for which the channel is responsible. In every other case, the channel sends no information. In population coding, by contrast, several of the available channels are used, so that, in all, more information about the signal is available. The same conclusion results from the observation that, for overlapping sensitivities, a difference in excitation of two channels can encode very small gradations in the overlap region. In interval coding, on the other hand, differences in channel activity contain very little information.

Population coding is a general principle of perception which operates not only in color vision but also in other contexts including directional hearing, place representation in the hippocampus, and motor signals in the generation of arm movements (Georgopoulos et al. 1982). Examples of interval coding, on the other hand, are few in number. Some examples of population coding mentioned in other chapters of this book are assembled in Table 5.2. On the theory of population coding, see Snippe (1996).

5.2   Color in images

5.2.1   Color appearance

The perception elicited by a beam of light with a given spectrum depends heavily on which colors are displayed at the same time in the vicinity of the test patch, and on which colors were previously displayed. Against a red background, a gray sheet of paper appears greenish; against a green background, it appears reddish. Conversely, if red and green backgrounds are placed next to one another, each with a sheet of paper on it, and the color of the two sheets of paper is adjusted to appear the same, the tristimulus values of the light reflected from the two pieces of paper can be very different. The apparent sameness of different tristimulus values ("chromatic induction") should not be confused with metamerism. While metamerism results from the restriction to three color channels, color induction results from interactions between the receptor excitations at various places in the image (cf. Fig. 5.7) or at different times.

The interactions between the colors of a scene and the illumination lead to a group of related phenomena whose names depend on the particular variables being considered:

Color constancy is the independence of the perceived color from the color of the light source. A first-order model of this phenomenon is that a tristimulus vector which corresponds to the average stimulus color is defined as white, and all other vectors are referenced to it by adaptation of the sensitivity of the receptors. This description is based on the simplifying assumption that the average color of a scene is gray or white, the "gray world assumption".

Successive color contrast: Color constancy is bound up with an adaptation to the predominant color of a scene. If the color composition of the scene changes suddenly, an aftereffect occurs. If, for example, the illumination changes suddenly from red to white, the scene at first appears greenish.

Simultaneous color contrast: As already mentioned, small gray areas appear greenish against a red background, but they appear reddish against a green background. Spatial summation by the opponent color cells (Fig. 5.7) is at least partly responsible for this effect. However, simultaneous color contrast is not simply an example of lateral inhibition, since it can be affected by the absence or presence of edges. Fig. 5.8 shows a gray ring, half against a dark and half against a light background. (the Koffka ring). In part b of the illustration, the ring is divided by a thin line which is a continuation of the boundary in the background. Lateral inhibition should lead to the same contrast increase in Fig. 5.8a and b. The actual contrast increase in b is significantly greater. If the edge is not present, the visual system attempts to assign a uniform gray value to the entire ring. Introducing the dividing line removes this necessity, and so the contrast increase is unimpeded (cf. Metzger 1975).

5.2.2 Posing the problem

As has already been shown in Chapter 2, image intensity is constituted of reflectivity and incident light, multiplied together:

$$I(\vec{x}, \lambda) = E(\vec{x}, \lambda) S(\vec{x}, \lambda). \tag{5.11}$$

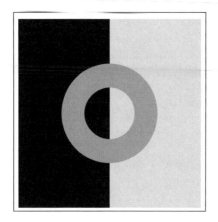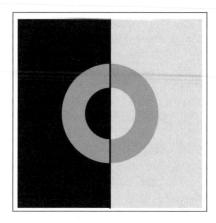

Figure 5.8
Koffka rings, illustrating the dependence of perceived intensities on edges. In both images, the gray ring is everywhere equally bright. While the ring at the left essentially appears that way, the two halves in the right-hand image appear to be of differing brightness: the part of the ring over the lighter background appears darker. This perception is generated by the added dividing line, which makes it easier to assign different gray values to the two halves.

Here, $E(\vec{x}, \lambda)$ is the irradiance at the place in the scene which is imaged at the point $\vec{x}$. $S(\vec{x}, \lambda)$ is the reflectivity of the surface at the same location; assuming that the surface is a Lambert radiator (Equation 2.5), then $S = c(\vec{n} \cdot \vec{l})$. Equation 5.11 holds independently for every wavelength λ. But if we proceed to the excitations in the color channels (Equation 5.1), the simple multiplicative structure no longer holds, since there is integration over ranges of wavelengths. The problem of color constancy is, then, to separate the two terms on the right side of Equation 5.11 and so to determine the characteristics of the surface $S(\vec{x}, \lambda)$ independently of those of the illuminant $E(\vec{x}, \lambda)$.

There is no general solution to this problem; besides, perception does not possess ideal color constancy either. If, however, there are enough different colored surfaces in the image, and if the illumination is not too unusual, there are satisfactory solutions.

5.2.3   Linear transformations

This section is based on work of Maloney & Wandell (1986). Real surfaces have only a rather limited variation in their absorption spectra, since absorption spectra are generally continuous and band-limited. In fact, only three to five base spectra $S_j(\lambda)$ can model most actual absorption spectra by linear combination. Therefore, S can be modeled as the sum

$$S(\vec{x}, \lambda) = \sum_{j=1}^{J} \sigma_j(\vec{x}) S_j(\lambda) \tag{5.12}$$

wherein the base spectra S_j are givens, and the coefficients σ_i represent the spatial dependency. We make the additional simplifying assumption that the spectral composition and intensity of the illumination are constant throughout the entire scene. If we substitute Equations. 5.11 and 5.12 into Equation 5.1, we obtain

$$e_i(\vec{x}) = \int E(\lambda) \sum_{j=1}^{J} \sigma_j(\vec{x}) S_j(\lambda) \varphi_i(\lambda) d\lambda. \tag{5.13}$$

wherein the index $i = 1, ..., 3$ represents the type of receptor, while j accounts for the degrees of freedom of the absorption spectra. If we denote the $J \times 3$ matrix by Λ_ϵ

$$\Lambda_\epsilon = \left\{ \int E(\lambda) S_j(\lambda) \varphi_i(\lambda) d\lambda \right\}_{(j,i)}, \tag{5.14}$$

then Equation 5.13 becomes the vector equation

$$\vec{e} = \Lambda_\epsilon \vec{\sigma}. \tag{5.15}$$

The matrix Λ_ϵ describes the role of illumination in the conversion from surface reflectivity, which is given by $\sigma_1, ..., \sigma_J$, to receptor excitation. The subscript ϵ indicates that the matrix also depends on the illumination E. It is interesting as an exercise to consider that metameric illuminations of the same scene can result in different illumination matrices and so in different patterns of excitation of the cones, i.e. different colors.

Fig. 5.9 gives an example. We will assume that the surface colors in the scene mostly vary with only two degrees of freedom. The matrix Λ_ϵ then has 2×3 coefficients, and the locations of all excitation vectors $\vec{e}$ in the receptor space construct a plane which passes through the origin of tristimulus space, according to Equation 5.15. The intersection of this plane with the chromaticity diagram is indicated by the straight line in Fig. 5.9. Different lighting results in different planes in the receptor space, and therefore, the different straight lines in Fig. 5.9.

The problem of color constancy is solved if the matrix Λ_ϵ has been determined and if, in addition, the illumination matrix Λ_o for white light is known. For any arbitrary excitation vector $\vec{e}$, the result in this case is the excitation vector $\vec{e}_o$ which the same surfaces would have produced under white lighting, and they are related as

$$\vec{e}_o = \Lambda_o (\Lambda_\epsilon^\top \Lambda_\epsilon)^{-1} \Lambda_\epsilon^\top \vec{e}. \tag{5.16}$$

Here, $(\Lambda_\epsilon^\top \Lambda_\epsilon)^{-1} \Lambda_\epsilon^\top$ is what is called the pseudoinverse* of Λ_ϵ, whose existence we can assume if the illumination is not too unusual. If Λ_ϵ is quadratic and can be inverted, the pseudoinverse becomes an ordinary inverse matrix.

Equation 5.16 describes the linear transformation of the color coordinates of Fig. 5.9b, c to those of Fig. 5.9a if the lighting of Fig. 5.9b (green) and c (red) is

---

*If Λ_ϵ is not quadratic, then we multiply both sides of Equation 5.15 from the left with the transposed matrix$\Lambda_\epsilon^\top$. The matrix $\Lambda_\epsilon^\top \Lambda_\epsilon$ is quadratic in any case. If its inverse exists, then Equation 5.15 can be solved for $\vec{\sigma}$. Substitution into $\vec{e}_o = \Lambda_o \vec{\sigma}$ results in Equation 5.16.

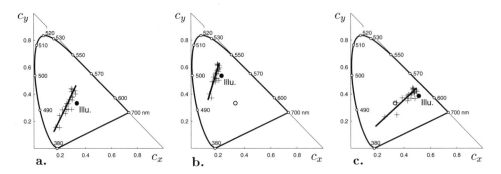

Figure 5.9
The influence of illumination on chromaticity. The illustration shows the chromaticities of a random sample of surface colors under differing illumination. **a.** White
illumination. The colors fall along a straight line in the blue-green region. **b.** Under
green illumination, the locations of the colors are correspondingly shifted. **c.** A shift
also occurs with red illumination. Illu.: color of the illumination. The open circle ○
indicates white. In **a.**, it coincides with the color of the illuminant.

used for the calculation of Λ_ϵ. It can be seen that the process described by Maloney
& Wandell (1986) does not simply position the average of the color coordinates of the
samples on the white point, but rather gives more precise results which make it possible for mostly monochromatic images (e.g. the image of a green meadow) to maintain
their dominant color after calculation of color constancy. If the average were simply
shifted to the white point, a green meadow would appear gray after being viewed for
a long time.

The problem still remains of determining the matrix Λ_ϵ from image data. Since
neither the base spectra of the surface colors S_j, the spectrum of the illumination
E, nor the absorption spectra of the receptors φ_i can be assumed to be known,
the only remaining approach is to solve the system of equations 5.15. Allowing J
degrees of freedom for the surface colors, Λ_ϵ has a total of $3J$ components, which
are all unknown. For each surface patch, Equation 5.15 generates three determinant
equations but also J additional unknowns, $\sigma_1(\vec{x}), ..., \sigma_J(\vec{x})$. A solution is therefore
only possible if $J < 3$, in other words, if the surface colors have only two degrees of
freedom. If, in this case, there are six colored surfaces with the spatial coordinates
$\vec{x}_1, ..., \vec{x}_6$, then the six coefficients of Λ_ϵ as well as the 2×6 coefficients of the surface
colors $\sigma_1(\vec{x}_1), ..., \sigma_2(\vec{x}_6)$ can be determined. If the surface colors have more than two
degrees of freedom, i.e. if their chromaticities do not fall on a straight line in the
chromaticity diagram, the estimate of Λ_ϵ is worse the greater the deviation from the
straight line. The rather narrow constellations of points in Fig. 5.9, for example,
would still give acceptable results.

There is an additional restriction on the matrix Λ_ϵ, of which Maloney & Wandell

(1986) do not make use: the transformation of Equation 5.16 may not lead outside the chromaticity diagram or the domain of the real colors. Especially when samples with large numbers of surface colors are used, this is a severe restriction, and can significantly improve the calculation of color constancy (cf. Forsyth 1990, Finlayson 1996).

A psychophysical comparison between the linear theory and human color constancy is given by Lucassen & Walraven (1996).

5.2.4 Piecewise constant surface characteristics

The retinex theory (Land & McCann 1971), developed by Edwin H. Land (1909 – 1991) is based on the importance of edges for color constancy. This theory counts as one of the seminal ideas in image processing. We will briefly discuss this historically important theory, despite its having been largely superseded both for modeling of human color vision and for computer processing of images (Brainard & Wandell 1986; cf. however Jobson et al. 1997). We will discuss not Land's original approach, but rather a version of the theory by Horn (1974) which is in many ways equivalent, but more clearly defined.

Let us consider a plane with piecewise constant reflectivity. Such excitation patterns are often called "Mondrians," referring to the Dutch painter Pieter Cornelis Mondrian (1872 – 1944)—though the similarities with his work are relatively minor. Using a suitable illumination pattern, an intensity profile like that in Fig. 5.10 may occur. We will consider the problem in only one dimension, i.e. for images like those in Fig. 5.10b. The retinex concept consists of:

1. finding the edges in $I(x)$,
2. eliminating the "slow" changes (i.e. smooth changes in illumination across the image), and
3. finally, reconstructing $S(x)$ from the edges.

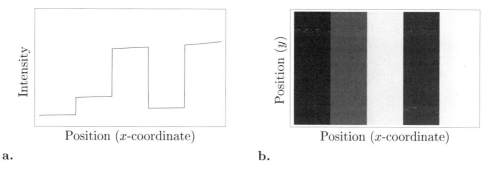

a.   b.

Figure 5.10
Gray value function of an image with piecewise constant reflectivity ("Mondrian pattern") under uneven lighting. **a.** Gray value profile. **b.** Image

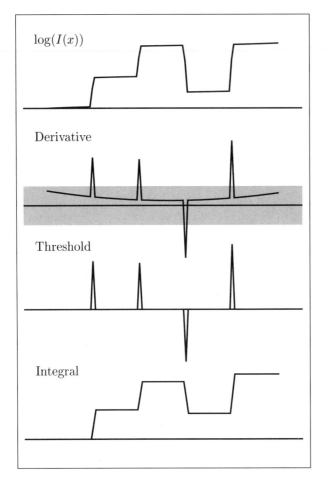

$\log(I(x))$

Derivative

Threshold

Integral

Figure 5.11
Illustration of the one-dimensional retinex process. First, the gray value profile (Fig. 5.10) is scaled logarithmically, and then the derivative is taken. An appropriate threshold operation may then remove the "slow" gray value changes. If the remaining spikes are integrated, the result is an estimate of the logarithm of surface reflectivity. Finally, the exponential function must be applied to reverse the logarithmic scaling (this step not shown).

Fig. 5.11 illustrates the basic concept which underlies the retinex process. The intensity distribution differs somewhat from that for surface reflectivity S, assuming this is piecewise constant. First, the logarithm of the intensities is taken, to convert the multiplication of surface reflectivity and illumination (Equation 5.11) into an addition of logarithmic quantities.[*]

---

[*]Brainard & Wandell (1986) point out that the spectral irradiance function $I(x, \lambda)$ is not known. This is the only function for which the multiplicative conversion is correct. Only the receptor excitation $e_i(x)$ is in fact known. Unlike multiplication, the taking of the integral in Equation 5.1 is not transformed into an addition by applying the logarithm, and so this fundamental concept of the retinex process is problematic. There is, nonetheless, an important special case in which taking the logarithm does serve the desired purpose. Consider illumination of the scene by a dim lamp. In this case, the spectrum of the illumination is the same everywhere in the scene, while the intensity falls off with distance from the lamp. The dependences of illumination on space and wavelength are therefore separable factors: $E(x, \lambda) = E_1(x)E_2(\lambda)$. The spatial dependence can, then, be removed from the integral in Equation 5.1, and taking the logarithm leads to the desired result.

The jumps between the individual colored surfaces in the image can be located by means of an edge detection process: after taking the logarithm and differentiating, the slow changes in intensity which result from lighting constitute an additive component which falls below a threshold and so can be filtered out. All components below the threshold are therefore set to zero; only the information in the step-like edges remains. Finally, the image must be reconstructed from these edges. In the one-dimensional case, the reconstruction requires a single integration to reverse the differentiation. The logarithm is then inverted by application of the exponential function, and the result is a piecewise constant intensity distribution, which in the ideal case reproduces the reflectivity of the surfaces.

The retinex process performs satisfactorily if the goal is to eliminate minor changes in illumination from the image (Jobson et al. 1997). The reconstruction of the colors brings about a normalization in which the average color is shifted toward the white point. The color shift results from the assumption that the average color of the world is approximately gray (the "gray-world assumption"). If this assumption does not hold, e.g. if a grassy meadow is the imaged scene, the retinex process is, as to be expected, inaccurate. A related problem is that the simultaneous color contrast which the process generates is much higher than that in human perception (Brainard & Wandell 1986).

Part III

Depth Perception

The reconstruction of depth from two-dimensional images is a classic problem in the field of information processing. Some of the means by which depth may be determined from images are as follows:

Type of image	Depth cue	cf. Chapter
Single image	Shading and shadows	7
	Texture gradients and perspective	8
	Occlusion	
	Size of known objects	
Pairs of images	Various types of disparities	6
Image sequences: motion	Motion parallax (Motion of the observer)	10
	Dynamic occlusion	
	Kinetic depth effect (Motion of an object)	(10)

The human visual system uses all of these depth cues. Each type of cue furnishes different types of "raw" data: shading and textures hold information about surface orientation, while binocular stereopsis allows absolute distances to be determined if the gaze directions of the eyes are known. Since isolated depth cues do not occur in nature, there is also an issue of *integration of depth cues*.

The expression "perceived depth" may refer to a number of rather different perceptions and sensory processes. Some examples are the perception of distances, of three-dimensional shapes, and of local characteristics of surfaces (e.g. orientation, curvature) or apparent size. From a more behavior-oriented point of view, it is also possible to regard the opening of the hand to grasp an object, or the direction and extent of the grasping motion, as expressions of perceived depth, and to use these in experiments. The following chapters, however, will only examine simple geometric concepts such as depth maps and surface orientation. In the next chapter, we will discuss stereoscopic depth perception; later chapters will cover shading and texture as examples of monocular, or pictorial, depth cues. Motion parallax and the kinetic depth effect will be discussed briefly in connection with optical flow.

Chapter 6

Stereoscopic vision

6.1   Differences between images due to parallax

Stereoscopic depth perception is based on the differences between the images in the two eyes (the half-images of a stereogram) which result from parallax. Fig. 6.1 illustrates the mirror stereoscope invented by Sir Charles Wheatstone (1838), which demonstrated the relationship between stereoscopic depth perception and differences between images. This device separates the images by means of two mirrors set at an angle to one another. Other stereoscopes separate the images by means of prisms, polarizing filters or colored filters (used with red and green images called *anaglyphs*). In computer graphics and in virtual reality applications, it is common to separate the images in time, displaying them alternately on the screen at a high frame rate

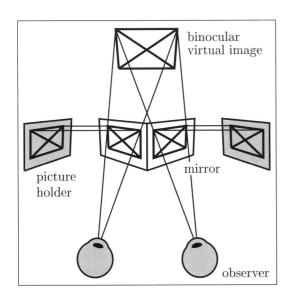

Figure 6.1
The mirror stereoscope as devised by Wheatstone. The two half-images are inserted into the image holders and observed in the two mirrors. A fused image results, with a strong stereoscopic impression of depth.

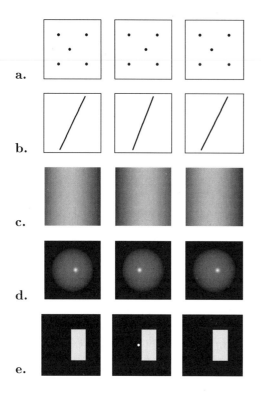

a.

b.

c.

d.

e.

Figure 6.2
Types of image differences. **a.** Point disparity. **b.** Orientation and point disparity. **c.** Gray value disparity. **d.** Photometric disparity (disparity in specular reflection). **e.** Monocular occlusion. To generate the stereoscopic effect, first cover the right column and place a white piece of cardboard vertically as a divider between the two left columns. Then look directly down on the illustration, with the tip of the nose exactly above the cardboard, so the left eye sees only the left column and the right eye sees only the middle column. For nearsighted observers, it may help to remove eyeglasses. If the left column is covered and the divider is placed between the middle and right columns, the same stereograms may be viewed with the two half-images exchanged right and left.

(for example, 60 per second) and observing them through eyeglasses with alternating shutters. An overview of stereoscopes and their design principles is given by Howard & Rogers (1995).

With some practice, it is possible to fuse two images which have been placed side by side. The left image is observed with the left eye and the right image, with the right eye (uncrossed free fusion). Fig. 6.2 describes this technique. Alternatively, free fusion can be crossed, in which case the left eye views the right image and vice versa. Large stereograms such as projected slides in lecture halls can be fused only by crossing the eyes.

There are different types of differences, or disparities, between images due to parallax:

1. *Horizontal disparity:* An isolated point in the three-dimensional world is imaged at a slightly different place in each of the half-images. The horizontal component of the difference between the distances to the center point of the respective image (or of the angles relative to the axis of vision) is called the horizontal disparity. (Fig. 6.2a).

2. *Vertical disparity:* When the axes of vision are not parallel but converge on some fixation point, vertical differences in position can also occur (see below); these are called vertical disparities (Rogers & Bradshaw 1993).

3. *Orientation of lines:* A slanted straight line in space is generally seen by each of the two eyes as having a different slope (Fig. 6.2b). Stereoscopic depth perception may make use of disparities of orientation, even though it is difficult to present one experimentally without also displaying point disparities. The projected motions of points can have similar disparities (Cagenello & Rogers 1993).

4. *Differences in shape and size:* Figures which have a spatial extent are distorted differently depending on different viewing angles and on different distances to the left and right eyes. In this way, for example, the two eyes can image the aspect ratio of rectangles or the eccentricity of ellipses differently.

5. *Shading disparity:* Even smooth, featureless surfaces reflect different amounts of light depending on their orientation to the light source (direction of incidence) and to the observer (direction of reflection). For example, if a sphere is observed by the two eyes, the gray value functions in the two images will have disparities. These occur because:

   (a) points on the surface imaged at corresponding points on the two retinas have different local orientations (Fig. 6.2c), and

   (b) if the surface is glossy, even the very same point may radiate different amounts of light in different directions (i.e. to the two eyes; Fig. 6.2d). This type of disparity results from the reflective properties of the surface, not from its geometry, and is called a *photometric* disparity.

Human perception uses both types of shading disparities (Arndt et al. 1995, Blake & Bülthoff 1991).

6. *Monocular occlusion:* At step edges, a part of the more distant surface is often only visible to one eye. Conversely, image elements which are present in only one half-image can serve as cues to the existence of such step edges (Fig. 6.2e; Anderson & Nakayama 1994, Nakayama 1996).

While the geometry of binocular imaging plays a role in all of the types of disparities just described, the materials characteristics of the imaged surfaces affect only shading disparities. If no monocular occlusion is present in the image—in other words, if the entire observed surface is visible to both eyes—the geometric problem can be formulated as follows: Let $I_l(\vec{x}')$ and $I_r(\vec{x}')$ represent the left and the right half-images. We want to find a vector function $\vec{d}(\vec{x}')$ satisfying the following equation

$$I_l(\vec{x}') = I_r(\vec{x}' - \vec{d}(\vec{x}')). \qquad (6.1)$$

We call the vector field $\vec{d}(\vec{x}')$ the *displacement field* of the stereogram. Its components are the horizontal and vertical disparities which have already been mentioned.

Equation 6.1 describes only one special case of stereoscopic vision, though it is a very important one. A few additional problems are:

1. *Depth discontinuities.* The assumption that the surface is entirely visible to both eyes is rarely valid. In most images, there are regions for which Equation 6.1 does not have a solution, at and near depth discontinuities or sufficiently steep depth gradients. Consequently, the displacement field $\vec{d}$ generally has discontinuities. Regions with depth discontinuities are the most interesting parts of a stereogram.

2. *Transparency.* When there are transparent objects, each point of one of the half-images must be mapped to more than one point of the other half-image. The different displacements then correspond to the depths of the transparent surfaces. Equation 6.1 does not account for transparency, since it only describes one displacement vector for each point in the image.

3. *Photometric effects.* As already mentioned, Equation 6.1 accounts only for geometry, not for the reflective characteristics of the surface.

6.2   Stereoscopic geometry (binocular perspective)

The most important cause of disparities, i.e. of differences between the two half-images of a stereogram, is the different position of the two cameras or eyes, along with possible different orientation of their axes. Internal camera parameters (focal length and position of the target with relation to the nodal point) should be the same for both cameras. In practice, this requirement can be a problem, since small errors in alignment of the camera targets can make the internal coordinate systems (x_l, y_l) and (x_r, y_r) differ slightly from one another. If disparities are to be quantified, the cameras must be very precisely calibrated. We will not pursue this problem further here.

We will distinguish two cases of imaging geometry:

1. Parallel camera axes: In this case, there are only horizontal disparities; however, there are no points without disparities.

2. Convergent camera axes: There are points with horizontal and/or vertical disparities, but also points without disparities. One such point, obviously, is the intersection of the visual axes. The set of all points in space which are imaged without disparities is called the theoretical horopter. It plays an important role in stereoscopic geometry.

6.2.1   Parallel camera axes

In the simplest case, the camera axes are set parallel to one another and the line which connects the nodal points of the cameras, the *base line b* of the stereo camera system, is at a right angle to them (Fig. 6.3). Let us consider the image of a point P at a distance z from the base line, measured in the direction of the camera axes. In the left image, this point should fall at the position x_l and in the right image, at the

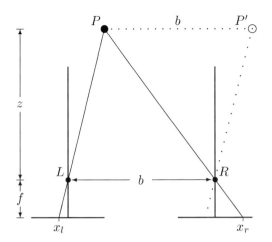

Figure 6.3
Horizontal disparities with parallel camera axes. The point P is imaged in the left and right images with the x coordinates x_l and x_r. The disparity is $d = x_l - x_r$. Parallel transposition of the left ray from P to P' and application of parallel proportionality theorem results in: $d = -f\frac{b}{z}$.

position x_r. A parallel transposition of the left ray LP and application of the parallel proportionality theorem yields:

$$d = \vec{d}_x := x_l - x_r = -f\frac{b}{z}. \tag{6.2}$$

The appropriateness of the minus sign in Equation 6.2 becomes apparent if we consider the case in which the camera axes converge. In this case, points closer than the fixation point have negative disparities, and points farther away have positive ones.

The *horizontal disparity* as a difference in image coordinates is the x component of the displacement field of Equation 6.1. It is inversely proportional to the distance of the point and increases with the focal length f and base distance b. In camera systems, very long base lines are sometimes used in order to improve the depth resolution. An extreme case is cartographic contour mapping from aircraft, in which a series of images is taken using a single camera. In this case, the distance which the aircraft flies between two photographs becomes the base line. If such stereograms are observed in a stereoscope, the objects they represent often appear remarkably small and unnatural. The physiological base line distance of $b \approx 6.5$ cm is responsible for this appearance. The large disparities appear to be those of a miniature landscape close to the observer. This phenomenon is called micropsia.

The geometry of Fig. 6.3 is preserved if P does not lie in the horizontal plane defined by L, R and the horizontal axis. The images of P therefore always have the same y components; if the camera axes are parallel, there are therefore no vertical disparities.

6.2.2 Convergent camera axes

Let us once more consider a stereo camera system with the base line b; however, now the optical axes intersect at a point F (the "fixation point"). If cameras (or eyes) are

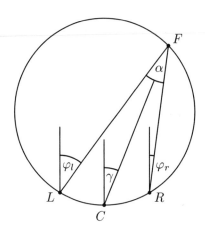

Figure 6.4
Binocular geometry with convergent camera alignment. The angle between the lines from the fixation point F to the two nodal points (L, R) is the vergence angle α. All points on the circle through L, R and F (Vieth-Müller circle) have the same vergence angle. The angles between the current direction of view and the rest position of the eyes ("straight ahead" relative to the orientation of the head) are φ_l and φ_r. C is the "cyclopean point," which bisects the arc between the two nodal points. The direction of view measured with reference to this point is called the angle of *version* and is denoted by γ.

movable, the existence of such a fixation point is not obvious, but within the scope of this introduction, we will always assume that one does exist.

Disparities vanish at the point where the visual axes intersect. More generally, the set of all points in space whose disparities are zero is called the *theoretical horopter*. It depends on the location of the fixation point. The *empirical horopter*, in contrast, includes all points which are perceived by the observer to be as far away as the fixation point.

Vergence and version

The angle at which the optical axes of the cameras intersect is called the *vergence angle* α (Fig. 6.4). It does not change if the axes of vision are fixed on another point on the circle which passes through L, R and F; this circle is called the Vieth-Müller circle. The equality of the apex angle for all points P on the Vieth-Müller circle is an application of the theorem of Thales (see Glossary, Fig. G.8). If, as shown in Fig. 6.4, the directions of view of the two eyes relative to the straight-ahead orientation of the head are designated as φ_l and φ_r, then:

$$\alpha = \varphi_l - \varphi_r. \tag{6.3}$$

Here, the angles φ_l and φ_r are each measured clockwise from straight ahead. The vergence angle is 0 if the camera axes are parallel to one another; i.e. if the fixation point is infinitely far away. If it is at a finite distance, the vergence angle is always positive.

The average of the two directions of view is called the version angle, γ:

$$\gamma = \frac{1}{2}\left(\varphi_l + \varphi_r\right). \tag{6.4}$$

An intuitive interpretation of this angle follows, once again, from the theorem of Thales: If C is the so-called *cyclopean point* (Fig. 6.4), which bisects the short arc

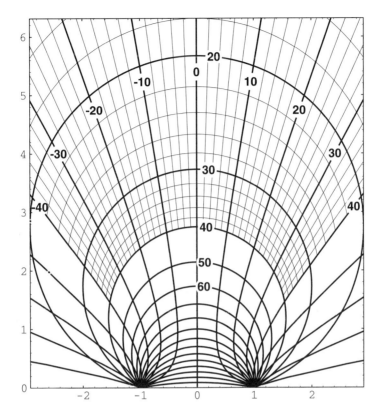

Figure 6.5
Hering coordinates in the horizontal plane. The circles are curves of constant vergence (Vieth-Müller circles), and the hyperbolas are curves of constant version (Hillebrand hyperbolas). The nodal points of the eyes are at $R, L = (\pm 1, 0)$; the proportions become those of the human visual system if all distances are multiplied by 3.25 cm. The thick lines form a 10° grid; the thin lines, a 2° grid. The coarser spacing with increasing distance from the nodal points corresponds to the decreasing accuracy of stereoscopic vision with increasing distance.

of the Vieth-Müller circle between the two nodal points, then the line $\overline{CF}$ is at the angle γ to the forward direction.

Version and vergence are known as Hering's coordinates of the plane which passes through the nodal points and the fixation point. The curves of constant vergence are circles which pass through the nodal points, i.e. Vieth-Müller circles for fixation points at different distances. The curves of constant version are called Hillebrand hyperbolas and each pass through one of the two nodal points. Both types of curves are shown in Fig. 6.5.

The terms vergence and version are used not only for the fixed angles α and γ, but also for binocular eye movements which lead to changes in these angles. Vergences,

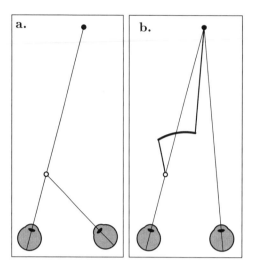

Figure 6.6
Vergence and version as internal variables of binocular eye movements (Hering's law). **a.** Both eyes fixate on the point indicated by ∘. Looking from the left eye, the next fixation point (•) lies directly behind the first one, so that no movement of the left eye is actually necessary. **b.** When moving fixation to the more distant point, the left eye first turns to the left, then to the right and again to the left, until it finally reaches the same position it had initially. The intersection of the axes of vision moves alternately along curves of constant version and of constant vergence.

or disjunctive eye movements, are therefore eye movements in opposite directions (convergence: both eyes turn toward the nose; divergence: both eyes turn toward the temples). Eye movements in the same direction (both eyes to the right or the left, conjugate eye movements) are called versions (cf. Section 2.4.2).

Why are the derived angles α, γ used in preference to the more directly observable directions of vision φ_l, φ_r? One advantage of Hering's system is that, as we will see in the next section, it allows a closed mathematical representation of the relationship between vergence and disparity. A physiological argument which is known as "Hering's Law" is that binocular eye movements break down kinematically into vergence and version components. Fig. 6.6 diagrammatically shows an eye movement between two fixation points, in which the direction of vision of the left eye ought not to have to change. But in fact, the eyes start to move slowly apart, i.e. they perform a divergence movement; version remains constant, and the intersection of the axes of vision moves away from the observer along a Hillebrand hyperbola. Somewhat later, a rapid version (saccade) occurs, in which both eyes move to the right with no change in vergence, so that the intersection of the visual axes follows a Vieth-Müller circle. When the required version is achieved, the saccade ends and the vergence movement is continued until the change of the point of fixation is complete. The kinematics of the eye movements (slow vergence, fast version) and the unnecessary movements of the left eye suggest strongly that physiological control of vergence and of version is separate. Precise experimental measurement, however, shows that the eyes only approximately conform to Hering's law. For example, saccades can include small vergence components (Collewijn et al. 1997, Enright 1998).

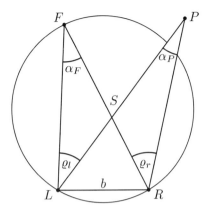

Figure 6.7
Calculation of horizontal disparity δ as an angle. $\alpha = \alpha_F$: vergence. P: any point which is present in the peripheral visual field while fixation is on F. α_P: Target vergence of P. ϱ_l, ϱ_r: Azimuth of the point P in camera-centered polar coordinates. S: Intersection of the straight lines $\overline{LP}$ and $\overline{RF}$. Simple trigonometry yields: $\delta = \varrho_r - \varrho_l = \alpha_F - \alpha_P$.

Horizontal disparity

If the camera axes converge, it is useful to describe the disparities as angles. Once again, we consider only the horizontal plane, and designate as ϱ the angle at which a point P appears when fixation is on F (Fig. 6.7). The quantities $\varrho_{l,r}$ are therefore the eccentricities of the images of the point P when fixation is on F. The horizontal disparity (for points in the horizontal plane) is therefore defined as the difference $\delta := \varrho_r - \varrho_l$. This quantity is positive if the point appears farther to the right as viewed by the right eye. Angular disparity can be derived from the apex angles α_F (the vergence angle) and α_P in Fig. 6.7 if we consider the sum of the angles of triangles $\triangle LFS$ and $\triangle RPS$. Since the angle at point S is the same in both triangles, it follows immediately that $\alpha_F + \varrho_l = \alpha_P + \varrho_r$, and therefore,

$$\delta = \varrho_r - \varrho_l = \alpha_F - \alpha_P. \tag{6.5}$$

The disparity therefore proves to be the difference between the apex, or vergence, angles.

Equation 6.5 has a number of important properties

1. The additivity of vergence and disparity in Equation 6.5 makes it possible to use a point's disparity directly to adjust vergence so as to fixate on that point. The Hering coordinates shown in Fig. 6.5 therefore may be used to determine disparities: no matter what point is fixated, the horizontal disparity of all other points is the difference in their α values.

2. The horizontal disparity of points on the Vieth-Müller circle is zero, $\delta = 0$. This circle is therefore called the (theoretical) horopter. Points inside the Vieth-Müller circle have negative disparities, and points outside this circle have positive disparities.

3. If the fixation point is in the median plane at the distance z, then for a point

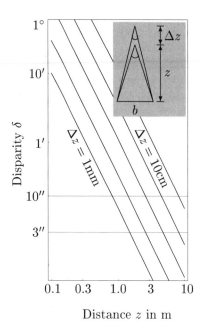

Disparity δ

Distance z in m

Figure 6.8
Relationship between depth and horizontal disparity in the median plane (Equation 6.6). Log-log scale. The lines show the disparity for a fixed depth offset Δz viewed at the distance z; this disparity decreases approximately as the square of distance. The base line is assumed to be $b = 6.5$ cm. The five lines correspond to the depth offsets $\Delta z = 1$ mm, 3 mm, 1 cm, 3 cm and 10 cm. The horizontal lines indicate the threshold of perception. At a distance of 3 meters, depth variations of less than 1 cm can no longer be resolved stereoscopically. The inset drawing shows the geometric construction which the main graph represents. The disparity corresponds to the difference between the two apex angles.

at a distance Δz behind the fixation point, the disparity is given by:

$$\delta(z, \Delta z) = 2 \left(\arctan \frac{b}{2z} - \arctan \frac{b}{2(z + \Delta z)} \right) \approx b \frac{\Delta z}{z^2}. \qquad (6.6)$$

The approximation holds well for large z and small Δz (Fig. 6.8).

4. Outside the median plane, disparities and depths are related in a complicated way to one another, as shown in Fig. 6.5. If the current vergence angle is α_F, a point P whose disparity is δ lies on a Vieth-Müller circle whose center $\vec{c}$ and radius r are given by:

$$\vec{c} = \left(0, \frac{b}{2} \cot(\alpha_F + \delta) \right)$$

$$r = \frac{b}{2 \sin(\alpha_F + \delta)}. \qquad (6.7)$$

The nodal points are at $(\pm b/2, 0)$. The actual distance of point P depends, therefore, not only on the vergence angle and the disparity, but also on the version and the "cyclopean" eccentricity $\frac{1}{2}(\varrho_l + \varrho_r)$. This relationship can not be simplified by defining disparity in terms of lengths rather than angles.

Vertical disparity and epipolar lines

The stereoscopic geometry of Fig. 6.3 and 6.4 applies as shown only to points in the plane defined by L, R and F, which is the horizontal plane if we assume that the

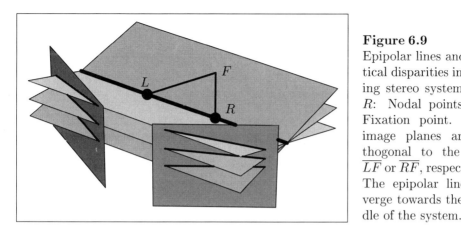

Figure 6.9
Epipolar lines and vertical disparities in verging stereo systems. L, R: Nodal points. F: Fixation point. The image planes are orthogonal to the lines $\overline{LF}$ or $\overline{RF}$, respectively. The epipolar lines diverge towards the middle of the system.

head does not tilt to one side or the other. If we consider a single point P_l in the left image, then any possible point P which is imaged as P_l lies on a straight line which passes through P_l and the nodal point of the left camera. If P_l is not itself in the horizontal plane, the line is slanted, and if the line is observed by the right camera, it is imaged as another line, also slanted, in the right image plane. P_r, the right image of P, is therefore displaced both horizontally and vertically relative to P_l, and the ratio between the horizontal and vertical disparity is a constant, the slope of the line in the right image plane.

Conversely, it is possible to observe with the left eye the straight line defined by the points imaged at P_r. The result is just the same, a slanted line. Both of these lines which have been described for the two eyes, as well as the rays used in their construction, lie in a plane which is defined by the two nodal points and the object point P (or one of the two image points P_l, P_r). This plane is called the *epipolar plane* of the point P. The lines where it intersects the two image planes are the two *epipolar lines* of that point. The stereoscopic counterpart of a point in one of the two eyes will always lie on the corresponding epipolar line in the other eye.

The geometry of the epipolar lines and planes is shown in Fig. 6.9. Since all epipolar planes include the two nodal points, they constitute a structure like that of a book whose pages have been spread open. The line between L and R is the "spine of the book." Since the image planes of a system with converging visual axes are not parallel to the base-line $\overline{LR}$ (the "spine"), the lines where the pages of the book intersect with the image planes are slanted so they diverge toward the middle of the stereo camera head. If the image plane is extended toward the outside until it intersects the base-line $\overline{LR}$, all of the epipolar lines cross at this same point. It is easy to understand that if the camera axes are parallel ($\alpha = 0$), the epipolar lines are horizontal (and so parallel to one another) and the vertical disparities vanish. Furthermore, the epipolar lines of the horizontal plane are always horizontal, and so vertical disparities can never occur in this plane. Finally, there are also no vertical disparities along the y axis of the image plane (the vertical meridian of the eye) if the

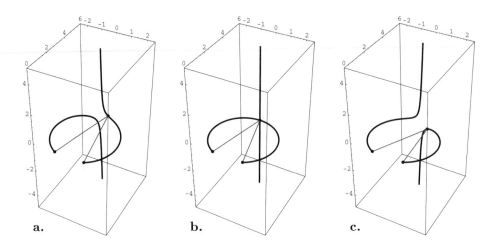

a.   **b.**   **c.**

Figure 6.10
The space horopter for a stereoscopic system with the nodal points $(\pm 1, 0, 0)^\top$. **a.** Fixation point $(0.5, 0.5, 4)^\top$. **b.** Fixation point $(0, 0, 4)^\top$. **c.** Fixation point $(0.5, -0.5, 4)$. Rotation of the eyes to the fixation points is carried out according to Listing's law.

vergence is symmetrical (if the point being fixated is in the median plane).

For a given vergence angle, vertical disparities stand in a fixed relationship to the horizontal disparity. It is therefore possible to use them to determine the vergence angle and, in turn, the absolute distances from the image. The possibility appears actually to be used in human perception (Rogers & Bradshaw 1993).

The space horopter

The (theoretical) horopter is defined as the set of all points in space which are imaged without a horizontal or vertical disparity by both cameras or eyes. If the fixation point is on the centerline of the horizontal plane, the space horopter consists of the Vieth-Müller circle and a vertical line through the fixation point (Fig. 6.10b). In general, the space horopter is a complicated curve (Fig. 6.10a, c), the analytical description of which is beyond the scope of this book (cf. Solomons 1975, Mallot 1999).

The curves in Fig. 6.10 are calculated based on the assumption that the eyes turn toward the fixation point as described by Listing's law (Section 2.4.1). In stereoscopic camera heads , the Helmholtz system is most commonly used, because it is more easily implemented. This system does not occur in nature (cf. Fig. 2.18). In the Helmholtz system, the space horopter is always of the form in Fig. 6.10b, but tipped forward or back by the applicable pitch angle.

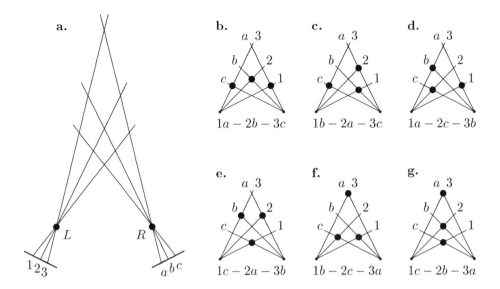

Figure 6.11
The correspondence problem of stereoscopic vision. **a.** The left image has features at the locations $1, 2, 3$, the right image at a, b, c. There are $3! = 6$ possible ways to match these three pairs of features (**b.** – **g.**), which meet the requirements of the uniqueness and completeness. Each match leads to a different spatial interpretation. L, R: Nodal points of the left and right eyes.

6.3 Stereo algorithms

6.3.1 The correspondence problem

The geometrical observations of the previous section show how depth can be inferred from disparities. However, an additional problem arises when disparities are to be determined in images: the problem of matching "corresponding" image features in the two half-images of a stereogram (cf. Fig. 6.11). Two image features "correspond" to each other when they are images of the same point in the outside world.* If the image features can not be distinguished from one another, there are $n!$ possible ways to match the n features in each half-image, and all lead to different spatial interpretations. Only when the correspondence problem has been resolved is it possible to determine the depths of the imaged objects by triangulation.

Fig. 6.11 shows an example based on the well-known double-nail illusion (Krol &

---

*The terminology here differs from that in optometry, in which two locations on the retinas are said to correspond if they have the same image coordinates. Corresponding points as described here can, however, be disparate, and are therefore not imaged onto corresponding locations on the retinas, as the term is used in optometry.

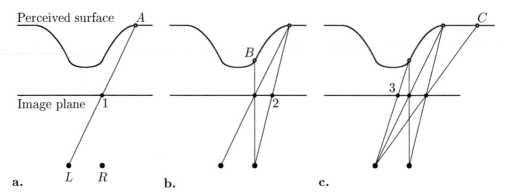

Figure 6.12
Illustration of the construction of an autostereogram. The goal is to generate the
"perceived surface" which is shown at the top. **a.** First, a point (1) is placed randomly
on the paper. As seen by the left eye, it corresponds to an object point A. **b.** The
image point (2) must then be placed on the paper, so as to correspond to the object
point A as seen by the right eye. Also from the right eye, image point 1 corresponds,
additionally, to an object point B. **c.** As seen by the left eye, image point (2)
must now be "accounted for," and so it generates the object point C. The imaging
of object point B results, in turn, in image point (3). An autostereogram of the
perceived surface is generated by many repetitions of this process.

van de Grind 1980, von Campenhausen 1993). If two nails are held one behind the
other in the median plane of the eyes, and if their ends are hidden by an opaque screen,
they appear to be side by side. The image of the left nail in the left eye is fused with
that of the right nail in the right eye, so that the correspondence problem is solved
in a way that is plausible even though it is physically incorrect. Another example of
the correspondence problem is the wallpaper illusion, in which the correspondences
are made between neighboring repetitions of a periodic pattern (for example, flowers
on wallpaper), and an illusionary depth is perceived. If the patterns are not exactly
periodic, but instead differ slightly from one another, additional depth variations are
perceived. Such images, which generate impressions of depth due to incorrect fusion,
are called "autostereograms" (cf. Fig. 6.12 and Tyler & Clarke 1990). They provide
an especially elegant demonstration of the correspondence problem of stereoscopic
vision.

The ambiguities of stereoscopic interpretation illustrated by the correspondence
problem and the described illusions provide yet another example of the general under-
defined status of visual perception: the "inversion" of optical imaging can not always
be performed in a satisfactory way.

Computer vision algorithms for determining depth from stereograms are concerned
mostly with the solution of the correspondence problem. An overview of the large
number of algorithms which have been proposed is given by Dhond & Aggarwal (1989),

Jenkin et al. (1991) and also Förstner (1993).

6.3.2 Correspondence of localized image elements

Research which builds on the classic work of Marr & Poggio (1979) formulates stereo algorithms in the following four steps:

1. Feature extraction. First, features such as edges, line terminations etc. (cf. Chapter 4) are extracted from the gray value image. The localization of these features is important, since disparities will be determined according to differences in position after the correspondence problem has been solved.

2. Solving the correspondence problem. Next, a correspondence between image elements is chosen from among the many conceivable ones. The resulting image match is only a plausible one and not necessarily the "correct" one. Various types of previous knowledge, constraints, and plausibility considerations are used at this stage:

(a) Search space
For an element in the left half-image, a matching element is sought only within a certain region of the right half-image. First of all, search can always be restricted to the corresponding epipolar line. A further restriction which can be assumed for reasonably smooth surfaces is that disparities are small. This assumption is especially useful in connection with the "coarse to fine" strategy mentioned below.

(b) Feature attributes
If the image elements can be distinguished from one another, then only those of the same type (edges, line terminations) and with the same characteristics (e.g., color, polarity of contrast) are matched.

(c) Ordering constraints
Once a match between two features has been established, the plausibility of other matches changes. Rules for interactions between correspondences are:

- The constraints of uniqueness and completeness: each element in the left half-image is assigned to exactly one element in the right half-image. This rule is based on the assumption that monocular occlusions and transparencies are rare. They are, however, entirely possible.

- Sequence: If a match (l_i, r_j) has been established, then an element to the right of l_i ought preferably to be combined with one to the right of r_j. In this way, solutions are preferred which assign similar depths to neighboring points (Fig. 6.13). Clearly, this rule reflects the fact that depths on surfaces in space change only continuously, while the boundaries of objects, where depth discontinuities occur, occupy only a few pixels in an image.

(d) Coarse-to-fine strategy
The complexity of the correspondence problem increases with the number of

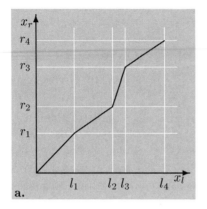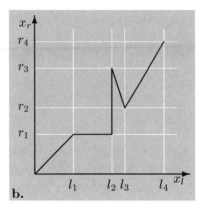

Figure 6.13
Search space for feature correspondence along two lines of the image (epipolar lines).
a. The interpretation shown conforms to the ordering constraints described in the text. **b.** This (entirely possible) interpretation violates the uniqueness constraint for image elements r_1 and l_2. In addition, the sequence is reversed from pair (l_2, r_3) to pair (l_3, r_2).

image elements. For this reason, the image is usually represented as a resolution pyramid (Chapter 3), and analysis begins at the coarsest resolution level. Once the relatively few features at this level have been matched, analysis proceeds to the next finer level, and the search space is displaced by the gross disparities which have already been found.

3. Triangulation. If the correspondences, and therefore the disparities, are known as differences in the positions of corresponding image elements, then if the camera geometry is also known, it is possible to determine depth through triangulation.

4. Surface reconstruction. Solutions to the correspondence problem which are restricted to localized image elements can generate depth values only for isolated points ("sparse data"). For this reason, the depth of a smooth surface must be calculated by interpolation through the data points in an additional step, e.g., by the use of two- dimensional spline algorithm (Grimson 1982).

6.3.3   Intensity-based stereopsis

In the matching processes, only the (symbolic) image features, possibly including some feature attributes, are considered at the binocular processing step. In intensity-based approaches, gray values also play a part. As a result, image data is less sparse, and a separate step of surface interpolation is generally unnecessary. For the sake of simplicity, we will consider one-dimensional "images" $I_l(x)$ and $I_r(x)$, for which we will specify a continuous disparity map $d(x)$. We will discuss two approaches, correlation and phase shift.

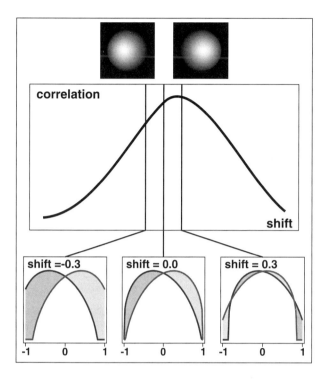

Figure 6.14
Diagram illustrating the correlation algorithm for determining disparities based on intensities. The lower inset graphs show intensity profiles along horizontal lines across the half-images (top) for different displacements or shifts s. The gray-shaded areas represent the difference between the two gray value functions. The correlation function shown in the larger graph is maximized when the displacement $s = 0.3$. Except for an additive constant, this function corresponds to the function $-\Phi_\infty(x, s)$ in Equation 6.8.

Correlation

In this case, disparity is defined as the relative displacement of two gray value functions which maximizes their similarity. The similarity is calculated through correlation, or better, through the mean square difference:

$$\Phi_\sigma(x, s) = \int w(\frac{x - x'}{\sigma}) \left(I_l(x' + \frac{s}{2}) - I_r(x' - \frac{s}{2}) \right)^2 dx'. \qquad (6.8)$$

Here, $w(x)$ is a suitable "window function", e.g., $w(x) = \exp\{-x^2\}$. By placing this window function at the location x, the local disparity at this location is measured. The resolution of measurement is limited by the width of the window function σ.

The disparity $d(x)$ at location x is defined as the shift s minimizing the mean square difference $\Phi(x, s)$:

$$d(x) = \text{argmin}_s \Phi(x, s). \qquad (6.9)$$

The more sharply defined the peak at this location, more reliable is the measurement of disparity.

Cepstrum procedures (Yeshurun & Schwartz 1989, Ludwig et al. 1994), which evaluate correlation across relatively large windows, are related to correlation processes. The use of cepstrum algorithms is motivated by the neuroanatomical finding that the inputs of the two eyes in many mammals are organized as separate "ocular dominance stripes" in the visual cortex, in such a way that the two half-images are "interlaced" with each other in a plane. The processing occurs in this plane.

Phase shift

If a plane image of a sinusoidal gray value function is moved in depth, stereograms result such that the same gray value function appears in both half-images at different phase angles. If the wavelength of the sinusoidal pattern is known, the phase difference corresponds to the disparity. This approach can in fact be used with any gray value functions, by filtering out all but one frequency band from the image (Sanger 1988). To this end, a symmetrical and an anti-symmetrical filter kernel are used. For example, the two filter outputs for I_l are:

$$I_{l,\sin,\sigma}(x,\omega) = \int w\left(\frac{x-x'}{\sigma}\right) I_l(x')\sin(\omega(x-x'))dx'$$

$$I_{l,\cos,\sigma}(x,\omega) = \int w\left(\frac{x-x'}{\sigma}\right) I_l(x')\cos(\omega(x-x'))dx'. \qquad (6.10)$$

If the window function is the Gaussian bell curve which has already been discussed, and if the ratio between ω and σ is a constant, then Equation 6.10 describes a convolution with Gabor functions.

The resulting local phase difference is:

$$\Delta\phi(x,\omega) = \arctan\frac{I_{l,\sin}(x,\omega)}{I_{l,\cos}(x,\omega)} - \arctan\frac{I_{r,\sin}(x,\omega)}{I_{r,\cos}(x,\omega)}. \qquad (6.11)$$

And, now, at each spatial frequency ω, we may calculate a disparity according to the formula

$$d_\omega(x) = \frac{\Delta\phi(x,\omega)}{\omega}. \qquad (6.12)$$

Because of the periodicity of phase angles, the phase difference in Equation 6.12 is determined only up to an additive constant $2n\pi$, where n is an integer. Comparison of phase shifts at the output of filters with different center frequencies ω can usually resolve this ambiguity. Generally, a consistent disparity value must be determined from the values at the individual spatial frequencies of the filters. The evaluation is equivalent to consideration of the entire scale space (cf. Theimer & Mallot 1994). For a formal comparison of the phase-based approach with other intensity-based stereo algorithms, see Qian & Mikaelian (2000).

Neither of the intensity-based procedures which have just been described solves the correspondence problem. If, for example, the correlation procedure is applied to the double-nail stereogram, a peak is obtained for each possible correspondence, and the height of the peak depends on the number of correspondences which lie in a particular disparity plane. This behavior is not a problem as long as the imaged surfaces are smooth. The usual way to design an intensity-based stereo algorithm is to start by

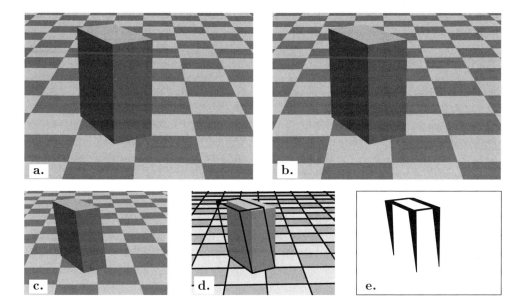

Figure 6.15
Obstacle avoidance by means of "inverse perspective". **a.,b.** Image of a scene as viewed by the left and right cameras. **c.** Prediction of the right image by inverse perspective mapping of the left image. **d.** Comparison of the actual right image (gray values) with the predicted one (lines). The two images coincide at floor level, but they diverge more and more with increasing height of the obstacle above the floor. **e.** Difference between the actual and the predicted image. The obstacle is separated from the background.

estimating local disparities according to correlation or phase-shift, and then reprocess the data in order to obtain a global surface estimate. Algorithms of this type have been developed for example in neural network theory, in which the local disparity detectors correspond to disparity-tuned neurons (Section 6.4).

6.3.4 Global stereopsis

The construction of depth maps is of great importance for the recognition and manipulation of objects. But on the other hand, there are tasks and behaviors for which high-resolution depth maps are not necessary. For example, the perception of an average depth for an entire object is sufficient when initiating the task of grasping the object: variations in the depth of the surface are of importance for the details of the actual grasping motion, but not for the arm motion which precedes it. Similarly, a global disparity is sufficient for the initiation of vergence eye movements (Theimer & Mallot 1994, Mallot et al. 1996c). In such cases, it is possible to apply Equation 6.8 with a very large window (in the extreme case $w(x) \equiv 1$) and so to obtain the required

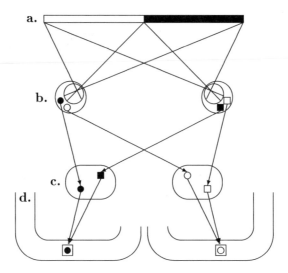

Figure 6.16
Scheme of the mammalian visual pathways. The visual field (**a.**) is imaged onto the
retinas (**b.**) of the two eyes. Two ganglion cells are indicated in each eye: ●, ○: left
eye. ■, □: right eye. ○, □: left visual field. ●, ■: right visual field. In the *chiasma
opticum*, the axons of the cells on the nasal sides of the eyes (○,■) cross over to the
opposite sides of the brain, where they enter the lateral geniculate nucleus (LGN) **c.**
The cells in the LGN are innervated by only one eye. Only as they are subsequently
projected onto the visual cortex (**d.**) do the signals converge onto *binocular* cells.

global depth value. Psychophysical evidence for global depth evaluation in this way
is to be found in Mallot et al. (1996a, c) and Mallot (1997).

It is possible entirely to avoid finding disparities if the task is simply to establish
whether a specific depth structure is present or not. Such is the case e.g., in obstacle
avoidance, in which the requirement is to identify deviations from the horizontal plane
in the forward direction of travel. In this case, it is possible to use the left camera
image to predict the image which is to be expected in the right camera. To this
end, the image from the left camera is projected onto the ground plane and then
observed from the point of view of the right camera ("inverse perspective", Fig. 6.15).
The resulting mapping of the left image plane onto the right yields an overall image
transformation known as "collineation" in projective geometry (Mallot et al. 1989,
1992, cf. also Equation 8.8 in Chapter 8). If the two images are subtracted, there is no
difference in regions which actually show the ground plane, but obstacles are distinctly
visible. This process tests for the presence of a particular surface; it constitutes a kind
of matched filter for this surface. In computer vision systems for obstacle avoidance,
for example for the control of vehicles on highways, processing of this type is widely
applied (Zielke et al. 1990, Košecka et al. 1995, Luong et al. 1995).

6.4 Neural networks

On the basis of psychophysical measurements, Richards (1971) postulated the existence of disparity-selective "channels" in human perception. Subsequently, a neurophysiological correlate of such channels has been confirmed: disparity-tuned neurons, which are present in all vertebrates with stereoscopic vision (e.g., salamanders, owls, mammals); a recent overview of disparity-tuned neurons in primates is given by Poggio (1995; cf. also Regan et al. 1990). Such neurons have two receptive fields, one in each eye, and so require a convergence of nerve fibers from corresponding locations on the retinas. In mammals, this convergence is accomplished by partial crossing of the retinal ganglion cell axons in the optic chiasm (therefore called an *incomplete chiasm*). The retinal fibers from the nasal side of each retina cross to the opposite side of the brain, while the fibers from the temporal side of each retina remain on the same side. Binocular cells, which receive inputs from both eyes, are not found until the visual cortex (Fig. 6.16).

In order for binocular neurons to be selective for specific disparities, the receptive fields of these neurons for the two eyes must be slightly different. If, for example, the retinal positions and therefore the directions of view are different, then the preferred disparity of the neuron is equal to the difference in positions (Fig. 6.17a). In this case, activity in disparity-tuned neurons can be modeled by similarity function Φ defined in Equation 6.8. An alternative suggestion has been that phase differences between receptive fields are the basis for disparity measurements, in which case Gabor functions describe the profiles of receptive fields (DeAngelis et al. 1995; cf. also Equation 6.10).

The excitation of a disparity-selective cell therefore indicates a particular disparity. Fig. 6.17b illustrates a hypothetical organization of disparity-selective neurons through a so-called Kepler* projection. Signal lines from locations on the two retinas connect to neurons whose binocular receptive fields cover these retinal locations. The map is only a geometric construction based on reverse projection of retinal points into rays, and does not show the actual arrangement of the disparity-selective cells in the brain. The set of disparity-tuned neurons constitutes a population code for disparity (Pouget & Sejnowski 1994).

Fig. 6.17b also shows that disparity selectivity alone is not sufficient to solve the correspondence problem. The two gray points in the visual field activate cells at the four locations indicated in the disparity map. The same four cells would also be excited if the objects were placed side by side rather than one behind the other. In order for the interpretation of depth by means of the disparity map to be unambiguous, appropriate activation dynamics is necessary. For example, it has been suggested that cells which respond to similar disparities might reinforce one another, while cells with different disparities might inhibit one another (Julesz 1971, Marr & Poggio 1976, Blake & Wilson 1991). By restricting the scope of inhibition, it is possible to accommodate several transparent depth planes (Pridmore et al. 1990). By means of appropriate neural network models, it has been demonstrated that the calculation

---

*The astronomer Johannes Kepler (1571 – 1630) gave one of the earliest accounts of binocular vision.

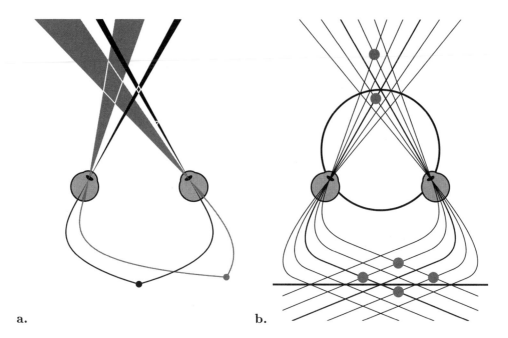

a.   b.

Figure 6.17
a. Disparity-selective neurons have slightly different receptive fields in the two eyes. Only when an object is within the quadrilateral bounded with white lines does a binocular excitation of the corresponding cell occur (cf. Poggio 1995). **b.** Hypothetical arrangement of disparity-selective neurons as a disparity map (the Kepler projection). Within the grid in the lower part of the illustration, the neurons' preferred disparity varies along the vertical axis, while the average ("cyclopean") direction of view varies along the horizontal axis. Mechanisms of stereoscopic vision are modeled as patterns of excitation in this disparity map.

of stereoscopic disparities can be achieved through cooperation and inhibition among disparity-selective neurons.

6.5 Psychophysics

Let us here briefly mention some of the important characteristics of human stereoscopic vision, especially as it compares to stereoscopic computer vision. A more thorough treatment is given by Arditi (1986), Westheimer (1994) and Arndt et al. (1995) as well as in the comprehensive review by Howard & Rogers (1995).

Fusion and single vision. Disparate images are fused into a single perceived image if the disparities are smaller than ca. ±12 minutes of arc (Panum's area). For sinusoidal intensity functions, the disparity range in which fusion occurs increases with

1	2	3	4	5	6	7	8
9	10	11	12	13	14	15	16
17			a	b	c	d	18
19			e	f	g	h	20
21			i	j	k	l	22
23			m	n	o	p	24
25	26	27	28	29	30	31	32
33	34	35	36	37	38	39	40

1	2	3	4	5	6	7	8
9	10	11	12	13	14	15	16
17	a	b	c	d			18
19	e	f	g	h			20
21	i	j	k	l			22
23	m	n	o	p			24
25	26	27	28	29	30	31	32
33	34	35	36	37	38	39	40

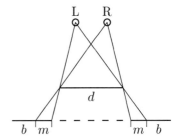

Figure 6.18
Construction of a random dot stereogram, after Julesz (1971). **Left:** Fields identified by the same numbers or letters in the left and right half-images are shaded with the same gray value (black or white). The blank fields are shaded randomly and independently in the two half-images. When the two half-images are observed stereoscopically, the fields identified by letters of the alphabet appear in front or behind the fields marked by numbers, depending on whether fusion is crossed or uncrossed. **Right:** three-dimensional interpretation when viewed stereoscopically. b: background region with zero disparity (numbers in the left part of the illustration) m: monocular regions occluded from the point of view of one eye (blank fields in the left part of the illustration) d: disparate region (letters in the left part of the illustration).

the period of the pattern (Schor & Wood 1983). Fusion includes the identification of corresponding points. If the disparities are too large, either double images appear or only one of the two images is perceived at any one time ("binocular rivalry").

Disparity and depth. Perceived depth corresponds to disparity only in Panum's area. When the disparity is greater (i.e., when image elements can not be fused), perceived depth falls away increasingly from the theoretical values, finally reaching zero. Surprisingly, depth values can be assigned to image elements which can not be fused.

Horizontal disparity can identify depth only with relation to the fixation point. For absolute depth to be perceived, the vergence angle must be known. In theory, it can be known through proprioception, through a copy of efferent nerve information, or through analysis of the distribution of vertical disparities. Absolute depth perception is much less precise than relative depth perception.

Resolution. The human visual system can resolve disparities between vertical lines down to as little as 3 – 10 seconds of arc (vernier resolution). As in the monocular case, this high resolution is an example of hyperacuity, since the width of receptors in the fovea is approximately 30 seconds of arc (cf. Chapter 3 and McKee et al. 1990). Resolution for variations in depth of smooth surfaces is markedly lower. Consider, for example, a sinusoidally varying surface (like a corrugated metal roof) displayed as a random dot stereogram with high dot density to allow for smooth depth variations. If

the wavelength is reduced while the amplitude remains constant, the perception of a
surface falls apart at approximately four periods per degree. At smaller wavelengths,
the perception of depth does not completely disappear, but rather is transformed into
a perception of transparency: a cloud or plate whose thickness is the amplitude of
the depth modulation (Tyler 1974).

Matching primitives (features used for image matching). Stereoscopic perception can occur with patterns of dots which appear random as observed with one
eye, but show meaningful forms defined by the distribution of disparity. This fact was
first demonstrated by the random dot stereograms developed by Bela Julesz (1971)
(cf. Fig. 6.18). Point disparities, therefore, are sufficient for the generation of the
stereoscopic impression of depth.

Variations in gray values which are not linked to localized image features (edges,
points), can also lead to stereoscopic perceptions, though with poor spatial resolution
(Mayhew & Frisby 1981, Bülthoff & Mallot 1988, Arndt et al. 1995). This observation
does not agree well with feature-based algorithms for stereoscopic vision, and points
rather to an intensity-based mechanism.

"Higher-order" disparities, i.e. disparities derived from complex image elements,
are also not simply ignored. As has already been pointed out in Fig. 6.2, characteristics such as line orientation or the perspective distortion of the corners of rectangles
can contribute to stereoscopic vision (Cagenello & Rogers 1993).

Correspondence. The double-nail illusion and the wallpaper illusion, which have
already been described, provide psychophysical demonstrations of the correspondence
problem. That the human visual system can successfully resolve the correspondence
problem even in difficult cases is shown by the random dot stereograms of Julesz
(1971; Fig. 6.18).

Not all of the assumptions and processes for resolving the correspondence problem
which were mentioned in Section 6.3.2 are actually used in perception. It can be
shown, for example, that the uniqueness constraint in relating image elements of
the right and left half-images does not always hold strictly (Weinshall 1991). The
exceptions permit the perception of transparency, i.e. of multiple depths at the same
location in the image; computer vision systems usually do not account for this. Color
is used to some degree as an indication of corresponding image elements (Jordan et
al. 1990). However, image elements of different colors can be fused even when there
is an interpretation in which objects of the same color correspond with one another
(e.g., Krol & van de Grind 1980). A color is then perceived which results from mixing
of the color stimuli of the two eyes (binocular color mixing).

Smaller disparities are favored in the image matching process. If, for example, a
periodic pattern is viewed with a fixation point slightly in front of the pattern, the
interpretation yielding the smallest disparity values may be the one matching the n-th
repetition of the pattern in the right eye to the $n + 1$-th repetition of the pattern in
the left eye (McKee & Mitchison 1988). This mismatch of the image features results
in an error in perceived depth known as the wallpaper illusion: the pattern appears

to float in front of the paper on which it is printed. A similar influence of the current vergence angle on the solution of the correspondence problem occurs with the double-nail illusion: matches are preferred which result in a perceived object close to the current fixation plane (Mallot & Bideau 1990).

The stereoscopic visual system has channels which operate at different resolutions, but which apparently are not used in a coarse-to-fine strategy (see discussion in Mallot et al. 1996b). Rather, channels seem to be combined in a maximum-likelihood scheme, as has been suggested for other channel coded systems as well. Vergence eye movements during the image matching process, as would be predicted by a temporal implementation of a coarse-to-fine sequence in image processing, could not be demonstrated in human observers (Mowforth et al. 1981).

Chapter 7

Shape from shading

Shading is variation of gray values in an image due to different orientations of the imaged surfaces relative to the light source and observer. The different ways in which reflections may depend on direction (dull, glossy) have been discussed in Section 2.1; Lambert's formula describes the most important case:

$$I = cI_o(\vec{n} \cdot \vec{l}) = cI_o \cos(\angle \vec{n}, \vec{l}). \tag{7.1}$$

Shading differs from cast shadows in that it results not from complete obstruction of the light source, but rather, from the surface orientation with respect to the incident light. Shading or "attached shadows" are thus generated by the shaded surface itself and not "cast" on a background surface.

Two important types of edges which are not determined by the intrinsic geometry of the imaged surfaces are shown in Fig. 7.1. The *self-shadow boundary* comprises the points on the surface at which the illumination is parallel to the surface, so that the light rays just graze it. The *occluding contour* comprises the points on the surface at which the ray to the nodal point of the imaging system is parallel to the surface.

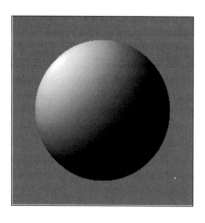

Figure 7.1
A shaded image of a sphere illuminated from above and to the left. The *self-shadow boundary* is the line where the direction of the illumination is at a right angle to the local surface normal. The outline of the sphere is an *occluding contour*, where the surface turns away from and out of view of the observer. Here, the local surface normal is at a right angle to the visual ray. If illumination is by a point source at the position of the observer, the self-shadow boundary and the occluding contour coincide.

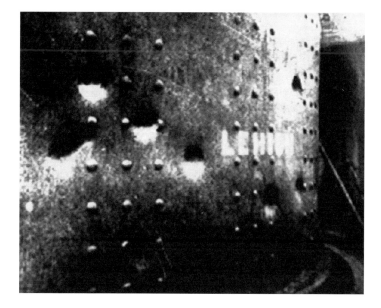

Figure 7.2
The effect of size on convex-concave inversion when interpreting shading. The large, round bulges in the wall of the boiler appear either raised or sunken, depending on the orientation of the image. The small rivets, on the other hand, almost always appear raised, regardless of the orientation of the image. If a *"common light source assumption"* holds, then both the bulges and the rivets must change appearance (after Ramul 1938; cf. also Metzger 1975).

Occluding contours can be outlines, but they can also occur in the interior of image regions, and have blind ends: for example, in the folds of curtains. Both types of edges provide information about the local surface orientation. This characteristic, important in the analysis of shading, distinguishes them from other types of edges, e.g., edges painted on a surface, or geometric edges such as those of a cube.

7.1 Psychophysics

Relatively little psychophysical research into shading has been conducted up to the date of this writing. One reason for this situation may be that it was difficult until quite recently to generate suitable test stimuli. The brightness of a surface is determined by its position, its orientation relative to the observer and to the light sources, its reflectivity, the brightness and spectral composition of the light sources, and interactions with other nearby surfaces. Only with the introduction of computer graphics did it become possible to generate such complicated stimuli under sufficiently controlled conditions. Some important observations and experimental results are as follows:

Quantification. Shading is a relatively weak depth cue; it furnishes data which is more qualitative than quantitative (Todd & Mingolla 1983, Bülthoff & Mallot 1988). For distant surfaces, shading does, however, gain in importance—probably due to the decreasing reliability of stereoscopic vision. Contrary to the results of Todd & Mingolla (1983), Koenderink et al. (1996), found that the local orientation of surfaces can be determined quite well from shading. The outline of the surface (the occluding contour), however, appears to play a major role (Mamassian & Kersten 1996).

Global ambiguity. Shading data is in many cases globally ambiguous in the sense that, for example, either concave or convex surfaces can be perceived, depending on assumptions about the position of the light source (the moon crater illusion, cf. Metzger 1975 and Fig. 1.4). Ramachandran (1988) postulates a *"common light source assumption"*, which holds for all objects in an image. A counterexample to this assumption has been presented by Ramul (1938; see Fig. 7.2 and Metzger 1975).

Light source. Information about the position of the light source appears to play a minor role. Correlation between the accuracy of depth estimates and estimates of light source position is very poor (Mingolla & Todd 1986). Shape constancy for different directions of illumination is also poor, i.e. the same surface appears to have different shapes when illuminated from different directions (Christou & Koenderink 1997). In ambiguous cases, the favored interpretation is that the light source is overhead. Hershberger (1970) showed that this assumption is innate in chicks, and can not be prevented by raising them in an environment which is lighted from below.

Gaussian curvature. The Gaussian theory of surfaces distinguishes between points of positive curvature (elliptical points) and those with negative curvature (hyperbolic points). The centers of curvature of all curves through elliptical points lie on the same side of the surface, while curves through hyperbolic points have centers of curvature on both sides of the surface (cf. Glossary, Fig. G.3). Mamassian et al. (1996) show that test subjects are able to distinguish elliptical and hyperbolic regions of a surface based on shading. It should be noted that this result is not in conflict with the convex/concave illusion, since both convex and concave points have positive Gaussian curvature.

Pre-attentive perception. Shading is of great importance for the qualitative interpretation of images. Ramachandran (1988) shows, for example, that concave shapes (holes) come immediately to attention in a group of spheres (bulges), and as a result of shading. If the shading at the self-shadow boundary is replaced by a sharp (binary) black/white edge, the impression of depth is lost and the holes are hard to find (see also Sun & Perona 1996). This immediacy is an example of what is called pre-attentive processing. This processing occurs simultaneously everywhere in an image, and without any particular need to look for the relevant image characteristics. Pre-attentive processing is to be distinguished from sequential, attention-driven processing, which seems to be necessary in order to evaluate the polarity of sharp black-white boundaries (cf. Treisman 1986).

Dull and glossy surfaces. Highlights improve the perception of shape from shading

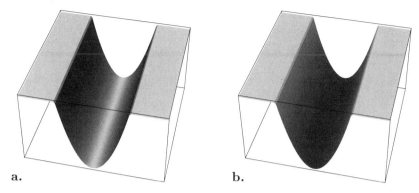

Figure 7.3
Shading with directional and non-directional lighting. **a.** Image of a valley with parallel illumination from above. The bottom of the valley appears bright, because the light impinges on the surface at a right angle. (Lambert reflection). **b.** If the illumination is diffuse, from a light source of large angular extent (a cloudy sky), the brightness of the surface is determined not by the direction of the normal, but rather, by the angle subtended by the valley rim. The valley bottom is in this case the darkest part. Langer & Zucker (1994) discuss this case under the heading *"Shape-from-shading on a cloudy day"*.

(Todd & Mingolla 1983). This effect is more pronounced with binocular vision (Blake & Bülthoff 1990; cf. the photometric disparities, Fig. 6.2d).

Outlines. Depth perception is strongly influenced by the outline of the shaded object (Barrow & Tenenbaum 1981). If, for example, a circular figure is cut out of a smoothly gradated gray value test strip, observers report that they see the surface curvature of a sphere. If, on the other hand, a long rectangle is cut out such that the brightness varies along its shorter dimension, observers report that they see a cylinder.

7.2   Problem statement

7.2.1   Local ambiguity

There have been a number of different approaches to the theory of shape from shading; for a recent review see Zhang et al. (1999). We will discuss here only the approach devised by Ikeuchi and Horn (1981), which is based on the inversion of the local reflectivity equation (see also Horn & Brooks 1989). An interesting alternative is found in the approach of Langer & Zucker (1994), which also considers nonlocal effects, in particular, the partial shading of a point by other areas of the surface when the light source has a large angular extent (cf. Fig. 7.3).

A typical case for analysis is that of viewing a uniform white surface under uniform illumination and without cast shadows. In this case, gray value variations in the image

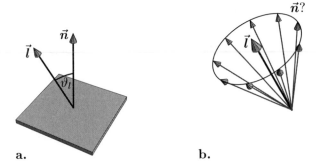

Figure 7.4
Local ambiguity of shape from shading with a Lambert surface with albedo 1. **a.** If $\vec{l}$ and $\vec{n}$ are known, the included angle ϑ_l, and therefore also the gray value of the corresponding point in the image, can be determined. **b.** If, conversely, only the gray value (i.e. the cosine of the angle ϑ_l) and the direction of the light source $\vec{l}$ are known, then any normal to the surface is possible as long as it lies in a conical shell around $\vec{l}$ whose apex angle is $2\vartheta_l$.

depend exclusively on variations in the surface normal. The relationship between the gray value and the direction of the normal is then described by a rule for local reflection, usually Lambert's formula (Equation 7.1 and Section 2.1).

The problem with this approach is that the normal at a point on the surface can not be unambiguously determined from the gray value measured at that point; Lambert's equation 7.1 can not be solved for $\vec{n}$ even if the direction of the illumination $\vec{l}$ is known (Fig. 7.4). This indeterminacy is not a characteristic of Lambert reflection, but rather applies to all models of shading which depend only on the local orientation of the surface and the direction of the illumination: the gray value, I, is a scalar quantity; measuring I does therefore not suffice to determine the vector quantity $\vec{n}$.

The assumptions which have been described (constant albedo, homogeneous parallel illumination, no mutual illumination of surfaces by one another) are of course very special. With respect to general gray value images, it is interesting to ask whether they can at all be the result of shading, or whether variations in surface albedo, i.e. a texture must be assumed. Obviously, albedo variations can mimic any type of shading, as a simple photograph of the shaded surface proves. Conversely, there are gray value patterns which cannot result from local shading of smooth surfaces. For example, given the assumptions listed above, there can be no smooth surface whose shaded image includes a dark spot on a bright background (e.g., $(I(r) = r^2/(1+r^2))$) (cf. Brooks et al. 1992). Nonetheless, the same image function does correspond to a smooth surface when the shading model of Fig. 7.3b applies.

One might conclude from the local ambiguity problem shown in Fig. 7.4 that shape from shading is an ill-posed inverse problem, which can be plausibly solved only if additional assumptions are made (regularization). But, strictly speaking, the indeterminacy arises only through the attempt to reconstruct the *orientation* of the

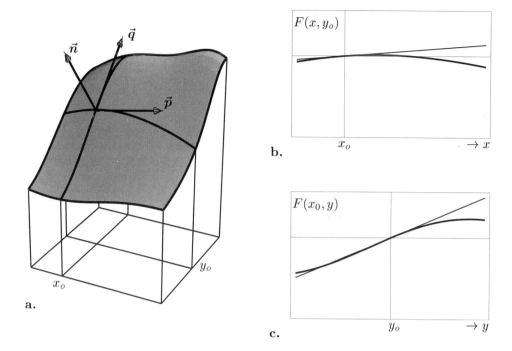

Figure 7.5
a. Representation of a fully visible surface by a function F. On the graph of F are shown the local normal to the surface, $\vec{n}$ at the point (x_o, y_o) as well as the two partial derivatives $\vec{p}$, $\vec{q}$ at this point. **b.**, **c.** Sections through the surface used in calculating the partial derivatives.

surface point by point. The surface itself is described locally by a *depth*, z, i.e. through a scalar quantity, i.e. one unknown per pixel, which can in principle be determined by point-by-point measurement of the gray value, another scalar quantity.

7.2.2   Mathematical notation

Surfaces

We represent the surface to be reconstructed as the graph of a function $F(x, y)$ in which (x, y) describes the image plane and $F(x, y)$ is the corresponding local depth value. This representation, which is different from the parametric representation of surfaces, is called either the graph or the Monge representation. Let the projection used for generating the image be parallel:

$$\begin{pmatrix} x \\ y \\ F(x, y) \end{pmatrix} \mapsto \begin{pmatrix} x \\ y \end{pmatrix}. \tag{7.2}$$

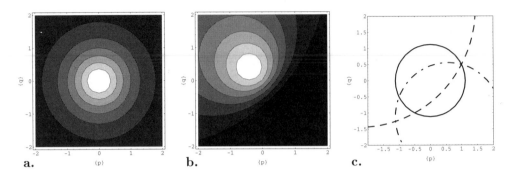

Figure 7.6
a. Contour lines of the reflectivity map $R(p, q)$ for a Lambert radiator when illumination is from the direction $\vec{l} = (0, 0, 1)^\top$. **b.** Similarly, when illumination is from the direction $\vec{l} = \frac{1}{\sqrt{3}}(-1, 1, 1)^\top$. **c.** Photometric stereo. If a point on a surface is illuminated sequentially from three different directions, then the normal to the surface can be determined as the intersection of corresponding contour lines of the reflectivity maps.

In order to derive the local surface normal $\vec{n}$, we first define two tangents to the surface with different directions, e.g.,

$$\vec{p}(x, y) = \begin{pmatrix} 1 \\ 0 \\ \frac{\partial F(x, y)}{\partial x} \end{pmatrix}, \quad \vec{q} = \begin{pmatrix} 0 \\ 1 \\ \frac{\partial F(x, y)}{\partial y} \end{pmatrix}. \tag{7.3}$$

The components

$$p := \frac{\partial F(x, y)}{\partial x}, \quad q := \frac{\partial F(x, y)}{\partial y} \tag{7.4}$$

are the partial derivatives of F with respect to x and y; they therefore correspond to the slopes of the tangents at the corresponding cross-sections through the graph of F (cf. Fig. 7.5). The normal to the surface is then calculated as the cross product (cf. Glossary), which is orthogonal to both of the vector multiplicands.

$$\vec{n} = \frac{\vec{p} \times \vec{q}}{\|\vec{p} \times \vec{q}\|} = \frac{1}{\sqrt{1 + p^2 + q^2}} \begin{pmatrix} -p \\ -q \\ 1 \end{pmatrix}. \tag{7.5}$$

Reflectivity

If the directions of illumination and of observation are fixed, reflection depends primarily on the local surface normal, $\vec{n}$. We represent the normal by the partial derivatives p, q of Equation 7.5 and describe the reflective characteristics of the surface in what is called the reflectivity map, $R(p, q)$, which gives the reflectivity for each orientation.

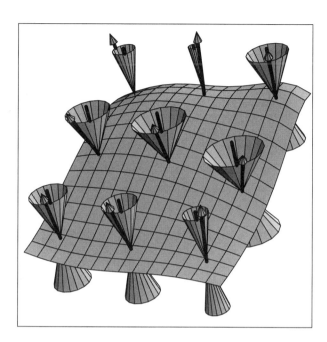

Figure 7.7
Geometric interpretation of the partial differential equation 7.7 using Monge cones. For every point in the space, the equation describes a cone in whose shell the local normal to the surface must lie. The axis of this cone is the direction of the illumination, and the cosine of one half of the apex angle corresponds to the local gray value. In the example solution given, the normals to the surface are shown as arrows. Each of these arrows must lie in the shell of the corresponding Monge cone.

For a Lambertian surface, the reflectivity map takes the form (Fig. 7.6):

$$R(p,q) = c(\vec{l} \cdot \vec{n}) = c \frac{l_3 - l_1 p - l_2 q}{\sqrt{1 + p^2 + q^2}}. \tag{7.6}$$

If the intensity of the image I at some point is measured, then the contour line $R(p,q) = I$ passes through all surface orientations (p,q) which are consistent with the measured gray value. The contour line, then, corresponds to the shell of the cone in Fig. 7.4b.

An example which is irrelevant to the modeling of human perception, but instructive, is that of *photometric stereo*. A point on the surface under consideration is illuminated from three different directions $\vec{l}_1, \vec{l}_2, \vec{l}_3$. For each gray value at the point, there is a constraint equation for (p,q), from which the orientation of the surface can be restricted to a contour line of the corresponding reflectivity map. The intersection of these three contour lines then identifies the orientation of that part of the surface (Fig. 7.6c).

7.2.3 The image irradiance equation

The mathematical representations which have just been introduced make it possible to formulate the basic equation for the analysis of shading. We call it the "image irradiance equation", after Ikeuchi & Horn (1981):

$$I(x,y) = R\left(\frac{\partial F}{\partial x}(x,y), \frac{\partial F}{\partial y}(x,y)\right). \tag{7.7}$$

The goal with this equation is to find the surface F whose partial derivatives reproduce the image I when inserted into the reflectivity map R. Equation 7.7 is a partial differential equation. For every point (x, y) of the image plane, there exists a gray value I, which corresponds to a cone of possible surface orientations by way of the corresponding contour line in the reflectivity map. This situation is illustrated graphically in Fig. 7.7. The surface illustrated is not the only possible solution: all surfaces whose normals lie in the shells of the Monge cones are valid solutions. Because of this indeterminacy, boundary conditions of the partial differential equations play an important role: these may be, for example, the boundary of the surface to be reconstructed, or the normals to the surface along the boundary. Boundary conditions are not shown in Fig. 7.7.

Equation 7.7 describes only simple reflection, as illustrated in Fig. 7.3. Light sources of large angular extent, illumination of different parts of the surface by sources from different directions, and differences in reflective characteristics at different points on the surface are not considered.

7.3   One-dimensional "images"

Let us consider one-dimensional gray value functions $I(x)$, which we can think of as sections through intensity surfaces which are constant in the y direction. In this case, only a depth profile $F(x)$, rather than a surface, need be reconstructed, with tangents $(1, F'(x))^\top$ and normals

$$\vec{n} = \frac{1}{\sqrt{1 + F'^2(x)}} \begin{pmatrix} -F'(x) \\ 1 \end{pmatrix} \tag{7.8}$$

(cf. Fig. 7.8). Here, the sign is chosen so as to make the normal always point upward (positive z component).

Let $\vec{l} = (\sin\varphi, \cos\varphi)^\top$ be the direction of the illumination, i.e. $\varphi = 0$ signifies that the illumination is from directly overhead (from the z direction). We assume that reflection from the surface obeys Lambert's formula and that the value of the constant c (the albedo) is 1. We obtain the image irradiance equation:

$$I(x) = (\vec{l} \cdot \vec{n}) = \frac{\cos\varphi - F'(x)\sin\varphi}{\sqrt{1 + F'^2(x)}}. \tag{7.9}$$

Here, the right side of the equation is the one-dimensional reflectivity map of a Lambert radiator with parallel illumination from the direction φ. In contrast to the corresponding two-dimensional Equation 7.7, the equation in this case is an ordinary differential equation in which the unknown F appears only as a first derivative. Squaring Equation 7.9 produces a quadratic equation, which can be solved for F':

$$F'(x) = \frac{1}{I^2(x) - \sin^2\varphi} \left(\pm I(x)\sqrt{1 - I^2(x)} - \sin\varphi\cos\varphi \right). \tag{7.10}$$

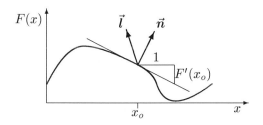

Figure 7.8
One-dimensional depth profile $F(x)$ with the local normal to the surface $\vec{n}$ and the derivative $F'(x)$. The intensity of the image of F can be determined according to Lambert's formula from the dot product $(\vec{l} \cdot \vec{n})$.

In the one-dimensional case, unlike the case illustrated in Fig. 7.4, the gray value determines the normal to the surface, except for the sign of the square root term in Equation 7.10. If $I(x) = 1$, then $F'(x) = -\tan\varphi$, i.e., the illumination locally falls at a right angle to the surface. If $I(x) = 0$, then $F'(x) = \cot\varphi$, i.e., the light grazes the surface.*

Possible profiles in this case result simply from integration of F'. Even if the direction of the light source is known, however, there are still some ambiguities. For one, the sign of the root in Equation 7.10 may be chosen at will. If smooth surfaces are assumed, the sign may be chosen at the start (i.e. one end of the gray value function) or at zero crossings of the term inside the root. Secondly, there is also an integration constant which allows the profile to be placed at any distance. This freedom is not surprising, since, conversely, the image is not altered by simply changing its distance: we have, after all, assumed parallel illumination and projection. Finally, we have also assumed that the normalization of I is known, for example, that $I(x_0) = 1$ indicates that the surface is illuminated at a right angle at the location x_0. If this is not the case, the surface has an unknown albedo, and there are additional difficulties.

Let us consider three special cases with illumination from above ($\vec{l} = (0,1)^\top$, $\varphi = 0$). Analytical solutions may be obtained through integration of Equation 7.10 and insertion of $\sin\varphi = 0$:

$$F(x) = F_o + \int_0^x F'(x')dx' = F_o + \int_0^x \pm\sqrt{\frac{1 - I^2(x')}{I^2(x')}}\,dx'. \qquad (7.11)$$

Fig. 7.9 also shows numerical solutions for the case in which the illumination is from diagonally to the right and above ($\vec{l} = (\frac{1}{2}, \frac{\sqrt{3}}{2})^\top$, or $\varphi = 30°$).

Case 1: $I(x) \equiv I = const.$ By substitution into Equation 7.11, it follows that:

$$F(x) = F_o \pm \sqrt{\frac{1 - I^2}{I^2}}\,x.$$

---

*In the two-dimensional case (Equation 7.7) the normal to the surface is only determined unambiguously if $I(x,y) = 1$; the cone in Fig. 7.4b degenerates into the line which is its axis. The case $I(x,y) = 0$ remains ambiguous; the cone of possible normals to the surface becomes a circular disk at right angles to the direction of the light, i.e., the surface may be at any orientation such that the light grazes it.

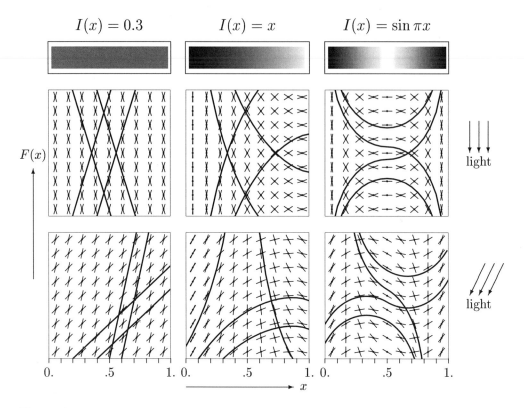

Figure 7.9
Reconstruction of one-dimensional depth profiles for three intensity distributions (shown as gray value strips) and two directions of illumination (from directly above, and from 30° to the left). The six panels show the tangent fields of the differential equation 7.10 as well as a few selected solutions. Additional explanations are to be found in the text.

In this case, the solution is therefore a straight line, i.e., a ramp which is closer at one end than at the other. Examples of solutions with orthogonal and oblique illumination are shown in the left column of Fig. 7.9.

Case 2: $I(x) = x$. Insertion into Equation 7.11 results in:

$$F(x) = F_o \pm \left(\sqrt{1 - x^2} - \log \frac{1 + \sqrt{1 - x^2}}{x} \right).$$

Examples are given in the middle column of Fig. 7.9.

Case 3: $I(x) = \sin \pi x$, $0 \le x \le 1$. In this case, analytical solutions are possible for all directions of illumination φ. Substitution into Equation 7.10 results in:

$$F'(x) = \frac{\pm \sin(\pi x)\cos(\pi x) - \sin\varphi\cos\varphi}{\sin^2(\pi x) - \sin^2\varphi} = \cot(\varphi \pm \pi x)$$

and, in turn by integration,

$$F(x) = F_o \pm \frac{1}{\pi}\log(\sin(\varphi \pm \pi x)).$$

At the location $x = \frac{1}{2}$, $I(x) = 1$, and so $F'(x)$ is orthogonal to the direction of illumination for both solutions. It follows that there are additional smooth solutions, which, for example, employ the positive sign in the general solution for $x < \frac{1}{2}$ and the negative sign for $x > \frac{1}{2}$. Fig. 7.9 (right column) gives examples for all possible combinations.

7.4 Shape from shading in two dimensions

7.4.1 Global indeterminacy and boundary conditions

In the two-dimensional case, the indeterminacy of shading analysis is even more serious. Fig. 7.10 shows a gray value image together with four different surfaces, all of which are possible spatial interpretations of the image and solutions of Equation 7.7. The indeterminacy differs from that in Fig. 7.4: here, if the type of surface can be determined at any one location, then the solution for the entire surface is determined; this type of indeterminacy is therefore called a *global* indeterminacy. In order to resolve this problem, additional information is necessary, e.g., about depth and orientation of the surface along the image boundaries. As a rule, two types of such *boundary conditions* are applied:

- If there is a shaded part of the image between edges, then the depth of the edges may be determined stereoscopically or in some other way. The shape of the surface between the edges may then be determined by solving the reflectivity equation with the edges as a boundary condition.

- Closed surfaces such as spheres or ellipsoids all have occluding contours, i.e, edges which are not those of the surface, but rather, which result from the "turning away" of the surface from the observer (e.g, the outline of a sphere: cf. Fig. 7.1). At occluding contours, the surface is locally parallel to the direction of observation. Therefore, the local orientation of the surface is known, though the depth along the occluding contour is not known.

Besides these boundary conditions, additional heuristics, e.g., about the likelihood of specific shapes of the surface, may be applied. One example is the *generic viewpoint assumption*, which also plays a role in connection with other depth cues. Fig. 7.11 illustrates this assumption for the problem of three-dimensional interpretations of line

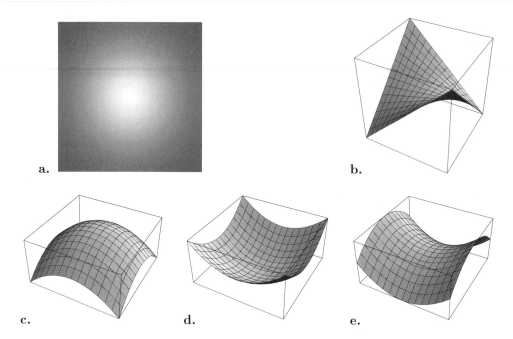

Figure 7.10
Global indeterminacy of shape from shading.   **a.**   Intensity image $I(x, y) = 1/\sqrt{1 + x^2 + y^2}$.   Under vertical illumination and with Lambert reflection, all of the following surfaces generate this image. **b.** Saddle-shaped surface (hyperboloid) $F(x, y) = xy$. **c., d.** Paraboloid $F(x, y) = \pm \frac{1}{2}(x^2 + y^2)$. **e.** Saddle-shaped surface (hyperboloid) $F(x, y) = \frac{1}{2}(x^2 - y^2)$. The two saddle-shaped surfaces can be transformed into each other by rotation around the vertical axis.

drawings: the outline of a cube can appear to be a hexagon (Fig. 7.11b) if the axis of view coincides with one of the cube's body diagonals. In actual observation of the cube, only a slight motion of the head changes the image qualitatively, for example, into the figure shown in Fig. 7.11a. Even without moving the head, the interpretation of Fig. 7.11b as a spatial object has little plausibility, since it is very unlikely that the axis of view and the body diagonal will coincide. In determining shape from shading, a similar situation occurs when observing a shaded cup (hollow hemisphere) exactly from above. Only from this point of view can it be confused with a sphere: from all other points of view, part of the outside of the cup will be visible, so that it no longer can be confused with a sphere.

The generic viewpoint assumption may be applied along with the Bayes theory of estimation (Freeman 1996). The assumptions about the likelihood of a point of view are in this case incorporated in the *a priori* part of the estimation.

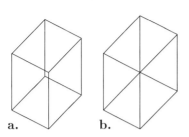

Figure 7.11
Generic viewpoint assumption: Both images can
be images of a cube. In **b.**, it must additionally be
assumed that the direction of view coincides exactly with one of the body diagonals of the cube.
Since this coincidence occurs only rarely, and can
be undone by small movements of the head, the
favored interpretation of **b.** is as a hexagon.

a.   **b.**

7.4.2 Solution of the reflectivity equation*

Given an image $I(x, y)$ and a reflectivity map $R(F_x(x, y), F_y(x, y))$, which gives the
reflectivity of the surface as a function of orientation, we will now attempt to solve
Equation 7.7; that is, we will attempt to find a surface $F(x, y)$, whose orientations
agree with the reflectivity map and result in the correct image.

Ikeuchi & Horn (1981) suggest that an unconstrained vector field $(p(x, y), q(x, y))$,
rather than a gradient field $(F_x(x, y), F_y(x, y))$, should be considered when beginning
an attempt to solve this problem. The partial differential equation 7.7 is thereby
transformed into an algebraic equation with two unknowns, p, q:

$$I(x, y) = R(p(x, y), q(x, y)). \tag{7.12}$$

Since this equation has the two independent unknowns p and q, it is under-defined. An
additional constraint, however, is that the vector field (p, q) must actually represent
a surface: i.e., that it must be integrable. This constraint may be formalized based
on the following observation: The quantities p and q are the partial derivatives of the
surface function F. Consequently, $p_y(x, y) = F_{xy}(x, y)$ and $q_x = F_{yx}(x, y)$. According
to Schwarz's theorem from calculus, partial derivatives may be evaluated in arbitrary
order as long as the function is differentiable for a sufficient number of times, i.e.,

$$p_y(x, y) = F_{xy}(x, y) = F_{yx}(x, y) = q_x(x, y). \tag{7.13}$$

The quantity $p_y - q_x$ is called the *curl* of the vector field (p, q). By inverting the
statement made in Equation 7.13, it can be shown that every smooth vector field
with zero curl is integrable.

Both equations (Equation 7.12, 7.13) together are equivalent to the equation with
which we started, 7.7, and, if boundary conditions are given, have unique solutions.
A practical problem when using the integrability constraint 7.13 occurs with sampled
image functions, with which no meaningful calculation of derivatives at the pixel level
is possible. For this reason, Ikeuchi & Horn (1981) replace Equation 7.13 with a
smoothness constraint. This approach is unsatisfactory in that smooth vector fields
are not necessarily integrable; if the smooth solutions for p and q are integrated
separately with respect to x and y, the result is, in general, not the same surface.

---

*This section may be skipped on first reading.

One way to apply the exact integrability constraint to sampled images is to apply the finite element method (Janfeld & Mallot 1992).

Now, let us briefly discuss the process described by Ikeuchi & Horn (1981). Since exact solutions are not to be expected, the problem is formulated as one of minimization of errors. For the sampled reflectivity equation 7.12, the following error term may be defined:

$$r_{ij} := (I_{ij} - R(p_{ij}, q_{ij}))^2. \qquad (7.14)$$

Here, r_{ij} is the intensity error per pixel, i.e., the deviation of the measured gray value from what it would be based on the assumed surface orientation (p_{ij}, q_{ij}). From the smoothness constraint, there arises an additional error term, in the form of the expression:

$$s_{ij} := \frac{1}{4} \left((p_{i+1,j} - p_{ij})^2 + (p_{i,j+1} - p_{ij})^2 + (q_{i+1,j} - q_{ij})^2 + (q_{i,j+1} - q_{ij})^2 \right). \quad (7.15)$$

If the surface is locally flat, then the values of p and q for neighboring pixels are equal, and the value of s is 0. Otherwise, s_{ij} measures the local curvature of the surface, or to put it more precisely, the deviation from an ideal smooth, that is, flat, surface.

The two error terms can be combined into a single error term e:

$$e := \sum_i \sum_j (\underbrace{s_{ij}}_{\text{smoothness}} + \lambda \underbrace{r_{ij}}_{\text{image data}}) \quad ; \lambda > 0. \qquad (7.16)$$

The number λ is called the regularization parameter; it can be chosen at will. This parameter determines the weighting of the data against the smoothness constraint; if the data is very noisy, a small value is assigned to this parameter.

By minimizing e as a function of p_{ij}, q_{ij}, the orientation at all locations on the surface may now be evaluated. With e minimized, the partial derivatives $\frac{\partial e}{\partial p_{ij}}$, $\frac{\partial e}{\partial q_{ij}}$ must vanish for all i, j. If n is the number of pixels in one dimension of the image, then there are $2n^2$ equations to solve for the $2n^2$ unknowns p_{ij}, q_{ij}. Taking the derivative results in

$$\frac{\delta e}{\delta p_{ij}} = \frac{1}{2}[(p_{ij} - p_{i+1,j}) + (p_{ij} - p_{i,j+1}) + (p_{ij} - p_{i-1,j}) + (p_{ij} - p_{i,j-1})]$$

$$+ 2\lambda(I_{ij} - R(p_{ij}, q_{ij})) \cdot \frac{\partial R}{\partial p}(p_{ij}, q_{ij})$$

$$\overset{!}{=} 0, \qquad (7.17)$$

and

$$\frac{\partial e}{\partial q_{ij}} = \frac{1}{2}[(q_{ij} - q_{i+1,j}) + (q_{ij} - q_{i,j+1}) + (q_{ij} - q_{i-1,j}) + (q_{ij} - q_{i,j-1})]$$

$$+ 2\lambda(I_{ij} - R(p_{ij}, q_{ij})) \cdot \frac{\partial R}{\partial q}(p_{ij}, q_{ij})$$

$$\overset{!}{=} 0. \qquad (7.18)$$

These two equations can not be solved directly for p_{ij} and q_{ij}, since the reflectivity term R which occurs in the second part of the sum (error minimization term) in each equation can not be inverted. We introduce the local averages,

$$p_{ij}^* := \frac{1}{4}(p_{i+1,j} + p_{i,j+1} + p_{i-1,j} + p_{i,j-1}) \tag{7.19}$$

$$q_{ij}^* := \frac{1}{4}(q_{i+1,j} + q_{i,j+1} + q_{i-1,j} + q_{i,j-1}). \tag{7.20}$$

An approximation that can be improved by iteration is given by:

$$p_{ij}^{n+1} = p_{ij}^{*,n} - \lambda(I_{ij} - R(p_{ij}^n, q_{ij}^n)) \cdot \frac{\partial R}{\partial p}(p_{ij}^n, q_{ij}^n) \tag{7.21}$$

$$q_{ij}^{n+1} = q_{ij}^{*,n} - \lambda(I_{ij} - R(p_{ij}^n, q_{ij}^n)) \cdot \frac{\partial R}{\partial q}(p_{ij}^n, q_{ij}^n). \tag{7.22}$$

Here, the superscript is the iteration index. If the series in p_{ij} and q_{ij} converge, then the limit value is a solution of the conditional equations 7.17 and 7.18. The initial conditions (p_{ij}^0, q_{ij}^0) follow from appropriate boundary conditions, e.g., the occluding contour of the object. As already mentioned, the smooth vector field (p, q) that is found may not be integrable.

The iterative process for solving the conditional equations corresponds to the standard procedure in numerical mathematics. More interesting here is the introduction of the regularization parameter λ, which can be viewed as a formalization of the concept of inverse optics: the smoothness constraint is an additional assumption which is introduced to make the solution of the under-defined, or "ill-posed" Equation 7.12 possible. The "regularization" of ill-posed problems by means of a smoothness constraint is widely used in image processing (Poggio et al. 1985). In shading analysis, however, exact solutions are also possible, without the need for regularization (see Oliensis 1991, Janfeld & Mallot 1992).

A further important consideration has to do with the role of boundary conditions: namely, the same intensity distribution can lead to entirely different evaluations of depth if the boundary conditions are different. This fact reflects a general problem in the treatment of partial differential equations. The importance of outlines for the perception of form from shading has already been pointed out in Section 7.1.

Chapter 8

Texture and surface orientation

8.1 Texture and texture gradients

Textures are more or less regular surface patterns composed of similar elements. These elements can be designs (differences in pigmentation) or variations in depth (e.g., corrugations), and are sometimes called "texels" (from texture elements). Most natural surfaces have textures. Examples are textiles (the origin of the word "texture"), grass or gravel surfaces, stone-work and many others. As a rule, the similarity of the texture elements is not complete, but rather, it is of a statistical nature.

In image processing as in perception, textures are used in two independent contexts:

- Image segmentation: Borders between textures, like borders between areas of different brightness or depth, can provide a basis for dividing an image meaningfully into regions. Conversely, in nature, surface patterns are also used to make segmentation more difficult; that is, for camouflage. Image segmentation will not be covered in this chapter.

- Depth perception: Continuous variation of textures provide an important depth cue, from which information about the orientation and curvature of surfaces can be obtained. Such variations in textures are called *texture gradients* (Gibson 1950).

In this chapter, we will consider three approaches to the extraction of depth information from texture gradients:

1. Identification of vanishing points
2. Density gradient of texture elements

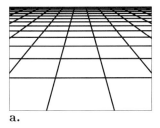 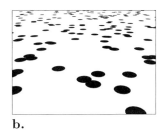 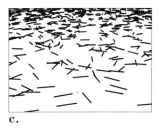

a.   b.   c.

Figure 8.1
Texture gradients in the perspective projection of a plane. **a.** Image of a plane with a slant of 68°. **b.** Disks on the plane are imaged as ellipses which become smaller and more eccentric with increasing distance. The orientation of the longer axis is parallel to the horizon. **c.** With increasing distance, the orientation of line segments becomes more and more horizontal.

3. Form gradient of texture elements; in particular, the distribution of orientations found in images of slanted isotropic patterns.

Perception of depth based on texture gradients (Fig. 8.1) is closely related to perspective projection, which leads to a reduction in image size with increasing distance, and therefore also to an increase in the density of texture elements. In parallel projection, images of plane surfaces, however slanted, do not contain texture gradients. Images of curved surfaces, on the other hand, lead to texture gradients even in parallel projection. In this case the occluding contour of the curved surface corresponds to the horizon of a plane in perspective projection. Psychophysical work on the perception of surface orientation based on textures shows that the different types of texture gradients are used in different ways (cf. Todd & Akerstrom 1987, Blake et al. 1993).

8.2 Regular patterns: Vanishing points

As was shown in Section 2.3.2, a vanishing point at the location $(x'_f, y'_f)^\top$ establishes the direction in space of straight lines which converge on it in the image. Each straight line whose image aims toward the vanishing point can therefore be represented parametrically as

$$g(\lambda) = \begin{pmatrix} a \\ b \\ c \end{pmatrix} + \lambda \begin{pmatrix} x_f \\ y_f \\ -1 \end{pmatrix} \tag{8.1}$$

where $(a, b, c)^\top$ is an arbitrary starting point on the line. If, then, two vanishing points for different bundles of straight lines in a plane are known (cf. Fig. 2.12b), then the orientation of the plane is completely defined. All vanishing points for other directions of straight lines in this plane lie along a line which passes through the two vanishing points that are already known—and this line is the horizon of the plane. The further question now arises of how vanishing points can be identified in images.

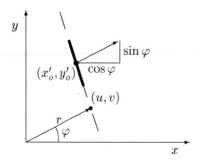

Figure 8.2
The extension of a line segment which is defined by the coordinates (x'_o, y'_o) and the orientation φ is described by the point (u, v), at which it passes closest to the origin. We will call (u, v) the "passage point" of the straight line.

Given an oriented edge element at the location $(x'_o, y'_o)^\top$, with the normal $(\cos\varphi, \sin\varphi)^\top$, let us designate the dot product of the position vector and the normal as r, $r = x'_o \cos\varphi + y'_o \sin\varphi$. The equation of the line g through the edge element derived by means of its normal is:

$$x' \cos\varphi + y' \sin\varphi = r. \tag{8.2}$$

We now proceed in four steps:

Step 1. We must first describe the line that is defined by an edge segment in a way which does not depend on the position of the edge element along the line. If the embedding line g does not pass through the origin of the coordinate system, then we can use the point at which the line passes closest to the origin. We designate this point the "passage point" (u, v) of the line. From Fig. 8.2, we can see that:

$$\begin{pmatrix} u \\ v \end{pmatrix} = r \begin{pmatrix} \cos\varphi \\ \sin\varphi \end{pmatrix} = \begin{pmatrix} x' \cos^2\varphi + y' \sin\varphi \cos\varphi \\ x' \sin\varphi \cos\varphi + y' \sin^2\varphi \end{pmatrix}. \tag{8.3}$$

For each edge element (x', y', φ), Equation 8.3 gives the "passage point" of the embedding line g. The representation of a line by its passage point it unique for lines not containing the origin; therefore, using the passage point (u, v) makes it possible to determine whether two edge elements lie along the same line.

   If $(u, v) = (0, 0)$ for an edge element, then simply enough, another point is chosen as the origin.

Step 2. The passage points of the lines which correspond to each edge segment are now assembled into a two-dimensional histogram ("Hough transform", cf. Fig. 8.3). Edge elements belonging to the same line appear as clusters in Hough space u, v. The description in terms of Hough space allows, on the one hand, the correction of minor errors of position and orientation of the edge segments, and on the other hand, the assembly of widely separated segments into a line. Usually, the Hough transformation is followed by a cluster analysis performed in Hough space, in order to identify the lines that correspond to the edge elements (cf. Rosenfeld & Kak, 1982, Vol. 2). Here, however, we are not interested in the lines themselves, but only in the vanishing points which they identify.

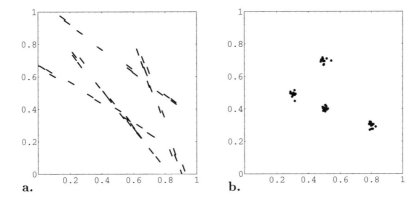

Figure 8.3
Hough transform. **a.** Edge segments identified by suitable preprocessing steps. **b.** Passage points of the lines of which the edge elements are segments (cf. Fig. 8.2). Four clusters are recognizable, corresponding to four lines in the original image.

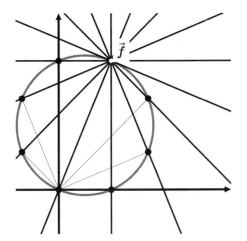

Figure 8.4
The passage points of all lines through a vanishing point $\vec{f}$ construct a circle through the origin and the vanishing point. The line which connects the origin to the vanishing point is a diameter of this circle. The passage points of some of the lines are identified.

Step 3. In order to find the vanishing point (x'_f, y'_f), we must first consider where the images of the lines through a given vanishing point in Hough space might be found. Clearly, the lines through a point (x'_f, y'_f) can all be characterized by an edge element (x'_f, y'_f, φ), if φ can take on any value in the range $[0, \pi]$.

In the (u, v) plane, these lines, or the corresponding passage points (u_φ, v_φ), form a circle through $(0, 0)$ and (x'_f, y'_f) whose diameter is $2r = \sqrt{(x'_f)^2 + (y'_f)^2}$ (cf. Fig. 8.4). This result follows from the theorem of Thales, according to which the angle at the apex of a triangle inscribed in a semi-circle is always $90°$. The problem of identifying the vanishing point is therefore reduced to one of finding circles through the origin in Hough space.

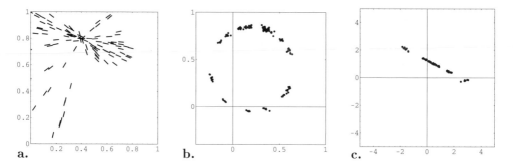

Figure 8.5
Identifying a vanishing point by applying the Hough transform. **a.** Edge segments.
b. The passage points of the lines which pass through the edge segments lie in a
circle. **c.** Evaluation of the parameters of the circle (center, radius) can be performed
through regression using an image transformed as in Equation 8.4.

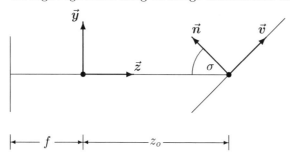

Figure 8.6
Imaging geometry of a
slanted plane. Explana-
tion in the text.

Step 4. In order to make it easier to find the center of the circle in Hough space,
the additional transformation

$$\begin{pmatrix} u \\ v \end{pmatrix} \longrightarrow \left(\frac{u}{u^2 + v^2}, \frac{v}{u^2 + v^2} \right) \tag{8.4}$$

(inversion with respect to the unit circle) can be performed. The circle is converted
into a straight line, which can be found through regression (cf. Fig. 8.5).

8.3   Stochastic patterns 1: Density gradient

Let us consider a plane surface on which texture elements are evenly distributed. We
designate the density of the texture elements (number per unit of area) as ϱ. An
area A of the surface therefore holds, on average, ϱA texture elements. A perspective
projection of this area is then imaged onto an area A' in the image plane, in which
the texture density is, then, $\varrho' = \varrho A/A'$. By determining ϱ' at different locations in
the image, it is possible to obtain information on the angle at which the plane is being
observed, and therefore on the slant of the plane.

8.3.1 Coordinates of a plane and its image

In order to apply and interpret gradients of texture density, we need first to work through some mathematical definitions and preliminary observations.

Fig. 8.6 shows a slanted plane in the camera coordinate system. The $\vec{x}$ axis of the camera coordinate system and the $\vec{u}$ axis of the plane's coordinate system are orthogonal to the page, and are not shown in the illustration. The angle between the direction of view (optical axis, $\vec{z}$) and the normal vector of the plane is called the slant angle, σ. Generally, the $\vec{u}$ axis of the plane is chosen as the intersection of the x, z plane of the camera coordinate system with the plane. The angle between the $\vec{u}$ axis when defined in this way and the projection of the optical axis onto the plane is called the tilt, τ. In the example shown, $\tau = 90°$. If the direction of view is described in a polar coordinate system aligned with the slanted plane (cf. Glossary: polar coordinates), then σ corresponds to the elevation ϑ and τ corresponds to the azimuth φ. The tilt angle may be changed without changing the slant by rotating the plane around the optical axis.

In what follows, we will consider only the case illustrated in Fig. 8.6 in which $\tau = 90°$. In this case, the coordinate system of the plane is:

$$\vec{u} = \begin{pmatrix} 1 \\ 0 \\ 0 \end{pmatrix}, \quad \vec{v} = \begin{pmatrix} 0 \\ \cos\sigma \\ \sin\sigma \end{pmatrix}, \quad \vec{n} = \begin{pmatrix} 0 \\ \sin\sigma \\ -\cos\sigma \end{pmatrix}. \tag{8.5}$$

This coordinate system assigns coordinates (u, v) to each point of the plane; the three-dimensional coordinates of such a point are:

$$\begin{pmatrix} x \\ y \\ z \end{pmatrix} = \begin{pmatrix} 0 \\ 0 \\ z_o \end{pmatrix} + u \begin{pmatrix} 1 \\ 0 \\ 0 \end{pmatrix} + v \begin{pmatrix} 0 \\ \cos\sigma \\ \sin\sigma \end{pmatrix} = \begin{pmatrix} u \\ v\cos\sigma \\ z_o + v\sin\sigma \end{pmatrix}. \tag{8.6}$$

If this point is projected onto the image plane, the coordinates of the plane are transformed into the image coordinates according to:

$$T : \mathbb{R}^2 \to \mathbb{R}^2$$
$$T \begin{pmatrix} u \\ v \end{pmatrix} = \begin{pmatrix} x' \\ y' \end{pmatrix} := \frac{-1}{z_o + v\sin\sigma} \begin{pmatrix} u \\ v\cos\sigma \end{pmatrix}. \tag{8.7}$$

Unlike perspective, which assigns a point in the image to each point in space, this transformation can be inverted, as long as $\sin\sigma \neq -z_o/v$, that is, for all points which are not on the horizon. This transformation plays an important role when inferring the local characteristics of planes from the image. We will use the same transformation again when analyzing optical flow. The inverse mapping (from the image into the plane) is as:

$$T^{-1} : \mathbb{R}^2 \to \mathbb{R}^2$$
$$T \begin{pmatrix} x' \\ y' \end{pmatrix} = \begin{pmatrix} u \\ v \end{pmatrix} := \frac{-z_o}{\cos\sigma + y'\sin\sigma} \begin{pmatrix} x'\cos\sigma \\ y' \end{pmatrix}. \tag{8.8}$$

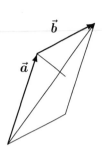

Figure 8.7

The surface area of a parallelogram. A parallelogram may be described by the vectors $\vec{a} = (a_1, a_2)^\top$ and $\vec{b} = (b_1, b_2)$. After dividing it into two triangles along the diagonal $\vec{a} + \vec{b}$, the surface area may be calculated as the base times the height. The length of the base is $\|\vec{a} + \vec{b}\|$. The normal vector in the direction of the height is $(-a_2 - b_2, a_1 + b_1)^\top / \|\vec{a} + \vec{b}\|$. The height may be obtained by projecting $\vec{a}$ onto this normal. Then the surface area may be calculated: $A = |a_1 b_2 - a_2 b_1|$.

This is exactly the "inverse perspective" shown in Fig. 6.15. The transformations T and T^{-1} in Equations 8.7 and 8.8 are examples of collineation (projective mappings).

8.3.2   Areal magnification

The density ϱ' which can be measured in the image, along with the relation $\varrho' = \varrho A / A'$ which has already been discussed, makes it possible to determine the magnification (or reduction) of surface area accomplished by the imaging process T. In order to make use of this data, we must also determine the relationship between the slant σ and the areal magnification.

We first note that the surface area of a parallelogram defined by the vectors $(a_1, a_2)^\top$ and $(b_1, b_2)^\top$ (cf. Fig. 8.7) is

$$A = |a_1 b_2 - b_1 a_2| = \left| \det \begin{pmatrix} a_1 & b_1 \\ a_2 & b_2 \end{pmatrix} \right|. \qquad (8.9)$$

The areal magnification of a linear mapping L,

$$L \begin{pmatrix} x \\ y \end{pmatrix} = \begin{pmatrix} a_{11} & a_{12} \\ a_{21} & a_{22} \end{pmatrix} \begin{pmatrix} x \\ y \end{pmatrix} = \begin{pmatrix} a_{11}x + a_{12}y \\ a_{21}x + a_{22}y \end{pmatrix},$$

can be determined by examining the square defined by the vectors $\vec{a} = (1, 0)^\top$ and $\vec{b} = (0, 1)^\top$ in the domain of the mapping. The area of this square is 1. Its image is the parallelogram defined by the vectors $L(\vec{a}) = (a_{11}, a_{21})^\top$ and $L(\vec{b}) = (a_{12}, a_{22})^\top$. According to the rule discussed above, its area is $|a_{11}a_{22} - a_{12}a_{21}|$. Since the area of the original square was 1, the new area is also the areal magnification of the linear mapping. This magnification is everywhere the same.

For a general (differentiable) mapping $T : \mathbb{R}^2 \to \mathbb{R}^2$, areal magnification can be determined by first finding a local linear approximation and than calculating the magnification of this linear mapping (cf. Fig. 8.8). A linear approximation (gray grid in Fig. 8.8) can be obtained from the matrix of the partial derivatives of the two components of the mapping T, that is, from the Jacobi matrix (see, for example

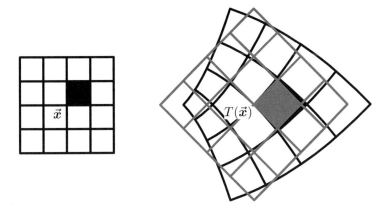

Figure 8.8
The definition of areal magnification of a general transformation T. Left: the domain in which T is defined. The center point of the grid is marked $\vec{x}$. Right: The image of the grid as transformed by T (black) and by $\mathrm{J}_T(\vec{x})$ (gray) which approximates T around the center of the grid, $T(\vec{x})$

Rudin 1976):

$$\mathrm{J}_T(x, y) := \begin{pmatrix} \dfrac{\partial T_1}{\partial x} & \dfrac{\partial T_1}{\partial y} \\ \dfrac{\partial T_2}{\partial x} & \dfrac{\partial T_2}{\partial y} \end{pmatrix}. \tag{8.10}$$

The linear approximation of a multidimensional mapping by means of the Jacobi matrix is equivalent to the approximation of a one-dimensional function by a tangent whose slope is given by the local derivative of the function. The determinant of the Jacobi matrix is the local magnification produced by the mapping T. In particular, the result for the projection of a plane, (Equation 8.8) is:

$$\frac{A'}{A} = \left| \frac{\partial x}{\partial u} \frac{\partial y}{\partial v} - \frac{\partial x}{\partial v} \frac{\partial y}{\partial u} \right| = \frac{z_o \cos \sigma}{(z_o + v \sin \sigma)^3} = \frac{\varrho}{\varrho'}. \tag{8.11}$$

8.3.3 The density gradient

Equation 8.11 for areal magnification allows us to determine the expected density gradient for a plane whose slant is σ. By solving the last equality in Equation 8.11 for ϱ' and observing that due to the assumption $\tau = 90°$, ϱ' depends only on y', we first obtain:

$$\varrho'(y') = \varrho \cdot \frac{(z_o + v \sin \sigma)^3}{z_o \cdot \cos \sigma}. \tag{8.12}$$

The expression on the right, however, depends on the coordinate v on the plane. (Here, the simplification $\tau = 90°$ is applied; for the general case of any tilt angle, u

also appears on the right side of Equation 8.12.) According to the inversion formula, Eq. 8.8,

$$v = \frac{-z_o y'}{\cos \sigma + y' \sin \sigma}.$$

(8.13)

If this is substituted into Equation 8.12, it follows that:

$$\frac{\varrho'(y')}{\varrho} = \frac{(z_o \cos \sigma)^2}{(\cos \sigma + y' \sin \sigma)^3}.$$

(8.14)

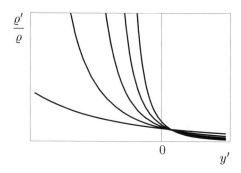

Figure 8.9
Expected behavior of the density gradient $\varrho'(y')/\varrho$ for $\sigma = 10°, 20°, 30°, 40°$ (from left to right). y' is the vertical image position. The curves have asymptotes at $y' = -\cot \sigma$, i.e., at the horizon of the plane. For $y' = 0$, they take on the values $z_o^2 / \cos^2 \sigma$.

Fig. 8.9 shows the expected behavior of the density gradient according to Equation 8.14. Since the images, as always, are upside down, the texture density increases for negative y', finally becoming infinite at the horizon, $y' = -\cot \sigma$. If, then, the texture density is measured as a function of the y' coordinate of the image, the theoretical curve may be fitted to the measured data, and σ may be evaluated on the basis of the best curve fit. More simply, σ may be determined from the location of the singularity which corresponds to the horizon of the plane, though more precise results may be obtained by considering ϱ'/ϱ for all available values of y'.

In the example illustrated in Fig. 8.9, the orientation of the plane is completely defined by the curve $\varrho'(y')/\varrho$. The same is not true in the general case, in which the tilt angle τ is unknown. In that case, ϱ'/ϱ depends on x' as well, and the orientation must be evaluated from the two-dimensional density function (Aloimonos 1988).

8.4   Statistical patterns 2: Shape gradient

8.4.1   Changes in the orientation of edges through projection

We follow in this section the approach developed by Witkin (1981). Let us consider once again the plane whose normal is $\vec{n} = (0, \sin \sigma, -\cos \sigma)^\top$ and whose coordinates are u, v, as in Section 8.3.1. Now, however, we will examine not the variation in texture as a function of image coordinates, but rather the probability distribution of line orientations at the origin of the coordinate system of the plane $(u, v) = (0, 0)$. We assume that at this point, the texture pattern contains an edge of unit length

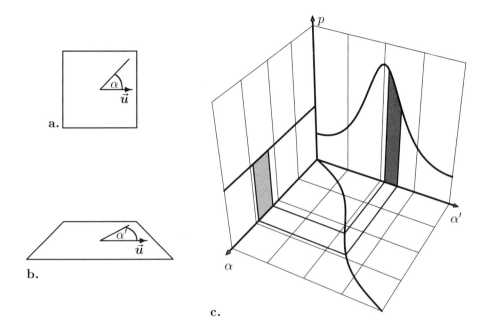

Figure 8.10
Change in orientation α of a line through projection. **a.** Orientation in the coordinate system of the plane. **b.** Orientation after projection of the slanted plane (cf. Equation 8.16). **c.** Probability density functions for α (left panel), α' (right panel) and their relation via the projection rule illustrated in a and b (bottom panel). For explanations see text.

oriented at the angle $\alpha \in [-\frac{\pi}{2}, \frac{\pi}{2}]$ to the $\vec{u}$ axis. The edge can be described by two points, its start point $(u, v) = (0, 0)$ and its end point $(u, v) = (\cos \alpha, \sin \alpha)$.

We would like to know the orientation of the image of this edge relative to the $\vec{x'}$ axis of the image plane. Therefore, we project the start and end points of the edge element into the image, by means of Equation 8.7, and obtain:

$$T \begin{pmatrix} 0 \\ 0 \end{pmatrix} = \begin{pmatrix} 0 \\ 0 \end{pmatrix}; \quad T \begin{pmatrix} \cos \alpha \\ \sin \alpha \end{pmatrix} = \frac{-1}{z_o + \sin \alpha \sin \sigma} \begin{pmatrix} \cos \alpha \\ \sin \alpha \cos \sigma \end{pmatrix}. \quad (8.15)$$

It follows that the orientation α' of the image of the edge is (cf. Fig. 8.10):

$$\alpha' = f(\alpha) := \arctan \frac{\Delta y'}{\Delta x'} = \arctan(\tan \alpha \cos \sigma). \quad (8.16)$$

Graphs of the function $\alpha' = f(\alpha)$ for various slant angles σ of the plane are shown in Figs. 8.10c, "floor", and Fig. 8.11a. If the plane is at a right angle to the direction of view (frontoparallel; $\sigma = 0$), then $\alpha' \equiv \alpha$. As the slant increases, the orientation of the edge as imaged diverges increasingly from the orientation of the edge in the plane.

8.4.2 Statistics of edge orientation

We now describe the edge orientation α as a random variable which can take on any value in the interval $[-\frac{\pi}{2}, \frac{\pi}{2}]$. We want to calculate the distribution of orientations in the image, given the distribution on the surface and the surface slant. The general idea is illustrated in Figure 8.10c: The shaded area on the left "wall" of this figure corresponds to a number of edges whose orientations fall into a certain interval. By Equation 8.16 (illustrated on the "floor" of Fig. 8.10c), this orientation interval is transformed into another interval of edge orientations in the image (right "wall" in Fig. 8.10c). Since the edge elements included in both intervals, either on the surface or in the image, are the same, the two shaded areas in Fig. 8.10c must be equal. From this condition, the curve $p(\alpha')$ can be derived.

In order to formalize this idea, we note that the distributions of *continuous* random variables are described by *probability density functions* $p(\alpha)$ or *distribution functions* $F(\alpha)$, for which:

$$\mathrm{P}\{\alpha \in A\} \quad = \quad \int_A p(\alpha)d\alpha \tag{8.17}$$

$$F(\alpha) \quad := \quad \mathrm{P}\{\beta \leq \alpha\} = \int_{-\frac{\pi}{2}}^{\alpha} p(\beta)d\beta. \tag{8.18}$$

We assume that all orientations are equally probable on the surface. Since probabilities always must add up to 1, $\int_{-\pi/2}^{\pi/2} p(\alpha)d\alpha = 1$, it follows that

$$p(\alpha) \equiv \frac{1}{\pi} \quad \text{and} \quad F(\alpha) = \frac{1}{2} + \frac{\alpha}{\pi} \quad \text{for} \quad \alpha \in [-\frac{\pi}{2}, \frac{\pi}{2}]. \tag{8.19}$$

We now want to find the distribution (or density) of the random variable α', i.e., the orientation of the image of the edge being examined. The distribution function is:

$$\mathrm{P}\{\alpha' \leq \beta\} = \mathrm{P}\{\alpha \leq f^{-1}(\beta)\} = \int_{-\pi/2}^{f^{-1}(\beta)} p(\alpha)d\alpha. \tag{8.20}$$

Here, f is the projection formula for orientations as given in Equation 8.16. We substitute $\alpha' = f(\alpha)$ inside the integral and obtain

$$\mathrm{P}\{\alpha' \leq \beta) = \int_{f(-\pi/2)}^{f(f^{-1}(\beta))} \underbrace{p(f^{-1}(\alpha'))}_{\text{const. } \frac{1}{\pi}} \frac{d\alpha}{d\alpha'} d\alpha' = \frac{1}{\pi} \int_{-\pi/2}^{\beta} (f^{-1})'(\alpha')d\alpha'. \tag{8.21}$$

By comparison with the definition of a distribution function, Equation 8.18 we find: $p(\alpha') = \frac{1}{\pi}(f^{-1})'(\alpha)$. In order to determine f^{-1}, we solve Equation 8.16 for α, and obtain:

$$f^{-1}(\alpha') = \arctan(\frac{\tan \alpha'}{\cos \sigma}) \tag{8.22}$$

and further, by the chain rule:

$$\frac{d\alpha}{d\alpha'} = \left(f^{-1}\right)'(\alpha') = \frac{1}{1 + \frac{\tan^2 \alpha'}{\cos^2 \sigma}} \cdot \frac{1}{\cos^2 \alpha' \cos \sigma} = \frac{\cos \sigma}{\cos^2 \sigma \cos^2 \alpha' + \sin^2 \alpha'}. \quad (8.23)$$

From this series of operations, it follows that:

$$p(\alpha') = \frac{1}{\pi} \frac{\cos \sigma}{\cos^2 \sigma \cos^2 \alpha' + \sin^2 \alpha'}. \quad (8.24)$$

Figure 8.11b shows the probability density functions $p(\alpha')$ for various values of σ. When $\sigma = 0$, the plane is orthogonal to the direction of view, and the density of α' is equal to that of α, i.e., constant. As the slant increases, orientations nearer the angle $\alpha' = 0$ become more and more probable. Clearly, this occurs because the vertical component of the image is shortened more than the horizontal component. This effect is also evident in Fig. 8.1c and 8.10.

The position of the peak in Fig. 8.11b applies only to the one case considered here, with a tilt angle τ of 90°. In general, the tilt angle can be read from the position of the peak: the greatest shortening is in the direction of the tilt angle.

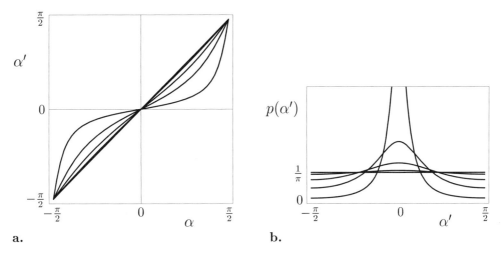

a.   b.

Figure 8.11
Orientation of the image of an edge element. **a.** Effect of projection on the orientation of individual edges (Equation 8.16). **b.** Effect of projection on the probability density function of edge orientations modeled as random variables (Equation 8.24). If $\sigma = 0$ (plane at right angles to the direction of view), then $\alpha' \equiv \alpha$; in the graph at the left, this situation corresponds to the diagonal, and in the graph at the right, to the straight line (uniform distribution) $p \equiv \frac{1}{\pi}$. As σ increases, the orientation in the image and the probability density function diverge increasingly from this. Curves for $\sigma = 0, 20°, 40°, 60°$ and $80°$ are shown.

8.4.3   Estimating σ from the probability density function

Equation 8.24 gives the expected distribution of orientations in the image if all orientations in the plane are equally probable and the slant of the plane is σ. If this assumption holds, it is possible to proceed as in the previous section, generating a histogram of all orientations and then fitting curves of the form in 8.24 to that histogram. But in this case, deviation in ranges in which the histogram is small—that is, in which few measurements are available—would be weighted the same as in ranges in which there are many measurements. A maximum likelihood estimation, which maximizes the probability of the measurement subject to the surface slant σ, is more satisfactory.

In order to perform the maximum likelihood estimation, we must first describe σ by means of a random variable. The probability density $p(\alpha')$ is replaced by what is called a "conditional density," since it depends on σ. It is written as $p(\alpha'|\sigma)$.

Furthermore, we will no longer look at a single measurement of α', but rather at a large number $n \in \mathbb{N}$ of such measurements. We assume that all of the orientations are independent of one another. We obtain, then, as the conditional probability density function of the n-dimensional random variable $(\alpha'_1, ..., \alpha'_n)$,

$$p(\alpha'_1, ..., \alpha'_n|\sigma) = \prod_{i=1}^{n} p(\alpha_i|\sigma). \tag{8.25}$$

The maximum-likelihood estimation is the σ which maximizes the conditional probability density function $p(\alpha'_1, ..., \alpha'_n|\sigma)$ for the given measurement $(\alpha'_1, ..., \alpha'_n)$.

If there are additional sources of information about the surface slant σ, then the Bayes rule may be used to obtain an improved estimate (Berger 1985). This formula is:

$$P(S|D) = \frac{P(D|S)P(S)}{P(D)}. \tag{8.26}$$

Here, S represents the scene to be reconstructed, which, in our example, is the slant of the surface, and D represents the available data. It is for the most part relatively easy to determine the distribution $P(D|S)$, i.e., the distribution of image data which is to be expected for a given scene; we have already done this for the orientation of edges in the image. The usefulness of the Bayes formula is in the ability to calculate, based on those probabilities, how likely a particular scene interpretation is in the light of the available data. This switch in the roles of S and D allows a conclusion about the scene based on the data without the need explicitly to invert the imaging process. The so-called *a priori* probability $P(S)$ in Equation 8.26 is a measure of the general plausibility of the scene, and may be based on the general viewpoint assumption discussed in Chapter 7, or foreknowledge from other measurements or data.

In the present case, we are applying the Bayes formula to probability densities p. We obtain:

$$p(\sigma|\alpha'_1, ..., \alpha'_n) = \frac{p(\alpha'_1, ..., \alpha'_n|\sigma)p(\sigma)}{\int_{-\pi/2}^{\pi/2} p(\alpha'_1, ..., \alpha'_n|\sigma')p(\sigma')d\sigma'}. \tag{8.27}$$

As with the maximum likelihood estimation, the estimated value of σ^* which best corresponds to a measurement $\alpha'_1, ..., \alpha'_n$ is found by looking for the maximum of this function. Both processes become the same if the *a priori* distribution is constant, $p(\sigma) = 1/\pi$, i.e., if there is no foreknowledge. We will not work through Equation 8.27 here; a thorough description of this process has been given by Witkin (1981) and Blake & Marinos (1990). Because of the general significance of Bayes methods to the understanding of images, we will point here to two important characteristics:

- Unlike in earlier chapters, no "inverse optics" process occurs; rather, the forward imaging process, from the scene to the image, is organized so as to give the orientation. The "inversion" from the image to the scene occurs indirectly, through the Bayes formula. This approach has the advantage that fewer assumptions need be made about the type of information to be applied and about image processing operations. As we have seen in connection with shading analysis, the formulation of mathematical theories of inverse imaging can be quite difficult. Moreover, Bayes estimation provides statistically optimal results given the measurements $(\alpha'_1, ..., \alpha'_n)$.

- The *a priori* distribution $p(\sigma)$ makes it possible elegantly to integrate foreknowledge about the surface. Such foreknowledge could, for example, result from an independently performed shading analysis. For more about the integration of visual cues by means of the Bayes formula, see Bülthoff & Yuille (1991) as well as Knill & Richards (1996).

Part IV

Motion

Little attention has been given to the time dependence of the image in earlier parts of this book, but now we will turn to the question of how temporal changes in the image can provide information about the motion of objects and of the observer. In motion detection, a distribution of local image displacements is estimated from a series of images, or more correctly, from a spatio-temporal intensity distribution. The result of motion detection is therefore a field of local displacement vectors, which we will call the "image flow." Chapter 9 examines various approaches used to determine such flow vectors.

If the observer is in motion, then systematic patterns of image motion arise; these are called "optical flow." These patterns play a large role in navigation tasks, such as, for example, steering and obstacle avoidance. Optical flow can provide information about the observer's own motion and also about the spatial structure of the outside world.

It has been suggested that the perception of motion represents an early, decisive step in the evolution of vision, which was the basis for other abilities such as figure-ground separation or the perception of shape and depth (Horridge 1987). The dominance of motion perception in biological visual systems is probably related to the fact that the image is, at least initially, temporally continuous, while space is sampled. In computer vision systems, the situation is exactly the opposite: the temporal sampling of the spatio-temporal intensity distribution into *sequences* of images makes it more difficult to analyze temporal changes.

Perception of motion takes on special significance in connection with eye movements and "active vision" (Bajcsy 1988, Ballard 1991), which involves, for one thing, the active choice of the direction of view to acquire specific information in the image. This type of activity in vision, i.e. acquisitory behavior, is closely related to the analysis of the optical flow generated as the observer moves. Some of the geometric and kinematic aspects of eye movements have already been examined in Section 2.4.

Optical flow is used for simple (instantaneous) navigational tasks such as course control, the measurement of the observer's motion or the detection of obstacles. In a narrower sense, the term "navigation" may be restricted to navigation to a goal, in which case memory of the goal and perhaps also of landmarks becomes a factor. This memory, too, can be organized visually. Autonomous navigation towards goals, based primarily on visual information is discussed in Chapter 11.

Chapter 9

Motion detection

9.1 Problem statement

9.1.1 Motion and change

Perception of change in the outside world is of the highest importance for all living beings. In the sense of vision, the great majority of changes in sensory excitation, that is, in the image, result from motion—of the light source, of the imaged objects or of the observer. Images also change very markedly when a light source is turned on or off, though this change can not be interpreted as motion.

A few examples will serve here to illustrate the relationship between image changes and motion. Ideally, motion detectors should be able to distinguish between the different cases described here, or should react selectively to only one of them.

- Spatio-temporal noise, such as is displayed, for example, by a television receiver tuned to an empty channel, should not be interpreted as motion, even though the image continually changes.

- Changes in lighting (shadowing, spotlights) change the image, but without local displacement of image components, and do not fall within a narrow definition of motion.

- When objects move against a background, parts of the image are coherently displaced with respect to the remainder. The moving parts need not be connected: consider the example of a flock of birds flying through a landscape. In fact, motion provides particularly strong evidence for the segmentation of an image into figure and ground (the *Gestalt* law of "common fate").

- If an object is in motion behind a picket fence and only visible in the gaps, then there is certainly motion within each gap—but at the edges of the pickets, new image elements are constantly appearing and disappearing. This situation should be interpreted as motion.

- Changes in the shape of objects: Motions are often not rigid, but rather, they include a change in the shape of the moving object. One example is a man walking; the individual parts are more or less rigid in their motion, while the overall shape changes periodically (articulated or biological motion, cf. Johansson 1973). Through changes in the direction of view, stiff movements in space often lead to changes in shape in the image: as an example, think of a flat stone thrown into the air with a spinning motion: the motion of the corresponding image is non-rigid.

- The normal to a surface in motion generally changes, and so the intensity of light reflected from the surface also changes. If a sheet of paper illuminated by parallel light is rotated around an axis in its own plane, then the intensity of the light in the image will change from bright (when the light impinges on the paper at a right angle) to dark (when the angle between the plane of the paper and the lighting is small). This effect is sometimes called "photometric motion;" it is not related to displacements of image parts, at least not in the interior of the region which images the sheet of paper. Complicated effects occur with glossy surfaces (cf. Blake & Bülthoff 1991).

- The observer's motion (and also eye motion) result in motion of large areas in the image. The interpretation of such "patterns of optical flow" will be discussed in the next chapter.

The result of the local evaluation of motion is a displacement vector $\vec{v}$. (In Chapter 10, this vector is designated as $\vec{v}^*$. For the sake of simplicity, the asterisk will be omitted here.)

Motion detection is fundamentally a non-linear operation. Imagine a dark dot moving to the right in front of a bright background. A motion detector is supposed to respond with some activity a to this signal. Conversely, when presented with a spatio-temporally constant signal, e.g. when looking at a white wall, the motion detector is supposed to produce zero output. If we subtract the two intensity distributions (white wall and dark moving dot), we obtain a bright dot moving again to the right. The output of a linear system to this difference signal would be $-a$, which is clearly not the desired behavior of a motion detector, since both motions were in fact the same. It follows from this observation that it is not possible to construct a motion detector using only linear elements. Linear operations are, however, very useful as preliminary steps in evaluation of motion. Mere changes in the image, on the other hand, can be detected very easily by a linear operation, i.e. by calculating the difference of subsequent images. This example illustrates, once again, the difference between motion and change in general.

An overview of motion algorithms used in computer vision is given by Barron et al. (1994). On the psychophysics of motion perception, cf. e.g., Nakayama (1985) and Thompson (1993).

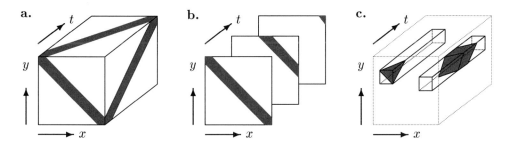

Figure 9.1
Possible representations of spatio-temporal "image sequences" using as an example
the motion of a gray diagonal stripe from the middle to the top right of the image.
a. Three-dimensional data cube. The cube is opaque, so that only the data in the
three planes ($t = 0$, $x = 0$ and $y = 0$) is shown. **b.** Sequence of images at discrete
times. **c.** Continuous functions of time at two positions in the image plane.

9.1.2 Formalization

In this chapter, we will consider the reconstruction of a field of local motion vectors $\vec{v}(x, y, t)$ from a series of images, or better, from a three-dimensional gray value
distribution $I(x, y, t)$. At least locally, it holds that

$$I(x, y, t) = I(x + v_x t, y + v_y t, 0), \tag{9.1}$$

i.e. that the current image at time t is a displaced version of the image obtained at
some previous instant $t = 0$. Not all conceivable motions conform to this definition of
displacement. Image motions which can not be modeled as displacements have been
discussed in the previous section; further examples are to be found in Section 9.5.

The approaches to motion calculation can be distinguished by the type of sampling
which takes place in a spatio-temporal cube of image intensities (cf. Fig. 9.1):

1. **Time-discrete:** The three dimensional gray value cube is dissected into individual "time slices" $I(x, y, t_i)$ (frames), such as the individual images of motion
   picture film or of video. A discrete sequence of images therefore exists, each of
   which represents a different moment in time. In research into perception, this
   approach is called sampled or apparent motion.

2. **Continuous change in the gray value at fixed locations:** The three-
   dimensional gray value cube is dissected into "columns" $I(x_i, y_j, t)$, each of
   which represents the temporal evolution of image intensity for one or a few
   pixels. This is also what is evaluated in the receptive fields of retinal ganglion
   cells or in the ommatidia of insect eyes.

Each of these two approaches leads to characteristic problems which are of great
importance in research on motion perception (cf. Marr & Ullman 1981, Hildreth &
Koch 1987).

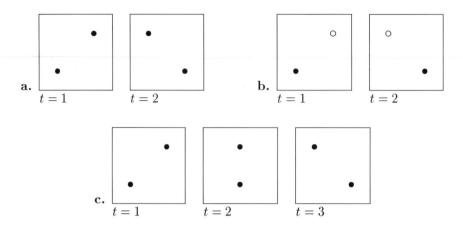

Figure 9.2
The correspondence problem in perception of time-sampled or "apparent" motion ("Schiller illusion", von Schiller 1933, Ramachandran & Anstis 1985). **a.** This sequence of images can be interpreted as a horizontal or a vertical motion. **b.** Marking the image elements does not solve the correspondence problem. Here, too, the perception may be of vertical motion. **c.** Increasing temporal resolution solves the correspondence problem. Here, only horizontal motion is perceived.

1. In the case of the discrete-time approach, image features must be followed from one image to the next, which is difficult if the time intervals are large. Consequently, a **correspondence problem** arises (Fig. 9.2). The search space is in this case truly two-dimensional, unlike that for the correspondence problem of stereoscopic vision: displacements can be in any direction, not only in the direction of epipolar lines. Only if the motion results from a known motion of the observer in a stationary environment can epipolar lines be defined, as they can with stereoscopic vision.

2. If the detector is strictly localized in space (and continuous in time), then the problem arises that the brightness variations at one point can be due to entirely different motions. In this case, the image is being observed, so to speak, through a small opening in a mask (aperture), and so this effect is called the **aperture problem**. Through such an aperture, it is possible to detect only the components of motion at right angles to the local edge orientation. The actual motion of an edge is ambiguous (Fig. 9.3).

   It the motion of a curved edge is considered, then the aperture problem can be solved by enlarging the aperture (the "weak aperture problem"). But if the image is locally one-dimensional (with straight edges), then the various motions indicated in Fig. 9.3c all generate the same spatio-temporal image $I(x, y, t)$. Information as to the true motion is, then, not actually present in the image (the "strong aperture problem").

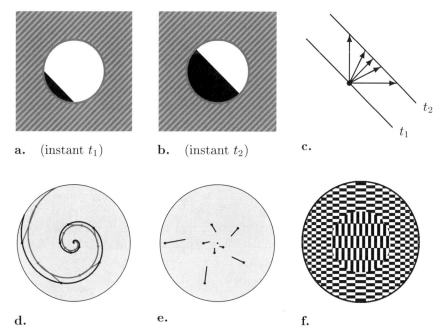

a. (instant t_1)   **b.** (instant t_2)   **c.**

d.   **e.**   **f.**

Figure 9.3
The aperture problem in motion perception. The motion (behind a mask with a circular opening) shown in **a.** and **b.** can result from various displacements. **c.** Only the component at a right angle to the edge is measurable; it is the same for all of the displacements shown. **d.** When a spiral is rotated, all points move along circular paths. **e.** Nonetheless, a radial motion is perceived, corresponding to the component of motion at a right angle to the edge. **f.** Ouchi illusion. If this pattern is moved along a diagonal line, the motion in the central field is perceived to be more nearly horizontal, and the motion in the surrounding area, more nearly vertical. This perception corresponds to the predominant orientation of edges in each part. The overall impression is of non-rigid motion (change of shape). (Drawing f after the cover illustration of the book by Spillmann & Werner 1990. Cf. also Hine et al. 1997)

Solutions which avoid both problems may be either not time-sampled or not completely local. Next, three approaches to the evaluation of motion in images will be discussed which solve these problems in different ways.

9.2 The correlation detector

Displacements of a pattern can be inferred by comparing the changes of intensity with respect to time at two points in the image. The correlation detector, or Reichardt detector which applies this principle was developed to explain the motion perception of flies and other insects (Hassenstein & Reichardt 1956, van Santen & Sperling 1985,

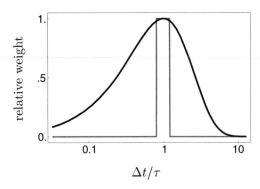

Figure 9.4
Examples of the weighting function $h(\Delta t)$ for the motion detector of Equation 9.5. Black line: first-order low-pass filter $h(\Delta t) := \Delta t \exp\{\Delta t/\tau\}$. Speeds near $v_o = 1/\tau$ are most heavily weighted. Gray line: Time delay by $\Delta t = \tau$. In this case, Equation 9.5 degenerates into Equation 9.3.

Borst et al. 1993), and the two points in the image model two ommatidia of the complex eye. However, the principle which underlies this process has widespread application in the study of human motion perception and in computer vision.

9.2.1   Local motion detection

Let us consider the change over time of a spatially one-dimensional gray value pattern at two points in the image $\vec{x}_1$, $\vec{x}_2$. The intensity variations can be written as $I_{\vec{x}_1}(t)$, $I_{\vec{x}_2}(t)$, or more simply, as $I_1(t)$, $I_2(t)$. The distance between the two points, described as a vector, $\Delta \vec{x} = \vec{x}_2 - \vec{x}_1$ is the base line of the detector. If, now, the pattern moves at the velocity $\vec{v}$ from $\vec{x}_1$ to $\vec{x}_2$, then:

$$I_{\vec{x}_1}(t - \Delta t) = I_{\vec{x}_2}(t) \quad \text{with} \quad \Delta t = \frac{\|\vec{x}_2 - \vec{x}_1\|}{\|\vec{v}\|}. \tag{9.2}$$

In order to determine whether the pattern has moved with the speed $\|\vec{v}\|$, we must observe the difference between $I_1(t - \Delta t)$ and $I_2(t)$. Since this analysis may result in errors, it is better to observe the correlation of the two signals over time rather than just looking for instantaneous equality:

$$\varphi_{\Delta t}(t) = \int_{-\infty}^{t} I_1(t' - \Delta t) I_2(t') dt'. \tag{9.3}$$

Correlation $\varphi_{\Delta t}(t)$ measures the similarity between inputs separated by a time interval Δt.

In general, the task is not just to decide whether a given speed $\|\vec{v}\|$ is present in the image, but rather, to find the actually occuring velocity vectors $\vec{v}$ from the sequence of images. To this end, many different measurements may be made using Equation 9.3 with differing values of Δt or of the base line distance $\Delta \vec{x}$, and the $\vec{v} = \Delta \vec{x}/\Delta t$ with the highest correlation may be selected. If the points $\vec{x}_1$ and $\vec{x}_2$ are fixed, then different possible speeds in the direction of the base line may be examined at the same time, by using in the comparison not the time-displaced signal $I_1(t - \Delta t)$ but instead, a weighted average of differently time-displaced signals. If the weighting is designated as $h(\Delta t)$, then the average (temporal convolution) is:

$$\tilde{I}_1(t) := \int_0^\infty h(\Delta t)I_1(t - \Delta t)d\Delta t. \qquad (9.4)$$

The bounds of integration are so chosen that for every point in time, only previous values of I_1 are used ("causality"). A possible function of $h(\Delta t)$ with a preferred speed $v_o = \Delta x/\tau$ is shown in Fig. 9.4. This function also establishes the speed selectivity of the detector. If $\tilde{I}_1(t)$ is substituted for $I_1(t - \Delta t)$ in Equation 9.3, then:

$$
\begin{aligned}
\varphi_+(t) &= \int_{-\infty}^t \tilde{I}_1(t')I_2(t')dt' \\
&= \int_{-\infty}^t \int_0^\infty h(\Delta t)I_1(t' - \Delta t)d\Delta t \; I_2(t')dt'. \qquad (9.5)
\end{aligned}
$$

The plus sign as a subscript of φ_+ in Equation 9.5 is intended to indicate that only motions in the direction from $\vec{x}_1$ toward $\vec{x}_2$ will register. If the pattern moves in the other direction, then Δt must formally take on negative values which are excluded in Equation 9.4. Motions in the reverse direction can be detected by a mirror symmetric device, for which:

$$\varphi_-(t) = \int_{-\infty}^t I_1(t')\tilde{I}_2(t')dt'. \qquad (9.6)$$

Lowpass filtering and time delay are in this case applied to the other input, I_2. Combining detectors for both directions of motion results in the complete Reichardt detector:

$$
\begin{aligned}
\varphi(t) &:= \varphi_+(t) - \varphi_-(t) \\
&= \int_{-\infty}^t \tilde{I}_1(t')I_2(t') - I_1(t')\tilde{I}_2(t')dt'. \qquad (9.7)
\end{aligned}
$$

In order to suppress output when structureless surfaces are being examined, the inputs are differentiated; $I'_{1,2}(t)$ is used instead of $I_{1,2}(t)$. A block diagram of the correlation, or Reichardt, detector is shown in Fig. 9.5.

With periodic input patterns, the algorithm has a correspondence problem of a sort: similarities at the inputs can be ambiguous. This problem is similar to the wallpaper illusion in stereoscopic vision. Spatio-temporal filters can be devised which suppress the motion signal output when the inputs are likely to be ambiguous.

In the version of the detector which has been described, the output signal $\varphi(t)$ depends not only on speed, but also on image contrast. If the input function I is amplified by a factor of two, the output is multiplied by a factor of four. If the purpose of the detector is to control an optokinetic response—i.e. a body turn canceling perceived image motion—this is no disadvantage, since a stronger input signal only strengthens the feedback and speeds up the cancellation process. The strength of excitation of the detector φ is used in this case less as a measurement of speed than

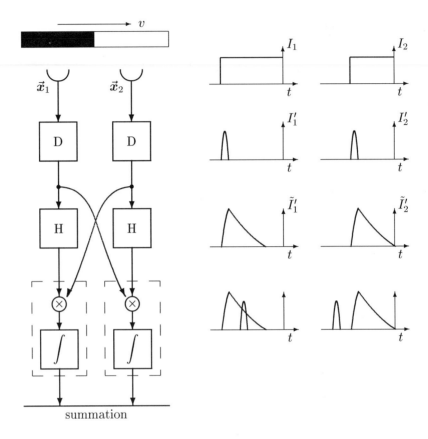

Figure 9.5
Block diagram of a correlation detector. A step edge moves from left to right past two brightness detectors, generating the signals $I_1(t), I_2(t)$. These signals are first differentiated in time (operation "D"). "H" represents the lowpass filtering of Equation 9.4. The actual correlation occurs in the areas enclosed by dashed lines: "$\int$" is the required integration, which can be realized neuronally as additional lowpass filtering. The graphs on the right side show the changes in the individual signals over time. Because of the multiplication, the only output is from the right detector (φ_+). The strength of this output corresponds roughly to the overlap of I_1' and $\tilde{I}_2'$.

as a measurement of confidence about its direction. This confidence does in fact increase as image contrast increases. If, however, the displacement field $\vec{v}(x', y')$ is to be measured, normalization of the output signal is necessary (see below).

The correlation detector was developed to model the optokinetic responses of various insects; the filter characteristics have been identified experimentally in great detail. In human motion perception, evidence for tuned, bilocal motion detectors based on correlation has been presented by van Doorn & Koenderink (1983).

9.2.2 Spatial integration

The direction of the vector of the measured motion is determined by the difference in position of the two inputs, $\vec{x}_2 - \vec{x}_1$. We will from now on consider only half-detectors, which respond only to a motion with a positive sign, i.e. motion from $\vec{x}_1$ to $\vec{x}_2$. Motions have to be measured in many different directions in the plane, and so it is no longer possible simply to assign positive and negative values to the different directions as in the one-dimensional case (Equation 9.7), and to add or subtract speeds. We will now discuss a simple and easily realizable suggestion for spatial integration in artificial vision systems (Bülthoff et al. 1989; see also Camus 1997). On spatial integration in the motion perception of flies, cf. Reichardt & Schlögl (1988) as well as the work already cited, by Borst et al. (1993). Spatial integration of motion in humans has been studied, e.g., by Fredericksen et al. (1994).

We start with the assumption that half-detectors are present at each location $\vec{x}$ in the image for a set of displacements $\vec{d} \in [-\delta, \delta]^2$. The half-detectors furnish a measurement of similarity

$$\varphi(\vec{x}, \vec{d}) = 1 - |I_1(\vec{x}) - I_2(\vec{x} + \vec{d})|. \tag{9.8}$$

The absolute difference between the signals is considered here, rather than their product as in Equation 9.3. Taking the differences has the advantage that surfaces without any structure do not contribute to the output.

The comparison occurs in only one time step, so the integration of Equation 9.3 is omitted. In order nonetheless to improve the comparison by averaging, spatial smoothing is performed for each direction $\vec{d}$ of displacement. To this end, we choose a neighborhood of $P_\nu(\vec{x})$ of $\vec{x}$ calculate:

$$\Phi(\vec{x}, \vec{d}) = \sum_{\vec{x} \in P_\nu(\vec{x})} \varphi(\vec{x}, \vec{d}). \tag{9.9}$$

This smoothing operation, which evaluates how often a particular displacement is "chosen" within the neighborhood, is called *voting*. With respect to each point $\vec{x}$, φ and Φ are local histograms of image displacement. Φ can be evaluated as follows:

- If $\Phi(\vec{x}_o, \vec{d})$ has a unique maximum at the location $\vec{d}^*$, then this displacement is accepted as the estimate of the local motion vector: $\vec{v}(\vec{x}_o) = \vec{d}^*$.

- If $\Phi(\vec{x}_o, \vec{d})$ has two maxima, then a boundary between areas of different motion is likely present in the image (motion discontinuity). The motions of the two surfaces correspond to the two maxima. This assumption can be used to segment images into areas of coherent motion.

- The variance of the correlation values Φ provides an additional measurement of confidence in the estimation of motion.

In effect, the summation in the one-dimensional case is replaced here by the calculation of maxima in the local motion histogram Φ. This calculation includes, at the same

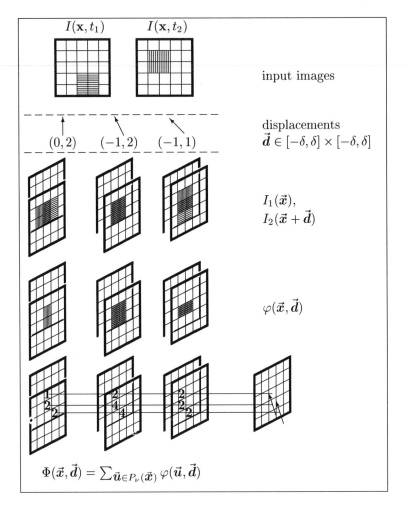

Figure 9.6
Diagram showing the correlation scheme of Bülthoff et al. (1989). The (possibly pre-processed) input images are each displaced by all vectors within the interval $[-\delta, \delta]^2$ and compared with the original image. The resulting local comparison values φ form a histogram which can then be suitably smoothed to generate another histogram of better estimates, Φ. Finally, the correlation values of all displacement vectors are compared pixel by pixel, and the one, $\vec{d}$, whose correlation value Φ is greatest, is chosen. (Revised, from Mallot et al. 1991)

time, the required normalization, since the value at the maximum, $\Phi(\vec{x_o}, \vec{d}^*)$ has no further application. More generally, $\Phi(\vec{x_o}, \vec{d})$ can be regarded as a population code for the displacement at the point $\vec{x_o}$.

9.3 The gradient detector

9.3.1 The aperture problem for continuous image functions

Let us consider a static gray value image $\tilde{I}(x,y)$, which is being displaced at the velocity (v_1, v_2). Its three-dimensional gray value volume is, then:

$$I(x,y,t) = \tilde{I}(x - v_1 t, y - v_2 t). \qquad (9.10)$$

The measured change in the gray value over time at a location (x,y), corresponds mathematically to the partial derivative $\frac{\partial}{\partial t} I(x,y,t)$. Before we relate this to the speed we are trying to find and to the static image $\tilde{I}$, let us first consider a simple example:

Example: linear gray value ramp. For our static image, we choose a linear gray value ramp:

$$\tilde{I}(x,y) = g_1 x + g_2 y.$$

The boundaries of the image and the constants g_1, g_2 are chosen so that $\tilde{I}(x,y) \in [0,1]$ holds everywhere in the image. The corresponding gray value map is a plane which slopes upward in the direction of the vector $(g_1, g_2)^\top$ (cf. Fig. 9.7). From Equation 9.10, we obtain the spatio-temporal image function:

$$I(x,y,t) = g_1(x - v_x t) + g_2(y - v_y t) = g_1 x + g_2 y - (g_1 v_x + g_2 v_y)t.$$

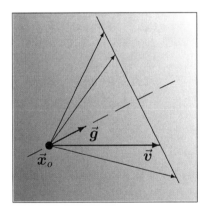

Figure 9.7
The aperture problem as it applies to continuous gray value functions. The image shows an intensity distribution $\tilde{I}(x,y) = g_1 x + g_2 y$. The gradient vector $\vec{g}$ points in the direction of the steepest slope in the gray value map. The pattern moves with the speed and direction $\vec{v}$. At the time $t = 0$, the observed gray value is $\tilde{I}(\vec{x}_o)$. After the time interval Δt has passed, the observed gray value is $\tilde{I}(\vec{x}_o + \vec{v}\Delta t)$. This gray value would also be reached by the other motions indicated with arrows, since the points of the arrows lie on a line of constant gray value.

The derivative can now be calculated very simply as:

$$\frac{\partial I}{\partial t}(x,y,t) = -(g_1 v_x + g_2 v_y) = - \begin{pmatrix} g_1 \\ g_2 \end{pmatrix} \cdot \begin{pmatrix} v_x \\ v_y \end{pmatrix}.$$

The last product here is a dot product. The vector $(g_1, g_2)^\top$ points in the direction of the steepest slope in the gray value map, i.e., the *gradient* of $\tilde{I}$. Since the gray value map is a slanted plane, the gradient does not depend on (x,y). The result indicates that the change in the gray value is equal to the length of the gradient vector multiplied by the projection of the velocity vector in the direction of the gradient.

In the general case, some calculus is necessary in order to derive this equation (cf. Rudin 1976). By introducing the transformation

$$V : \mathbb{R}^3 \to \mathbb{R}^2, \quad \begin{pmatrix} x \\ y \\ t \end{pmatrix} \longrightarrow \begin{pmatrix} x - v_1 t \\ y - v_2 t \end{pmatrix} \tag{9.11}$$

we can write $I(x,y,t) = \tilde{I}(V(x,y,t))$. The derivative may now be found, using the chain rule:

$$\mathrm{grad}I(x,y,t) = \mathrm{grad}\tilde{I}(x - v_1 t, y - v_2 t) \cdot \begin{pmatrix} 1 & 0 & -v_1 \\ 0 & 1 & -v_2 \end{pmatrix}. \tag{9.12}$$

The grad-function indicates, as usual, the vector described by the partial derivatives. In the example above (a linear gray value ramp) $\mathrm{grad}\tilde{I}(x,y) = (g_1, g_2)$. The desired result is obtained from the third component of the vector equation 9.12,

$$\frac{\partial I}{\partial t} = -(v_1 \cdot \frac{\partial I}{\partial x} + v_2 \cdot \frac{\partial I}{\partial y}) = -(\mathrm{grad}\tilde{I} \cdot \vec{v}). \tag{9.13}$$

If the motion vector is constant, then the change in the gray value at the location (x,y) is equal to the (length of the) projection of the motion vector onto the direction of most rapid gray value variation (the direction of the gradient) multiplied by the length of the gradient vector (slope of the gray value ramp). The measured change in the image intensity can, therefore, result from the slow motion of a steep gray value ramp, or from the rapid motion of a gently sloping gray value ramp. The projection (dot product) is maximized when $\vec{v}$ and $\mathrm{grad}\tilde{I}$ are parallel.[*]

In order to apply Equation 9.13 to intensity edges, we note that edges are locations normal to which there are especially large gray value gradients. Equation 9.13 is, therefore, the analytical formulation of the aperture problem (cf. Fig. 9.3). It is not possible, even if one factor (in this case, the gray value gradient) is known, to reconstruct the other one unambiguously from the dot product of two vectors.

Equation 9.13 is called the Horn constraint equation (Horn & Schunk 1981). An algorithm for the estimation of displacement fields from the local temporal derivatives

---

[*]This follows from the Cauchy-Schwarz inequality, cf. Glossary.

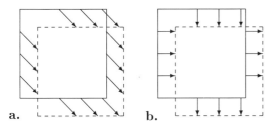

Figure 9.8
a. Diagonal displacement of a square. The true displacement vector is the same everywhere.
b. components of the displacement vector at right angles to the edges.

and the spatial gradients of the gray value function is also to be found in the cited work of Horn & Schunk (1981). Recent developments are described in the works of Uras et al. (1988) and Nagel (1995). Here, only a special case will be discussed, in which assumptions about the distribution of displacement vectors along a curve are used in the reconstruction of the displacement field from the temporal derivatives and the gray value gradients.

9.3.2   Integration of motion along edges

As a consequence of the aperture problem (Equation 9.13), gradient detectors measure only the component of motion at a right angle to the edge, or in the direction of the gray value gradient. If only these measurements are considered, the most plausible hypothesis is that the actual motion was in the direction of the gradient:

$$\vec{v}_g = -\frac{\partial I}{\partial t}\frac{\mathrm{grad}\tilde{I}}{\|\mathrm{grad}\tilde{I}\|^2}. \tag{9.14}$$

The agreement between this assumption and measurement can easily be tested by substitution into Equation 9.13: $-\mathrm{grad}\tilde{I}\vec{v}_g = \partial I/\partial t$. All other estimates of $\vec{v}$ make unsupported assumptions about components of motion at a right angle to the direction of the gradient. Fig. 9.8a shows the motion of a square together with the actual displacement vectors $\vec{v}$; Fig. 9.8b shows the displacements which can be measured using the gradient approach, i.e. $\vec{v}_g$ as in Equation 9.14. An additional example is shown in Fig. 9.3d, e.

Expected similarities between neighboring displacement vectors may be applied in order better to estimate the displacement field $\vec{v}(x, y)$. Additional assumptions are made in this case about the expected vector field. In the context of the idea of "inverse optics" which was introduced in Section 1.3.1, information which was not present in the available data is replaced by heuristics. The replacement is not theoretically necessary in the case of motion perception, since other detectors (e.g., the correlation detector) generate better output data. A suggestion by Hildreth (1984) for the integration of motion along edges will be presented here.

We designate as γ a curve in the image plane, i.e., a function $[0, S] \to \mathbb{R}^2$ interpreted such that s is the length of the curve measured from its start $\gamma(0)$ and $\gamma(s) = (\gamma_x(s), \gamma_y(s))$ are the coordinates of a point which is at a distance of s from the start point, measured along the curve. Since the parameter s also measures

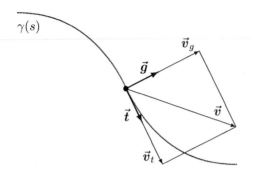

$\gamma(s)$

Figure 9.9
Mathematical notation for the integration of motion along curves. A curve γ moves such that the actual displacement vector is $\vec{v}$. The unit vectors $\vec{g}$ and $\vec{t}$ point in the directions of the gradient and of the tangent; $\vec{v}_g = \vec{g}(\vec{g} \cdot \vec{v})$ is the component of $\vec{v}$ in the direction of the gradient and $\vec{v}_t$ is the component in the direction of the tangent.

the length of the curve, the curve γ is said to be regular (cf. do Carmo 1976 and Section 10.3.3). The tangent vector of such a curve is given by the derivative (by components): $\vec{t}(s) = \gamma'(s)$, $\|\vec{t}(s)\| \equiv 1$. Orthogonal to this is the normal vector, which, by analogy to the previous section, will be designated as $\vec{g}$; in components: $\vec{g}(s) = \pm(\gamma'_y(s), -\gamma'_x(s))^\top$. If a point $\gamma(s)$ of the curve moves at the speed $\vec{v}$, then the locally measurable speed is, as in Equation 9.14, $\vec{v}_g(s) = \vec{g}(\vec{g} \cdot \vec{v})$ (note that $\|\vec{g}\| \equiv 1$).

Let us now assume that the curve γ is known, e.g., by means of a suitable edge detector. Edge detection also identifies the local direction of the gradient $\vec{g}(s)$. Let us also assume that the projections of the actual displacement vectors onto the directions of the gradient have been measured. We want to find a final estimate $\vec{v}^*(s)$ among all possible vector fields $\vec{v}(s)$, which

1. is consistent with the data, i.e. $(\vec{v}^*(s) \cdot \vec{g}(s)) = (\vec{v}(s) \cdot \vec{g}(s))$ and

2. fulfills one of the following additional conditions:

   - $\vec{v}^*(s)$ is constant, i.e., the motion is a pure translation in the image plane.

   - The line is rigid, but can rotate, so that $\vec{v}(s)$ need not be constant.

   - $\vec{v}^*(s)$ changes as little as possible with respect to s, and so is a smooth field. This condition is attained by minimizing a suitable index of smoothness, e.g., the integral over the magnitude of the variation of $\vec{v}^*(s)$ along the curve:

$$\int \|\frac{d}{ds}\vec{v}^*(s)\|ds. \tag{9.15}$$

   This approach allows non-rigid as well as rigid motion.

Fig. 9.10 shows how a rigid motion can be estimated from the components orthogonal to the curve. Fig. 9.10a shows the motion, and b shows the locally measured displacements. If all of the displacement vectors $\vec{g}(\vec{g} \cdot \vec{v})$ are assembled in one plot, with the same origin, then their ends lie on a circle whose diameter corresponds to the actual displacement vector $\vec{v}$; the center of the circle is $\vec{v}/2$ (Fig. 9.10c). This is because the measurable component and the corresponding tangential component form

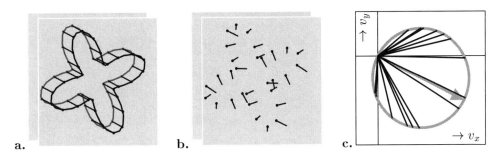

Figure 9.10
Motion integration for pure translation in the image plane (constant displacement field). **a.** Two images in a sequence showing actual displacements. **b.** Components of the displacement field in the direction of the local gradients. **c.** Representation of all displacements in b as a histogram. As in the Hough transform of straight lines through a vanishing point (Fig. 8.5), all end points lie on a circle of Thales. The diameter of the circle which starts at the origin is the actual displacement.

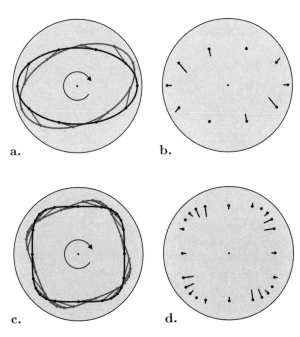

Figure 9.11
a. Actual displacement field for a rotating ellipse. **b.** Components in the direction of the gradient. It can be seen that the displacement field in b is smoother than the actual field. Since some of the vectors point inwards and others, outwards, b corresponds to a change in shape. **c.,d.** similarly for the curve of Equation 9.16. In d, the transition between inward and outward motion occurs four times, corresponding to a complicated change in shape. A figure that folds and unfolds is perceived. (a, b after Hildreth 1984, c altered, after Spillmann, personal communication).

the legs of a rectangular triangle whose hypotenuse is the actual displacement. The circle is therefore, the circle of Thales for the displacement vector (cf. Section 8.2).

Fig. 9.11 shows the effects of applying the smoothness constraint to two rotating curves. Fig. 9.11 a, b shows an ellipse, and Fig. 9.11 c, d a rounded square defined by the equation:

$$\left(\begin{array}{c} x \\ y \end{array} \right) := \left(\begin{array}{c} \mathrm{sgn}(\cos s)\sqrt{\cos s} \\ \mathrm{sgn}(\sin s)\sqrt{\sin s} \end{array} \right) \quad \text{where} \quad \mathrm{sgn}(x) := \left\{ \begin{array}{rcl} -1 & \text{if} & x < 0 \\ 0 & \text{if} & x = 0 \\ +1 & \text{if} & x > 0 \end{array} \right. \quad (9.16)$$

In both cases, the actual vector field is less smooth (as that term is defined by Equation 9.15) than the components in the direction of the gradient. These components, however, alternately point inward and outward, corresponding to a change in shape of the object. Under experimental conditions, the predicted change in shape is actually perceived (Hildreth 1984, Bressan et al. 1992). In the case of the rounded square, it is perceived as a folding and unfolding of the figure in three-dimensional space. For the ellipse, the perception is similar to the illusion described by Mach (1922, section X.17) in which a rotating egg rolled over its long axis is perceived as non-rigid. It can be concluded from these examples that the human visual system favors the assumption of smoothness over that of rigidity of motion, even if a rigid interpretation exists. In *Gestalt* psychology, this observation is taken as evidence for the *Gestalt* "laws" of nearness and parsimony (Metzger 1975, p. 571).

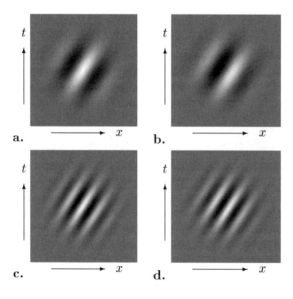

Figure 9.12
Gabor functions which can be used as kernels of filters to enhance oriented image components. **a., c.** Symmetrical (even, cosinusoidal) Gabor function (Equation 9.17). **b., d.** Antisymmetric (odd, sinusoidal) Gabor functions (Equation 9.18). Orientation (speed): $v = 2/3$. The functions in the upper and lower panels differ by a doubling of the center frequency ω of the filter passband.

9.4 Orientation in the spatio-temporal image

9.4.1 Motion energy

The approaches which have been described up to this point estimate motions on the basis of spatially and temporally sampled image data which describe the complete spatio-temporal data cube of Fig. 9.1 only very incompletely. If, however, more complete data is available, then motions and edge orientations in the spatio-temporal data cube can be described and measured. To this end, for example, an (x, t) section through the data cube makes it possible to observe the temporal change along a horizontal row of pixels in the image (a single value of y). If edges are found in this (x, t) image, then their slope corresponds to the x component of image velocity. The top of the data cube in Fig. 9.1 provides an example of such a section.

Let us now consider a one-dimensional motion in the x direction, i.e., motion detection in (x, t) images. We also assume, as an additional simplification, that we are not too close to the margins of the spatio-temporal data space, in other words, that we want to estimate motions which have been in progress for some time. This assumption has the advantage that we can evaluate all parts of the spatio-temporal image over a substantial range both backward and forward in time. To detect a spatio-temporal edge, we will apply Gabor functions as used already for ordinary edge detection (Section 4.2.3). The spatio-temporal form of these equations is

$$g_c(x, t) \quad := \quad \cos(2\pi\omega(x - vt)) \exp\left\{-\frac{x^2 + t^2}{2\sigma^2}\right\} \tag{9.17}$$

$$g_s(x, t) \quad := \quad \sin(2\pi\omega(x - vt)) \exp\left\{-\frac{x^2 + t^2}{2\sigma^2}\right\}. \tag{9.18}$$

Here, v is the velocity to which the filter is tuned, i.e., the orientation in the (x, t) image (cf. Fig. 9.12). The center frequency ω determines the spatial frequency range in which we search for the oriented edge. The size of the window, finally, is given by σ. In practice, sampled versions of these functions with masks of finite size are of course used, so that the infinite extent of the Gaussian function does not present a problem in the time dimension either.

If, now, the spatio-temporal image is filtered using the two masks of Equation 9.17 and 9.18, the output includes all components of the image whose spatial resolution is passed by the Gabor filter, and which move with the velocity v. Both filters are necessary, since the cosine filter responds only to line edges, and the sine filter only to step edges (cf. Section 4.2.3). The combination of an even (cosine) and an odd (sine) filter is called a *quadrature pair*. The Gaussian bell-shaped window guarantees the locality of the measurement.

The square of the intensity of the spatially and temporally filtered image may be used to measure the strength of the motion of velocity v at the image location x and time t:

$$\varphi(x, t) \quad := \quad [(g_c * I)(x, t)]^2 + [(g_s * I)(x, t)]^2$$

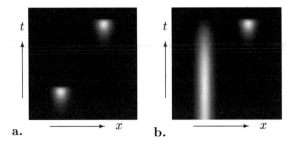

Figure 9.13
Reichardt detectors and motion energy. The illustration shows the filter masks g of
Equation 9.20 for different temporal parameters h_1, h_2. **a.** Both lowpass filters have
the same, short time constant, but h_1 has a time delay. **b.** Lowpass filter h_1 with a
long time constant but with no delay.

$$= \left(\iint g_c(x - x', t - t') I(x', t') \, dx' \, dt' \right)^2 \qquad (9.19)$$

$$+ \left(\iint g_s(x - x', t - t') I(x', t') \, dx' \, dt' \right)^2 .$$

Here, φ is called the *motion energy* (Adelson & Bergen 1985, Heeger 1987). This
expression is unrelated to the concept of kinetic energy in mechanics, but rather, was
chosen on the basis of analogies from signal theory. If φ is integrated over the entire
image, then the local motion energy corresponds to the combined variance of the two
images of edges (cosine and sine).

9.4.2   Comparison with Reichardt's correlation detector

The motion energy detector, like Reichardt's detector, uses a multiplicative nonlinearity, which appears in the form of the squared term in Equation 9.19. In fact, both
approaches are very closely related, as the following consideration shows. Instead of
the filters g_c and g_s, we use filters of the form

$$g(x, t) := d(x - x_1) h_1(t) + d(x - x_2) h_2(t). \qquad (9.20)$$

to enhance the oriented edges in the spatio-temporal image. In Equation 9.20, $h_{1,2}$
represents the lowpass filter of Equation 9.4, but with different time constants. The
function d describes the directional characteristic of the two ommatidia, i.e., the spherical angle within which each ommatidium is sensitive to light. As an approximation,
therefore, $\int I(x, t) d(x - x_o) dx = I(x_o, t)$. Unlike in Equation 9.4, we use a temporal
lowpass filter for both points in space x_1 and x_2, but the filter for x_2 should have
a very short time constant. As an approximation, then, $\int I(x, t) h_2(t) dt = I(x, 0)$.
For a fixed point $x = 0$, then, the filter of Equation 9.20 evaluates two points in

space separated by $x_2 - x_1$, and the signal of the first of these is delayed or lowpass filtered by the temporal weighting function h_1. The resulting motion energy of this spatio-temporal filter at the location $x = 0$ is:

$$
\begin{aligned}
\varphi(0,t) &:= (I * g)^2(0,t) \\
&= \left(\tilde{I}(x_1,t) + I(x_2,t) \right)^2 \\
&= (\tilde{I}(x_1,t))^2 + (I(x_2,t))^2 + 2\tilde{I}(x_1,t)I(x_2,t). \quad (9.21)
\end{aligned}
$$

The symbol $\tilde{I}$ is used as in Equation 9.4, to represent the lowpass filtered or time-delayed signal. In the time average, the first two terms do not depend on the direction of the motion. The third, product term on the right side corresponds exactly to the correlation in the half-detector in Equation 9.5, except for this time averaging. Fig. 9.13 shows, once again, the analogy to the motion energy process. Both filter masks respond most strongly to spatio-temporal orientations which correspond to the speed 2/3.

9.4.3   Integration of motion energies

Equation 9.19 defines a confidence value for each point in the image, and for each filter which is tuned to a specific speed and spatial resolution. This value indicates the strength of the evidence for the filter's preferred speed at the specified point. This leads to the problem of determining a unique estimate of speed for this point in the image based on all available speeds and their confidence values (energies). This problem becomes even more difficult in the two-dimensional case, with Gabor filters for various directions of motion. These filters are subject to the aperture problem and so respond to motions in directions which diverge from the intended ones.

Typically, a bank of spatio-temporal filters is chosen whose spatial components are organized as a resolution pyramid (cf. Section 3.4.2), and which sample the possible orientations (speeds) evenly. Rather than choosing the filter with the highest energy, it is better first to consider the expected results from all of the filters in response to a given speed. The final estimate is then calculated by means of a least squares or maximum likelihood procedure to fit the expected outputs to the data. Details of this process and also of the extension to the case of two-dimensional motion are to be found in the already mentioned works of Adelson & Bergen (1985) and Heeger et al. (1987), as well as Jähne (1997).

The spatio-temporal energy approach has become very important in connection with the neurobiology of, at least, vertebrates, since the motion energy of Equation 9.19, with suitable parameters for the filter functions, accurately describes the receptive fields of motion-selective neurons in the visual cortex. Surveys are given by Albright & Stoner (1995) and Heeger et al. (1996). The integration of the motion energies coded by individual neurons is studied using what are called *plaid* stimuli (named after the patterns of Scottish tartans), which have motion energy in two different spatial frequency channels. An example is given in Fig. 9.14. Fig. 9.14a shows a low-frequency pattern which moves toward the upper left. Fig. 9.14b shows

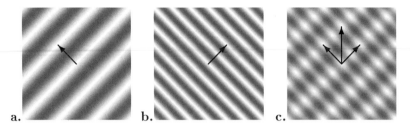

Figure 9.14
Integration of motion energy ("plaid motion"). **a.** A low-frequency pattern moves toward the upper left. **b.** A higher-frequency pattern moves toward the upper right. **c.** If the two patterns are superimposed, then a coherent upward motion is perceived which would have been a possible interpretation in both of the original cases, given the aperture problem. Under certain conditions, the individual motions of the two components are also perceived, but they then appear to be at different depths.

a higher-frequency pattern which moves toward the upper right. If both patterns are superimposed, the result is the image in Fig. 9.14c. The question of interest in connection with this pattern is whether the two directions of motion in the image are perceived separately, or whether a coherent motion in the direction of the vector sum of the components is perceived. This vector sum is consistent with both of the individual motions, given the aperture problem. It would seem likely that the simple vector sum solution to the aperture problem of 9.14a, b would be chosen by the visual system. Actually, however, if there are large enough differences in contrast, speed or spatial frequency, the individual striped patterns are seen moving in different directions. This perception is connected with one of transparency, i.e., the two component patterns are perceived to lie at different depths (Adelson & Movshon 1982). Neurophysiologically, cells are found which respond to the individual motion components, as well as others which indicate the direction of the coherent pattern's motion. The latter cells are found in the medio-temporal (MT) area of the visual cortex of primates. They may represent the neuronal correlate of the solution of the aperture problem.

9.5 Second-order motions

All motion perception processes described up to this point are based on the definition formulated in Equation 9.1, according to which motion is the coherent displacement of a part of an image. Not all motions, however, fit this definition. In the case of a wave generated by wind blowing across a field of grain, for example, the individual stalks move equally far and strongly in both directions. This problem could be regarded as one of the level of resolution (in a blurry image, the peaks of the waves actually move), yet it is possible to construct stimuli which have no motion energy as this is defined in Equation 9.19 but in which motion is still perceived.

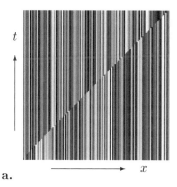 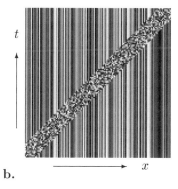

Figure 9.15

Spatio-temporal diagram of second-order motions. The images are best viewed through a narrow horizontal slit which is moved up or down the page. **a.** In a static noise pattern, the value of one pixel at a time from left to right is replaced with a new, random value. **b.** A window in which there is a dynamic, random pattern moves to the right in front of a static noise pattern. In both cases, human observers see motion, although the detectors discussed in Sections 9.2 – 9.4 do not respond.

Fig. 9.15 shows two examples of such patterns. In Fig. 9.15a, a "process" which sets a new value for one pixel at every time step moves from left to right across the image. There is therefore no correlation between neighboring pixels to be evaluated by a correlation detector. Spatio-temporal orientation does not work either, since linear edge detectors can not locate the edge in Fig. 9.15. Nonetheless, such stimuli result in a strong impression of motion in human observers. In Fig. 9.15b, a window is moved across a static background. Ever-changing random noise is displayed inside the window. Here, too, there is no correlation between the functions of time at neighboring pixels, and there is no orientation which can be measured by a linear detector. The effect illustrated by these examples is called a "second-order motion" or, somewhat unhappily, "non-Fourier-motion"; stimulus patterns of the type in Fig. 9.15 are also called "drift-balanced random patterns" (Chubb & Sperling 1988).

The simplest explanation for the described effects is that the motion detectors do not operate directly on the intensity, but rather, operate on a pre-processed image. The perception of motion immediately becomes understandable if, for example, the spatio-temporal image is first differentiated with respect to time, and only the absolute value of the derivative is considered. This operation converts Fig. 9.15a into a diagonal line, and Fig. 9.15b into a diagonal band. Both examples now contain oriented temporal-spatial structures to which the detectors that have been described can respond. It is important in this context that taking the absolute value introduces a nonlinearity into the preprocessing. As a consequence, second-order motion stimuli can be used as tool for the investigation of nonlinearities in the visual system (cf. Wilson 1994).

Chapter 10

Optical flow

The displacement vector field as defined in the previous chapter contains a large amount of information which is of great interest, particularly in connection with navigation, and the control of behavior in general. The observation that the observer's own motions are responsible for stimulus patterns which contain information about the outside world is of great importance to the ecological approach in psychology, and also for the idea of active vision. The concept of "optical flow" is one of the ideas that led to the foundation of ecological psychology (Gibson 1950).

This chapter will begin with a description of the characteristics of optical flow. Though fairly difficult mathematical analysis is involved, an attempt will be made to describe concepts clearly through simple examples and illustrations. Section 10.4 will examine how some important types of information can be reconstructed from the motion in the image. Introductions to the extensive literature in computer vision, psychophysics, and neuroscience are given by Horn (1986), Koenderink (1986), Hildreth (1992) and Lappe et al. (1999).

10.1 Information in the optical flow

A survey of the problems covered in this chapter may be given by looking at the sources of information in optical flow along with the conclusions which can be reached by evaluating this information. Two questions may be asked:

On what does the two-dimensional displacement field depend?

1. The observer's own motion generates characteristic motion patterns in the observer's visual image.

2. The shape and position of visible surfaces affects this pattern.

3. Motions of objects disturb this pattern.

4. The motion detector which is applied and the local contrast of the image determine which motions are at all measurable, and which systematic errors occur in the measurements.

What is to be calculated?

1. Reconstruction of the observer's own motion (*"egomotion"*): In the psychophysical literature, three perceptions are most commonly studied, those of posture, heading and vection, i.e. the sense of being transported (Warren & Kurtz 1992). In neuroethology, the primary object of study in connection with these concepts is the control and stabilization of the flight of insects; Srinivasan (1998) provides an overview of this topic.

2. Image segmentation based on relative motions of different parts of an image plays a large part in perception. Examples are the grouping of unconnected image elements which move consistently with one another (the Gestalt law of common fate); and dynamic occlusion, in which an object moves in front of a background, such that elements of the background disappear and reappear.

3. Depth perception based on the pattern of image motion.

   (a) image motion resulting from movements of the observer: motion parallax

   (b) image motion resulting from movements of objects: kinetic depth effect, structure from motion.

   Motion parallax and structure from motion are of great importance in depth perception, and especially so for animals whose eyes are close together, and which therefore do not have good stereoscopic vision. If the evaluation of motion is at discrete times, then the distance covered between two images corresponds to the base line in stereoscopic vision.

4. The time which remains until reaching an object (time to contact) provides a measurement which combines spatial structure of the outside world and observer motion. This is also the case for other schemes for obstacle avoidance based on optical flow.

10.2 Motion vector fields

10.2.1 Mathematical terminology

Optical flow is described by means of spatio-temporal distributions, or fields, of motion vectors. We will here first put aside the dependence of the motion field on time, and consider only stationary flows. Later, we will also examine some non-stationary flows. Three fields may be distinguished:

1. The three-dimensional field $\vec{w}(x,y,z) \in \mathbb{R}^3$ describes the relative motion between the observer (camera nodal point) and a point in space $\vec{x} \in \mathbb{R}^3$. If the observer is moving in pure translation in a stationary environment, $\vec{w}$ is constant.

2. Projection of this field onto the image plane generates the optical flow, $\vec{v}(x',y') \in \mathbb{R}^2$. From the field which encompasses all space, $\vec{w}$, vectors are first chosen which correspond to points to be imaged (visible surfaces); only these vectors are then projected into the image plane. In addition to $\vec{w}$ and the camera geometry, the varying depth of the visible surfaces also plays a part in this process.

3. In this context, the measurable displacement field in the image plane is called the image flow, $\vec{v}^*(x',y') \in \mathbb{R}^2$. The image flow is generally not the same as $\vec{v}$ and depends on local image contrast and the motion detector which is used. Algorithms for determining $\vec{v}^*(x',y')$ were discussed in Chapter 9*.

Only the first of the two of the fields just mentioned will be considered here; that is, we assume an ideal motion detector. Characteristics of the optical flow which can be determined robustly even with less than ideal evaluation of $\vec{v}$ are discussed by Verri & Poggio (1989).

10.2.2 The three-dimensional vector field $\vec{w}$ for egomotion

Let us now briefly recall a few results from classical mechanics; a thorough description of them is given by Goldstein (1980), among others. The most important conclusion in this section is that of Equation 10.6, for which Fig. 10.1 illustrates the geometric reasoning. The following mathematically more satisfactory derivation can be skipped on first reading.

The motion of an observer or of a camera coordinate system is the motion of a rigid body. According to theorems of Euler and Chasle, motion of a rigid body can always be decomposed into a translation and a rotation. The translation is described by the path $\vec{k}(t)$ of the nodal point of the camera, which has three degrees of freedom. The rotation corresponds to multiplication of the position vector $\vec{k}(t)$ by an orthonormal matrix A with determinant +1; the rotation also has three degrees of freedom, which can be represented as Euler's angles or as the direction of the axis of rotation (two degrees of freedom) plus an angle of rotation. If we note that both translation and rotation have a time dependence, then we obtain as the coordinates of a fixed point $\vec{p}_o$ in the camera coordinate system:

$$\vec{p}(t) = \mathsf{A}(t)(\vec{p}_o - \vec{k}(t)). \tag{10.1}$$

Without loss of generality, we can assume that A(0) is the unit matrix E and $\vec{k}(0) = 0$. The three-dimensional motion vector in camera coordinates is then obtained by taking

---
*Note that the symbol for the measurable displacement fields in Chapter 9 is $\vec{v}$.

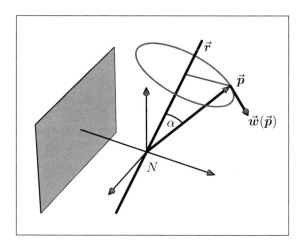

Figure 10.1

Three-dimensional motion field of a rotation around the axis $\vec{r}$ through the camera nodal point N. For a point in space $\vec{p}$, a motion vector $\vec{w}(\vec{p})$ can be found by observing that $\vec{w}(\vec{p})$ is orthogonal to both $\vec{r}$, and $\vec{p}$. The absolute value of $\vec{w}$ is proportional to the absolute value (length) of $\vec{p}$ and the sine of the angle α between $\vec{r}$ and $\vec{p}$. From these observations, it follows that $\vec{w}(\vec{p}) = \omega \vec{r} \times \vec{p}$. (Cf. Equation 10.6.)

the derivative with respect to time:

$$\vec{w}(\vec{p}(t)) = \mathsf{A}'(t)(\vec{p}_o - \vec{k}(t)) - \mathsf{A}(t)\vec{k}'(t). \tag{10.2}$$

Here, the derivatives of vectors and matrices are to be taken one component at a time, and the product rule holds. Since we are interested only in instantaneous motion fields, we can restrict ourselves to the instant $t = 0$. At that instant, then:

$$\vec{w}(\vec{p}_o) = \mathsf{A}'(0)\vec{p}_o - \vec{k}'(0). \tag{10.3}$$

The derivative of the path $\vec{k}'(0)$ is simply the translational component of the motion; we designate it as $v\vec{u}$, in which $\vec{u}$ is the unit vector in the direction of the translation.

Interpretation of the expression $\mathsf{A}'(0)$ is more difficult, since it involves an "infinitesimal rotation", as studied in classical mechanics (Goldstein 1980). The Taylor series expansion about $t = 0$ of the rotation A is $\mathsf{E} + \mathsf{A}'$. We use the symbol $\mathcal{O}^2$ to represent the second-order remainder term of the Taylor expansion. Since $(\mathsf{E} - \mathsf{A}')(\mathsf{E} + \mathsf{A}') = \mathsf{E} + \mathcal{O}^2$, $\mathsf{E} - \mathsf{A}'$ is the (infinitesimal) inverse of $\mathsf{E} + \mathsf{A}'$. Due to the orthogonality of the rotation, on the other hand, $(\mathsf{E} + \mathsf{A}')^{-1} = (\mathsf{E} + \mathsf{A}')^{\top}$, so so that, in all, $\mathsf{E} - \mathsf{A}' = (\mathsf{E} + \mathsf{A}')^{\top}$ and therefore $-\mathsf{A}' = \mathsf{A}'^{\top}$. If we represent the components of A' as a'_{ij}, then the most recently described relationship becomes $a'_{ij} = -a'_{ji}$, and from this it follows that the diagonal elements vanish. There remain, then, only three independent variables, which we describe as ω_1 through ω_3. These correspond to the three degrees of freedom of the rotation. We write:

$$\mathsf{A}' = \begin{pmatrix} 0 & \omega_3 & -\omega_2 \\ -\omega_3 & 0 & \omega_1 \\ \omega_2 & -\omega_1 & 0 \end{pmatrix}. \tag{10.4}$$

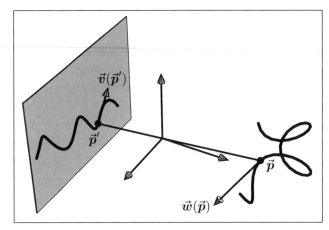

Figure 10.2
Illustration of projection of velocities. An object moves along the three-dimensional curve on the right side of the figure. The image of this object moves along the illustrated plane curve in the image plane. The momentary velocity of this object $\vec{w}(\vec{p})$ is imaged as the optical flow vector $\vec{v}(\vec{p}')$. Cf. Equation 10.10.

By transforming the vector $\vec{x}$ with the matrix A', we obtain:

$$\mathsf{A}'\vec{x} = \begin{pmatrix} x_2\omega_3 - x_3\omega_2 \\ x_3\omega_1 - x_1\omega_3 \\ x_1\omega_2 - x_2\omega_1 \end{pmatrix} = \vec{x} \times (\omega_1, \omega_2, \omega_3)^\top. \tag{10.5}$$

The vector $(\omega_1, \omega_2, \omega_3)^\top$ is the axis of the infinitesimal rotation A'; we have $\mathsf{A}'(\omega_1, \omega_2, \omega_3)^\top = 0$. We denote its norm as ω and the unit vector in the direction of the axis as $\vec{r}$. We can now combine this with Equation 10.3 to generate the equation for the three-dimensional vector field of egomotion:

$$\vec{w}(\vec{x}) = -v\vec{u} - \omega\vec{r} \times \vec{x}. \tag{10.6}$$

Now we can assemble the parts of the analysis. The three-dimensional vector field $\vec{w}(\vec{x})$ which is generated by the observer's motion can be separated at each moment into a translational component and a rotational component. The translational component is the same everywhere in space, while the rotational component is described by the cross product of the point in space with the momentary axis of rotation. The two components superimpose additively. Fig. 10.1 illustrates the rotational term of Equation 10.6.

10.2.3   Projection of $\vec{w}$

Let us consider a point in the imaged scene whose path in space relative to the camera coordinates is described by the vector function $\vec{p}(t) = (p_1(t), p_2(t), p_3(t))^\top$. The momentary velocity at the time $t = 0$ is, then, identical with the value of the three-dimensional velocity field $\vec{w}$ at point $\vec{p}(0)$:

$$\frac{d}{dt}\vec{p}(0) = \vec{w}(\vec{p}(0)). \tag{10.7}$$

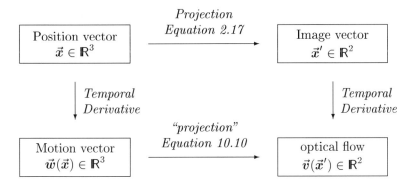

Figure 10.3
Overview of the rules for projection of positions and velocities.

The projection of the path onto the image plane can be calculated point by point as in Equation 2.17:

$$\vec{p}'(t) = -\frac{1}{p_3(t)} \begin{pmatrix} p_1(t) \\ p_2(t) \end{pmatrix}. \tag{10.8}$$

Here, the prime mark in $\vec{p}'$ indicates the projection of $\vec{p}$, not its derivative. By taking the derivative of the projected path with respect to time at $t = 0$, we obtain the *projection formula* for a motion vector $\vec{w}$ which is located at a point $\vec{p}$ in space. We calculate the first component according to the quotient rule:

$$\frac{d}{dt} p_1'(t) = \frac{d}{dt}\left(-\frac{p_1(t)}{p_3(t)}\right) = -\frac{1}{p_3}\left(\frac{dp_1}{dt} + p_1'\frac{dp_3}{dt}\right). \tag{10.9}$$

The second component is calculated in the same way; note that $\frac{d}{dt}\vec{p}(0) = \vec{w}$. The projection formula for motion vectors is thereby obtained:

$$\vec{v} := -\frac{1}{z}\left(\begin{pmatrix} w_1 \\ w_2 \end{pmatrix} + w_3 \begin{pmatrix} x' \\ y' \end{pmatrix}\right). \tag{10.10}$$

It can be seen that the projection formula is linear with respect to the three-dimensional motion $\vec{w}$. The flow fields generated by different components of egomotion therefore superimpose linearly. Fig. 10.3 gives an overview of the rules of projection for positions and motions.

In the stationary case, the projected paths $\vec{p}'(t)$ of individual points are the *flow lines* of optical flow, that is, they are also solutions of the differential equation $\frac{d}{dt}\vec{x}' = \vec{v}(\vec{x}')$. This relationship was used here in calculating $\vec{v}$. In the non-stationary case, the flow lines and the solutions of the momentary motion field are not identical, but the flow lines may be used to illustrate the optical flow graphically. (cf. Fig. 10.11).

Let us note three important characteristics of the projection formula 10.10:

1. As with the projection formula for positions, there is a division by the z-component of the point in space to which the velocity vector refers. The division

reflects the fact that the same motion at a greater distance results in a smaller motion in the image. This effect occurs, for example, in the pattern of apparent relative motion of trees observed through the side window of a moving automobile.

2. It follows from this depth dependence that the motion in the image is not simply the projection of the three-dimensional vector field. Rather, the motion in the image also depends on the points in space at which the external motion can be observed. The optical flow therefore contains information not only about motion in space, but also about the geometry of the visible surfaces and objects.

3. The projection formula 10.10 is linear with respect to the components of the three-dimensional vector field $\vec{w}$. The vector fields of different motion components therefore superimpose linearly in the projection as well as in space. As a consequence, for example, the projected vector field of a curved path is the sum of its translational and rotational components (see below).

4. Spatial motion and geometry can be determined from the optical flow only up to an indeterminate constant factor. It can be seen easily that multiplying $\vec{x}$ and $\vec{w}$ by such a factor has no effect on $\vec{v}$. If $\vec{w}$ results from a motion of the observer, then distances can only be given as multiples of the distance the observer covers in a given time. This distance plays the same role in motion parallax as the base line of the eyes plays in stereoscopic vision. Conversely, the perceived speed of the observer depends on the assumed distance of the imaged objects, and so, for example, drivers of motor vehicles often underestimate their speed on wide roads.

10.3   Flow fields for observer motion

10.3.1   Rotation of the observer

Let us consider a camera which rotates around an axis $\vec{r}$ through the camera nodal point N with the angular velocity ω. We set $\|\vec{r}\| = 1$. The three-dimensional motion field is therefore (cf. Equation 10.6, and Fig. 10.1):

$$\vec{w}(p_1, p_2, p_3) = -\omega \vec{r} \times \vec{p} = -\omega \begin{pmatrix} r_2 p_3 - r_3 p_2 \\ r_3 p_1 - r_1 p_3 \\ r_1 p_2 - r_2 p_1 \end{pmatrix}. \tag{10.11}$$

In the case of pure rotation around a nodal point, the point of view does not change; and so, neither does the "optical array" of the observer. It is therefore not surprising that rotation fields contain no information about the three-dimensional structure of the surrounding scene. In order to confirm this point formally, let us calculate the projection of the rotational field of Equation 10.11 using Equation 10.10.

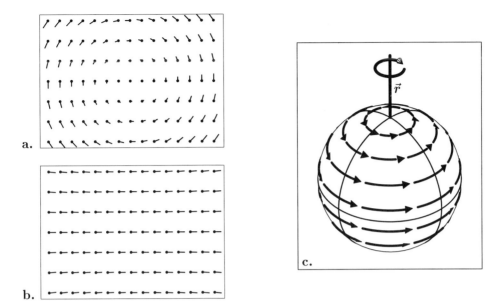

Figure 10.4
Projected motion field for rotation around an axis $\vec{r}$ through the camera nodal point.
a., b. projection onto the image plane (Field of view in the x direction of approximately 40°, corresponding to a normal focal length of a photographic lens). **a.** Rotation around the optical axis. **b.** Rotation around the elevation axis (y axis). Shown are "needle plots": that is, the raster points are the starting points the vectors, not their tips. **c.** Projection onto the surface of a sphere surrounding the observer. Relative to the poles defined by the axis of rotation, the flow lines are curves of latitude. If rotation is around a different axis, the entire pattern is relative to that axis. The optical flows in Fig. **a.** and **b.** correspond to parts of this flow field in the vicinity of a pole and of the equator.

We first project $\vec{w}(\vec{p})$ onto the image plane:

$$\vec{v} = \frac{\omega}{p_3} \left(\begin{pmatrix} r_2 p_3 - r_3 p_2 \\ r_3 p_1 - r_1 p_3 \end{pmatrix} + (r_1 p_2 - r_2 p_1) \begin{pmatrix} x' \\ y' \end{pmatrix} \right). \tag{10.12}$$

It can easily be seen that the spatial coordinates (p_1, p_2, p_3) appear here only in the form of the quotients $x' = -p_1/p_3$ and $y' = -p_2/p_3$. All points in space which lie along a ray extending from the camera nodal point therefore generate the same motion vector $\vec{v}$ in the image. We can therefore completely replace the external coordinates with the image coordinates $(x', y') = -(p_1/p_3, p_2/p_3)$, and we so obtain:

$$\vec{v}(x', y') = \omega \left(-r_1 \begin{pmatrix} x' y' \\ 1 + y'^2 \end{pmatrix} + r_2 \begin{pmatrix} 1 + x'^2 \\ x' y' \end{pmatrix} + r_3 \begin{pmatrix} y' \\ -x' \end{pmatrix} \right). \tag{10.13}$$

Special cases:

a. Let us consider the axis of rotation $\vec{r} = (0,0,1)$, that is, the optical axis of the camera, around which the camera turns with the angular velocity $\omega = 1$ (as in roll of an aircraft). By insertion into Equation 10.13, we obtain:

$$\vec{v}(x',y') = \begin{pmatrix} y' \\ -x' \end{pmatrix}.$$ (10.14)

b. If the observer rotates around the y axis of the camera system, it follows that $\vec{r} = (0,1,0)$ (yaw movement). If $\omega = 1$, then:

$$\vec{v}(x',y') = \begin{pmatrix} 1 + x'^2 \\ x'y' \end{pmatrix}.$$ (10.15)

Illustrations of both of these fields are shown in Fig. 10.4.

In the case of projection onto an image plane, the flow lines are conic sections; in Fig. 10.4a they are circles, and in Fig. 10.4b they are parabolas. If on the other hand, projection is onto the surface of a sphere with the nodal point at its center, the flow lines form a system of circles of latitude, and the intersections of the axis of rotation with the sphere are at the poles (Fig. 10.4c). This pattern is the same for all axes of rotation, and so it follows that mapping onto the surface of a sphere is often preferable to a plane image.

10.3.2   Translation

Flow lines, foci of contraction and of expansion

Let us consider the a pure translational motion of the observer, for which the translation vector is $v\vec{u}$; the speed is v; and the unit vector $\vec{u}$ gives the direction. The three-dimensional velocity field is then constant:

$$\vec{w}(p_1, p_2, p_3) = -v\vec{u} = -v(u_1, u_2, u_3)^\top.$$ (10.16)

Substitution into the projection formula for motion vectors (Equation 10.10) results in:

$$\vec{v}(x',y') = \frac{v}{p_3}\left(\begin{pmatrix} u_1 \\ u_2 \end{pmatrix} + u_3 \begin{pmatrix} x' \\ y' \end{pmatrix} \right).$$ (10.17)

In the case of translational motion, the flow field depends on the depth p_3 of the imaged object; conversely, it is possible to use translation to obtain information about the spatial structure of the surroundings (motion parallax). Let us first, however, consider a characteristic of translation fields which is independent of the spatial structure of the surroundings. Namely, it can easily be shown that if $u_3 \neq 0$, there is always a point in the image plane at which the projected vector field vanishes, $\vec{v}(x',y') = 0$:

$$\vec{v} = 0 \quad \Rightarrow \quad u_1 + u_3 x_o' = 0 \, , \ u_2 + u_3 y_o' = 0$$

$$\Rightarrow \quad \begin{pmatrix} x_o' \\ y_o' \end{pmatrix} = -\frac{1}{u_3}\begin{pmatrix} u_1 \\ u_3 \end{pmatrix} =: \vec{F}.$$

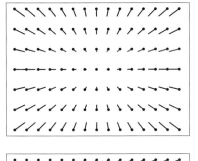

a.

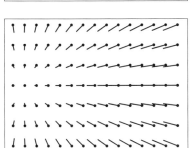

b.

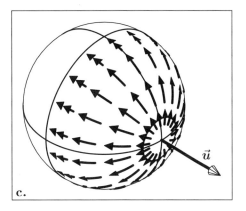

c.

Figure 10.5
Projected motion field for translation and the focus of expansion. The case shown is of direct approach toward a wall. **a., b.** Projection onto an image plane behind the nodal point (field of view in the x direction ca. 40°, corresponding to a normal focal length in photography). **a.** Motion in the direction of view. The focus of expansion lies at the middle of the image. **b.** Motion forward and toward the right; the focus of expansion lies in the left side of the image. **c.** Projection onto a sphere. The flow lines are arcs of great circles which pass through the foci of expansion and of contraction.

$\vec{F}$ is called the *focus of expansion* (f.o.e) or, if u_3, is negative, the *focus of contraction*. This is the vanishing point which corresponds to the direction in space determined by (u_1, u_2, u_3), i.e., the "point" toward which the observer is moving. (Of course, no point in the outside world need correspond to this point in the image plane, as is also the case with the horizon.) Since $\vec{F}$ is also the vanishing point corresponding to the direction of translation $\vec{u}$, the following relationship is to be expected:

In the translation field, all $\vec{v}$ vectors point away from the focus of expansion, or toward the focus of contraction, or in other words, the flow lines are straight lines through the focus of expansion or of contraction.

In order to prove this, it must be shown that for all $(p_1, p_2, p_3)^\top \in \mathbb{R}^3$, there is a $\lambda \in \mathbb{R}$, such that

$$\underbrace{\begin{pmatrix} x' \\ y' \end{pmatrix}}_{\text{image point}} + \lambda \underbrace{\left(\frac{1}{p_3} \left(\begin{pmatrix} u_1 \\ u_2 \end{pmatrix} + u_3 \begin{pmatrix} x' \\ y' \end{pmatrix} \right) \right)}_{\vec{v}} = \underbrace{-\frac{1}{u_3} \begin{pmatrix} u_1 \\ u_2 \end{pmatrix}}_{\text{f.o.e.}}.$$

By rearrangement, the requirement follows that:

$$\left(\frac{\lambda}{p_3} + \frac{1}{u_3} \right) \left[\left(\begin{array}{c} u_1 \\ u_2 \end{array} \right) + u_3 \left(\begin{array}{c} x' \\ y' \end{array} \right) \right] = 0,$$

which can always be satisfied by $\lambda = -p_3/u_3$ given that $u_3 \neq 0$. It is thereby shown that a consistent solution for both components of the conditional equation exists, and consequently, that all flow vectors lie on straight lines through the focus. The length of the flow vectors, nonetheless, depends on the distance of the image points.

The flow field is shown on the surface of a sphere in Fig. 10.5c. The flow vectors here lie on great circles ("meridians" or "circles of longitude"), whose intersection is given by the direction in space of the translation vector $\vec{u}$.

The flow field of a plane in translational motion

While the directions of the flow vectors in a translational field are fixed by the above requirement, their length depends on the spatial structure of the outside world: that is, on the distances of the imaged objects. If the visible outside world can described as a surface, then $\vec{v}(x', y')$ can be calculated in three steps:

1. *Ray tracing:* The point in space $(p_1, p_2, p_3)^\top$ which corresponds to a point (x', y') in the image, is found at the intersection of the visual ray $\lambda(x', y', -1)^\top$ with the visible surface.

2. *Three-dimensional motion field:* The relative velocity for $(p_1, p_2, p_3)^\top$ is found by evaluation of $\vec{w}$.

3. *Projection:* $\vec{v}(x', y')$ is calculated as a projection of $\vec{w}(\vec{p})$ as in Equation 10.10.

This process is clearly not limited to translational motions. We will, however, here considered only one example, namely translational motions when the imaged surface is a plane. Since the rotational field does not depend on the distances of objects, it can simply be added to the translational field, and the above results may thus be generalized.

Let us recall the mathematical notations introduced in Section 8.3.1, in which planes in space and their imaging characteristics were considered. Here, as in that section, a plane in space is uniquely defined by a normal vector $\vec{n}$ and its distance d from the origin (Fig. 10.6). All points $\vec{p}$ of the plane conform to the equation

$$(\vec{p} \cdot \vec{n}) = d \geq 0. \tag{10.18}$$

Let $\vec{x}' := (x', y', -1)^\top$ be a point on the image plane, described in the three-dimensional coordinate system. All object points which are imaged onto that point lie on the ray

$$\vec{p} = \lambda \vec{x}' \text{ with } \lambda < 0. \tag{10.19}$$

We next construct the flow field in the steps described above:

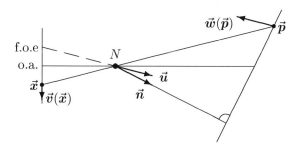

Figure 10.6

Geometry of approach to a plane. $\vec{n}$: normal to the plane; the distance of the plane from the camera nodal point N is d. $\vec{u}$: Translation vector of observer motion. The corresponding vanishing point is the focus of expansion (f.o.e.). A point in space $\vec{p}$ moves as $\vec{w}(\vec{p}) = -v\vec{u}$ relative to the nodal point. Its image $\vec{x}$ moves in the image plane with the velocity $\vec{v}(\vec{x})$.

1. *Ray tracing:* Find the intersection of the plane with the visual ray through $\vec{x}'$:

$$(\lambda\vec{x}' \cdot \vec{n}) = d \quad \Rightarrow \quad \lambda = \frac{d}{(\vec{x}' \cdot \vec{n})} = \frac{d}{x'n_1 + y'n_2 - n_3}. \tag{10.20}$$

Of course, this only works if $\vec{x}'$ is not orthogonal to $\vec{n}$. Otherwise, the visual ray is parallel to the plane, and either lies entirely inside it ($d = 0$) or does not intersect it at all ($d \neq 0$). Except in this case,

$$\vec{p} := \frac{d}{(\vec{x}' \cdot \vec{n})} \cdot \vec{x}' \tag{10.21}$$

is the point where the visual ray intersects the visible surface.

2. *Motion of the external point $\vec{p}$:* Let us consider a pure translational motion with $v\vec{u} = v(u_1, u_2, u_3)^\top$. In this case, $\vec{w}(\vec{p})$ is constant, and $\vec{w}(\vec{p}) = -v\vec{u}$ for all $\vec{p}$.

3. *Projection:* Application of Equation 10.10 results, finally, in the relationship:

$$\vec{v}(x', y') \;=\; -\frac{v(\vec{x}' \cdot \vec{n})}{d} \left(\begin{pmatrix} u_1 \\ u_2 \end{pmatrix} + u_3 \begin{pmatrix} x' \\ y' \end{pmatrix} \right). \tag{10.22}$$

Special cases:

1. $v\vec{u} = (0, 0, 1); \vec{n} = (0, -1, 0)$: Travel in a straight line above a horizontal plane. The directions of view and of motion are the same.

$$\vec{v}(x', y') = \frac{y'}{d} \begin{pmatrix} x' \\ y' \end{pmatrix}. \tag{10.23}$$

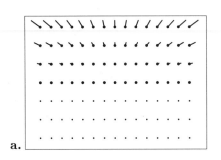

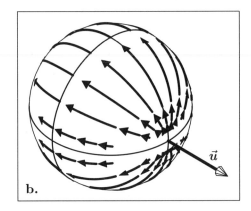

Figure 10.7

Optical flow for translation over a horizontal plane. **a.** Projection onto the image plane. The lengths of the y' component of the flow vectors does not depend on x' (cf. Equation 10.23). The small points in the lower part of the image correspond to locations at which the plane is not imaged. **b.** Projection onto the surface of a sphere. The flow for translation between two planes is shown so the complete field is visible.

For $y' < 0$, $(\vec{x} \cdot \vec{r})n$ is here negative, corresponding formally to the imaging of a point which lies behind the camera nodal point. In fact, the line $y' = 0$ is the horizon of the plane, and the plane is actually imaged only in the part of the (inverted) image above $y' = 0$. Fig. 10.7a therefore shows only this meaningful part of the vector field from Equation 10.23. The spherical projection in Fig. 10.7b shows the flow for a path between two parallel planes.

2. $v\vec{u} = (0,0,1), \vec{n} = (0,0,1)$: Frontal motion toward a wall.

$$\vec{v}(x',y') = \frac{1}{d} \begin{pmatrix} x' \\ y' \end{pmatrix}. \tag{10.24}$$

This time, flow vectors are present throughout the visual field (radial field). This field has already been illustrated in Fig. 10.5a, b. In this case, the distance of the plane, d, changes with time. The flow field is therefore not stationary; the flow vector which is present at a given time t_o at a given point in the image is different from the one which is present at the same point at a different time. In this case, the difference is only in the length of the vectors, not in their direction.

10.3.3   Curved path in the plane

Combinations of translations and rotations occur, for example, in curved paths. Let us consider the case of a circular motion of the observer, and use the camera coordinate system at the time $t = 0$ as the external coordinate system. Let the camera nodal point move along a path in space $\vec{k}(t)$:

$$\vec{k}(t) = R \begin{pmatrix} 1 - \cos 2\pi\omega t \\ 0 \\ \sin 2\pi\omega t \end{pmatrix}. \tag{10.25}$$

Here, R is the radius of the circular path. We assume that the camera is rigidly connected to the device which transports it along this path, such that the direction of view is always the same as the direction of translation. At the time $t = 0$, this direction is simply the $\vec{z}$ axis of the coordinate system, $\vec{u} = (0, 0, 1)^\top$, and the speed of translation is $v = 2\pi\omega R$. The momentary rotational axis is the vertical axis of the system, $\vec{r} = (0, 1, 0)^\top$ and the angular velocity is ω.

The travel along a curved path is above a horizontal plane, such that the distance d between the camera nodal point and the plane is constant; the translation field therefore is of the form of Equation 10.23. The rotation field also has already been described, in Equation 10.15. Super-imposition gives the result:

$$\vec{v}(x', y') = v\frac{y'}{d} \begin{pmatrix} x' \\ y' \end{pmatrix} + \omega \begin{pmatrix} 1 + x'^2 \\ x'y' \end{pmatrix}. \tag{10.26}$$

It is easy to see that the vector field of a curved path in a plane does not vanish at any point. This is, however, true only for projection into an image plane orthogonal to the direction of view. In this image plane, the center of a circular path, whose image naturally is immobile, can not be imaged. The complete situation is shown in Fig. 10.8, using a projection onto the surface of a sphere. In order to make the illustration clearer, a path between two parallel, equidistant planes. rather than with relation to only one plane, is shown.

When curved paths occur in the presence of vertical walls, foci of expansion also occur, which are displaced laterally in comparison with those of Fig. 10.5.

General description of motion along curves

A few results from differential geometry are assembled here in preparation for a discussion of general curved paths. This section may be skipped on first reading.

Let us assume that the observer moves along a smoothly curved path $\vec{k}(t)$, always looking in the direction of motion and carrying out no unnecessary roll motions around the axis of vision and motion. To state this differently, the camera is rigidly attached to the observer, and the motion, like that of a point-like object, has only three degrees of freedom. In this case the camera coordinate system is defined at the time t by the "moving" or "Frenet" trihedral of the curved path, which consists of the direction of the tangent to the curve, the direction of curvature, and the normal to the "osculating" plane which is defined by the two other vectors (cf. do Carmo 1976).

This coordinate system is defined by first parameterizing the curved path according to the length along the curve,

$$s = \int_{t_o}^{t} \left\| \frac{d}{dt'}\vec{k}(t') \right\| dt'. \tag{10.27}$$

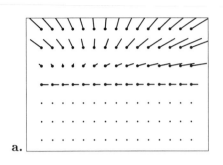 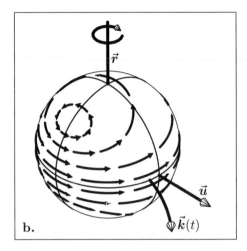

Figure 10.8
Flow field for a curved path in a plane. **a.** Projection onto the image plane. **b.**
Projection onto a sphere. For the sake of clarity, the motion is once again shown
between two parallel planes in **b**.

The curve $\vec{k}(s)$ is then "regular", that is, it has the characteristic that

$$\|\frac{d}{ds}\vec{k}(s)\| \equiv 1.$$

Parameterizing according to the length of the path is not necessary if the motion
along the curve is at the constant speed 1. In this case, the curve is already regular.

The first vector of our local coordinate system is, then, $\vec{t} = \vec{k}_s(s)$; the subscript
signifies that this is a derivative with respect to the length of the path s. $\vec{t}$ is the
normalized tangent vector of the curved path, that is, the instantaneous direction of
translation; it corresponds to the $\vec{z}$ vector of the camera coordinate system. Because
of the parameterization by the path length, the equation $\vec{t}^2(s) = 1$ is everywhere
valid. The second vector of the local coordinate system is obtained by taking the
derivative of this equation with respect to s. It follows from the chain rule that

$$\vec{t}\vec{t}_s = \vec{k}_s\vec{k}_{ss} = 0,$$

i.e., the second derivative of $\vec{k}$ is orthogonal to the first. We denote the normalized
second derivative of the path vector as $\vec{n}$. Except for the sign, this corresponds to the
$\vec{x}$ axis of the camera coordinate system. The plane defined by $\vec{t}$ and $\vec{n}$ is called the
"osculating plane" of the curved path; if the curve is plane, it lies entirely within this
plane. The norm of the second derivative is the local curvature of the curved path,
that is, the inverse of the radius R of a circle approximating the curve at a given
point.

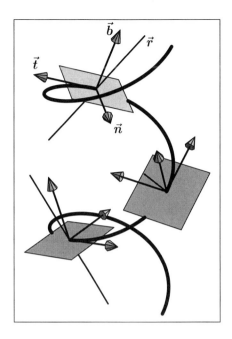

Figure 10.9
Moving (or Frenet) trihedral of a space curve (helix). $\vec{t}$: tangent vector; $\vec{n}$: normal vector; $\vec{b}$: binormal vector. For each instant, the vectors $\vec{t}$ and $\vec{n}$ define the osculating plane. The instantaneous axis of rotation is denoted by $\vec{r}$; it is the axis of the rotational flow component seen by an observer whose direction of view is straight ahead ($\vec{t}$).

The third vector of the moving coordinate system is the cross product of $\vec{t}$ and $\vec{n}$. It is defined simply as orthogonal to the two other vectors, and therefore it is called the "binormal vector" $\vec{b} = \vec{t} \times \vec{n}$. The derivative of the binormal vector is parallel to $\vec{n}$; the equation $\vec{b}_s = -w\vec{n}$ defines what is called the torsion w of the curve, which indicates how fast and in which direction the curve emerges from the osculating plane. For plane curves, $w \equiv 0$.

The moving trihedral defined in this way is a right-hand coordinate system ($\det[\vec{t}, \vec{n}, \vec{b}] > 0$), contrary to our usual convention; this difference has no significance to our further discussion.

The coordinate transformations related to motion, as in Equation 10.1, can be obtained by using the basis vectors of the moving coordinate system as columns of the transformation matrix B, $\mathsf{B}(t) := [\vec{t}(t), \vec{n}(t), \vec{b}(t)]$. In order to determine the momentary axis of rotation, we consider the expression

$$\mathsf{B}^{-1}(0)\mathsf{B}'(s)\big|_{s=0} = \begin{pmatrix} 0 & -1/R & 0 \\ 1/R & 0 & -w \\ 0 & w & 0 \end{pmatrix}. \tag{10.28}$$

The momentary optical flow is therefore described by the translation $v\vec{u} = \vec{t}$ and the axis of rotation $\omega\vec{r} = \vec{n}/R + w\vec{u}$ (see Fig. 10.9).

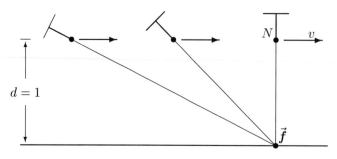

Figure 10.10
Egomotion parallel to a plane with simultaneous fixation of a point $\vec{f}$ in the plane ("slow nystagmus phase").

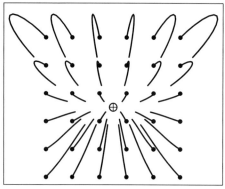

Figure 10.11
Non-stationary optical flow $\vec{v}$ for the slow nystagmus phase (Equation 10.30). Illustrated are the curved paths of certain points of the fixated plane as imaged for a time interval $t < 0$ (i.e., during the approach to $\vec{f}$). If the trajectories are extended to times $t > 0$, the result is reflected around the horizontal axis. The symbol $\oplus$ indicates the fixation point.

10.3.4   Fixation and egomotion

Let us consider an observer who moves with a velocity v at a constant distance $d > 0$ above a ground plane with a normal vector $\vec{n} = (0, 1, 0)^{\top}$. In the plane, there is a fixation point $\vec{f}$, toward which the optical axis remains directed during the entire time interval (Fig. 10.10). For the sake of simplicity, the observer is directly over $\vec{f}$ at the time $t = 0$. The origin of the external coordinate system is at $\vec{f}$, its $\vec{z}$ axis is the direction in which the observer is moving, and its $\vec{y}$ axis is the normal to the plane. If $\vec{a}, \vec{b}, \vec{c}$ are the axes of the camera coordinate system which changes over time, then:

$$N = (0, d, vt)^{\top}; \quad \vec{a} = \begin{pmatrix} 1 \\ 0 \\ 0 \end{pmatrix} \tag{10.29}$$

$$\vec{b} = \frac{1}{\sqrt{d^2 + (vt)^2}} \begin{pmatrix} 0 \\ vt \\ -d \end{pmatrix}; \quad \vec{c} = \frac{1}{\sqrt{d^2 + (vt)^2}} \begin{pmatrix} 0 \\ -d \\ -vt \end{pmatrix}.$$

If, now, $(p, 0, q)^{\top}$ is a point in the plane, its image $(p', q')^{\top}$ describes a curve in the image plane, and this curve can be calculated point by point using the projection formula for any camera coordinate system (Equation 2.18). Then:

$$\begin{pmatrix} p'(t) \\ q'(t) \end{pmatrix} = \frac{h}{d^2 + (vt)^2 - qvt} \begin{pmatrix} p\sqrt{d^2 + (vt)^2} \\ -qd \end{pmatrix}. \tag{10.30}$$

Fig. 10.11 illustrates the curved paths as projected onto the image in this case. Unlike with translational or rotational motions of the observer at a constant rate, this field changes during the approach; that is, the field is not stationary. In Fig. 10.11, for example, different directions of motion occur at points in the image plane where the trajectories intersect. The type of motion described here, which is the fixation of a point, is the most frequent pattern of eye movement during motion of the observer. A well-known special case of this is the slow phase of nystagmic eye movement, which consists of the alternation of fixations and jumps, such as when looking out the window of a moving railroad train.

10.3.5 Summary

The important conclusions about the characteristics of flow fields will be summarized here.

Vector field equation. Each motion of a rigid observer can be decomposed into a translation and a rotation. Insertion of Equation 10.6 into Equation 10.10 results in the general equation for optical flow resulting from egomotion:

$$
\vec{v}(x',y') = \frac{v}{z}\left(\begin{pmatrix} u_1 \\ u_2 \end{pmatrix} + u_3 \begin{pmatrix} x' \\ y' \end{pmatrix}\right) + \tag{10.31}
$$
$$
\omega\left(-r_1\begin{pmatrix} x'y' \\ 1+y'^2 \end{pmatrix} + r_2\begin{pmatrix} 1+x'^2 \\ x'y' \end{pmatrix} + r_3\begin{pmatrix} y' \\ -x' \end{pmatrix}\right).
$$

Here, $(u_1, u_2, u_3)^\top$ is the translational component, $(r_1, r_2, r_3)^\top$ is the momentary axis of rotation and ω is the angular velocity of the rotation around this axis. Due to the linearity of the projection formula 10.10 in $\vec{w}$, Equation 10.31 is simply the sum of Equations 10.17 and 10.13; the rotational and translational components therefore superimpose additively.

Dependence on the spatial structure of the surrounding scene. Pure rotational fields such as occur in connection with rotations around axes which pass through the camera nodal point do not depend on the distances of the imaged objects. They therefore provide no information about the spatial structure of the surroundings.

Singularities. If the surrounding scene is a smooth surface—that is, if there are no depth discontinuities, sharp edges or points—and the optical flow resulting from egomotion is projected onto a sphere around the camera nodal point, then there are always at least two points at which the flow vector vanishes (Poincaré's theorem; cf. do Carmo 1976). Several types of singular points exist: Figs. 10.4 and 10.8 show vortices, or rotations around poles. The foci of expansion and contraction (Fig. 10.5, 10.7 and 10.11) are examples of umbilical points. If the surrounding scene consists of more than one surface and the transitions between the surfaces are not smooth, then Poincaré's theorem no longer applies. In particular, each object which moves toward the observer has its own focus of expansion.

Stationary and non-stationary flows. Stationary flows are those with flow fields that do not change over time: the condition $\vec{v}(x', y', t_1) = \vec{v}(x', y', t_2)$ holds for all x', y', t_1, t_2. Examples for which this condition is completely fulfilled are rotation with a constant rate and axis, and translation and circular curved paths above a plane. In the case of translation toward a plane, the flow lines and therefore also the directions of the flow vectors are constant, but their length changes. Finally, in the example of translation while also fixating on a point, stationariness is completely lost: at different times, different flow vectors are present at the same place in the image.

Analogy with hydrodynamic flow. The term optical flow implies an analogy to hydrodynamics which is sometimes useful. Nonetheless, two basic limitations should be noted. For one, Horn's equation (Eq. 9.13) does not fully correspond to the continuity equation of hydrodynamics. The continuity equation implies that the flowing liquid does not change volume as it flows (incompressibility). In optical flow, surfaces may turn away from the observer, changing both the size of their images and their brightness. As a result, the corresponding flow field is in fact compressed or expanded. The second difference is that the optic flow is generally not differentiable, or not even continuous. Discontinuities occur at edges between objects at different depths, and are often the most interesting parts of a flow pattern. Globally, therefore, the theory of differential vector fields can not be applied.

10.4   Recovering information from optical flow

We consider here only three examples of the information mentioned in the introduction to this chapter which can be obtained from optical flow: namely, 1) the reconstruction of egomotion; 2) the remaining time until striking a target (*time-to-contact*); and 3) simple obstacle avoidance.

10.4.1   Reconstruction of egomotion

Direct approach

As was shown in Section 10.2.2, motion of the observer is generally described by six unknowns, of which three are degrees of freedom in translation and three are degrees of freedom in rotation. If an optical flow has been measured, then solutions for the six movement parameters may be obtained from Equation 10.31; this equation, however, contains not only the six unknowns, but also the depth values z of the point at which each flow vector originates.

Therefore, if n vectors of optical flow, $\vec{v}(x'_i, y'_i), i = 1, ..., n$ have been determined, the two vector components in Equation 10.31 generate $2n$ conditional equations for the $6 + n$ unknowns $vu_1, vu_2, vu_3, \omega r_1, \omega r_2, \omega r_3, z_1, ..., z_n$. A solution should be possible if at least six flow vectors have been determined. As has already been mentioned, a scaling factor must remain indeterminate, since the flow field does not change if the observer moves through surroundings which are p times larger at p times the speed.

The system of equations to be solved is nonlinear and has no closed solution; nonetheless, the standard procedures of numerical mathematics may be applied. A review is given by Zhuang and Haralick (1993).

Exploiting depth variations

Only the translational field depends on the distance z_i of moving points in the image, while the rotational field does not. If, instead of a few flow vectors at isolated points, a more or less dense flow field is available, that fact can be used in the reconstruction of translation and rotation. If the flow vectors at two points in the image which are very close to one another are observed, it can be assumed that the difference of these flow vectors depends primarily on the difference in depth of the corresponding object points. Since the rotational component does not depend on depth, the difference vector points toward the focus of expansion (or, depending on the sign of the difference in depth, toward the focus of contraction) of the translational component. From many such difference vectors, it is possible to identify a focus of expansion at the intersection of lines through these vectors. One way to identify the intersection of the line segments is to apply the Hough transform, which was introduced in Chapter 8 (Fig. 8.3). The locations of large variations in depth can be identified as discontinuities in the optical flow itself, or through other cues (for example, stereoscopic vision).

Perceptual experiments with human subjects have shown that egomotion in fields with depth variations is evaluated better than in fields without such variations (Hildreth 1992, Crowell & Banks 1996). The cited papers also give an overview of how to make use of depth variations when evaluating egomotion.

Matched filters

While solving the optical flow equations for egomotion is difficult, the expected flow field for any type of motion can easily be determined by applying Equation 10.31. Determining the expected flow is especially easy if reliable assumptions can be made about the surroundings. Clouds in the sky, for example, generate an optical flow whose translational component can be neglected to a good approximation, since their distance, and therefore the denominator of the flow equation, is very large. When the observer is flying high enough above the terrain, the same is also true of the ground below.

In such a situation, it is possible to determine egomotion by calculating a number of flow fields expected for different types of motion, and then testing which of these corresponds best to the flow field actually measured. The logic of this process resembles that of the Bayesian theory of estimation already mentioned in Chapter 8. The reconstruction of egomotion is performed not by means of inverse optics (as in the case of direct solution, i.e., inversion of the flow equations), but rather by comparison with an expected stimulus pattern.

In neurophysiological experiments on flies, a group of visual neurons has been identified which react specifically to different optical flow patterns (Krapp & Hengstenberg 1996). Fig. 10.12 shows the distribution of motion specificity in the visual

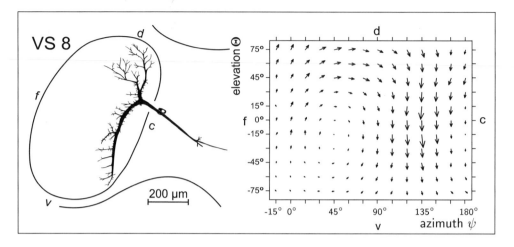

Figure 10.12
Distribution in the visual field of the motion sensitivity of a visual neuron ("VS8") of
the fly *Calliphora*. The receptive field of the neuron encompasses almost the entire
visual field. The forward direction is at the azimuth $\psi = 0°$ and elevation $\theta = 0°$.
When the fly rotates around an axis with $\psi = 45°$ and $\theta = -15°$, the cell is excited
everywhere in the visual field by motion in its preferred direction. This rotation
therefore leads to maximal reaction of the cell. The inset drawing at the left shows
the location of the neuron in the lobula plate, a part of the fly's brain. f: frontal; c:
caudal; v: ventral; d: dorsal. (From Krapp & Hengstenberg 1996; with permission of
Nature, ©1996 Macmillan Magazines Ltd.)

field for one such cell. The structure of a rotational field is clearly recognizable; this
cell reacts most strongly when the fly is rotating around a specific axis. Such cells are,
more or less, detectors or matched filters (cf. Horridge 1992, Franz & Krapp 2000)
for specific flow patterns. The fly has a total of ten such cells specialized for rotation
around different axes, and three for translations. By comparing the relative excitations of the individual neurons, egomotions can be measured which are not directly
represented by single cells (population coding).

Similar receptive fields specialized for specific flow patterns are also found in the
temporal lobes of the cerebral cortex of primates. These fields are, however, markedly
smaller and appear, rather, to analyze only parts of the flow pattern. An overview is
given by Lappe et al. (1996).

10.4.2   Expansion rate and "time to contact"

As already explained, the observer's velocity and the distance from objects can both
be determined only up to a multiplicative factor. If we consider the relationship of
distance and speed, that is, the time to contact with an imaged object, then this
factor cancels out. We may ask whether the "time to contact," represented here by

the symbol τ_C, can be determined from the flow pattern.

It is immediately clear that in the case of pure translational motion, contact will be with the point which is imaged at the expansion point in the image plane. As the observer approaches, and the remaining time to contact decreases, the size of the image of an area around this point will increase faster and faster. In the limit case, when the nodal point reaches the imaged surface, the image of this area becomes infinitely large.

Example: Let us now examine a special case in which motion is in the z direction of the camera coordinate system. In front of the observer at the distance d is a plane whose normal is $(0, 0, 1)^\top$: that is, a vertical wall. The time to contact at the time $t = 0$ is in this case $\tau_C = d/v$. It is easy to understand that, in agreement with Equation 8.11, the local image magnification at the focus of expansion is $M = 1/d^2$. As a result of the motion with $v\vec{u} = (0, 0, v)^\top$, it follows that on the one hand $\tau_C = (d - vt)/v$ and on the other hand,

$$M(t) = \frac{1}{(d - vt)^2}. \tag{10.32}$$

The change in image magnification with time is, then:

$$\dot{M}(t) = \frac{2v}{(d - vt)^3}, \tag{10.33}$$

where the dot denotes the temporal derivative. The expansion rate, finally, is the change in magnification relative to the current magnification:

$$\left.\frac{\dot{M}(t)}{M(t)}\right|_{t=0} = \frac{2v}{d} = \frac{2}{\tau_C}. \tag{10.34}$$

The time to contact with the expected point for this example can therefore be determined from the momentary expansion rate.

In the general case, the same result can be demonstrated by examining what is called the divergence of the vector field $\vec{v}$,

$$\text{div } \vec{v}(x', y') := \frac{\partial v_1}{\partial x'} + \frac{\partial v_2}{\partial y'}. \tag{10.35}$$

According to Liouville's theorem (cf. Arrowsmith & Place 1990), the divergence is equal to the expansion rate $\dot{M}/M$. In hydrodynamics, the divergence is also called the "source density", since it identifies how much of a fluid is entering at each point of a source region. In what follows, the formal relationship between divergence and time to contact will be described mathematically.

Equation 10.22 describes the optical flow for the approach to a plane. In the general case, $\tau_C = d/(v\vec{u} \cdot \vec{n})$. In this formula, $(\vec{u} \cdot \vec{n})$ is the motion component in the direction of the normal vector of the plane, $\vec{n}$, and d is the distance in that direction. We now calculate the divergence of the flow field generated by approaching a plane. Taking the derivative of Equation 10.22, we obtain:

$$
\begin{aligned}
\operatorname{div} \vec{v}(x', y') &= -\frac{v}{d}\left[n_1 u_1 + n_2 u_2 - 2n_3 u_3 + 3n_1 u_3 x' + 3n_2 u_3 y'\right] \\
&= -\frac{v}{d}(\vec{n} \cdot \vec{u}) + 3u_3(\vec{n} \cdot \vec{x}'), \qquad\qquad (10.36)
\end{aligned}
$$

where $\vec{x}' = (x', y', -1)^{\top}$ is the image point in camera coordinates. Let us now consider the divergence in the image of the anticipated landing point, i.e., the focus of expansion $(x', y') = -1/u_3(u_1, u_2)^{\top}$. By substitution, it follows that:

$$
\operatorname{div} \vec{v}(-\frac{u_1}{u_3}, -\frac{u_2}{u_3}) = \frac{2v}{d}(u_1 n_1 + u_2 n_2 + u_3 n_3) = \frac{2}{\tau_C}. \qquad (10.37)
$$

The divergence of the projected vector field $\vec{v}$ therefore provides an absolute measurement for the time to contact with the surface.

In the psychophysical literature, the expansion rate is often called *looming*. It would seem desirable to construct "looming detectors," to calculate the divergence, a scalar quantity, without first having to find the under-determined two-dimensional motion vector field. Unfortunately, this idea only works when the focus of expansion is known. The focus of expansion can not be determined from the distribution of divergence alone. Consider, for example, the divergence generated by the approach to a plane, Equation 10.36. Except for an additive constant, divergence depends linearly on the image coordinates (x', y'); thus, divergence is not greatest at the focus of expansion, nor is there any other way to infer the position of the focus from the distribution of divergence.

The existence of neural looming detectors, that is, of neurons which react selectively to specific expansion rates, is contested. In psychophysical experiments, Regan & Beverly (1978) show that channels adaptable for changes in depth and the expansions which are related to it exist in humans (cf. also Regan & Vincent 1995). However, the star-shaped pattern of outwards-pointing flow vectors appears to play a large role, and this pattern may occur also in places where divergence is low.

An application of the expansion rate in computer vision (assistance to automobile drivers) is described by Zielke et al. (1993).

10.4.3   Obstacle avoidance

An important application of optical flow is in obstacle avoidance. As with time to contact, this involves a combined estimation of egomotion and scene structure, since objects only become obstacles when they are in the anticipated path of the observer.

A simple approach to obstacle avoidance is to examine the optical flow in the left and right halves of the visual field separately, and then to turn toward the direction in which the optical flow is smaller. Since the length of flow vectors decreases with the distance of objects, the observer will then always turn toward the direction in which there is more room to maneuver. This behavior has the effect of centering an observer who is traveling down a corridor, and occurs, for example, in bees; a more thorough analysis shows that it in fact depends on the mechanism just described (Srinivasan et al. 1996).

In general, obstacle avoidance includes a simple form of image segmentation: in other words, it includes the recognition of regions of the image which are obstacles and regions which correspond to unobstructed paths. An example of a segmentation scheme is the inverse perspective mapping which has been discussed in connection with stereoscopic vision (see Fig. 6.15); applications related to optical flow are described by Mallot et al. (1991) and Campani et al. (1995). Experiments with human subjects show that the interaction of body movements and eye movements plays a large role, and that potential obstacles are often fixated (cf. Cutting et al. 1995). In doing this, patterns with motion in opposite directions in front of and behind the obstacle are generated.

Chapter 11

Visual navigation

One of the most important behavioral competencies supported by the visual system is navigation. Navigation is needed for locomotion, that is, behavior which leads to a change in the observer's position. Obstacle avoidance and the estimation of the observer's egomotion, which are of great importance in controlling the change of position, have already been discussed in earlier chapters. Navigation is defined more narrowly as comprising motions which are carried out with the purpose of arriving at a destination. The simplest case of navigation in this sense is return to the starting point of a trip or *homing*, which can be achieved by path integration, or by a visual search. The use of search mechanisms assumes that the destination can be recognized, for example by its visual markings or landmarks. Advanced navigation systems can make use of other information which is not related to the destination in order to navigate toward it. Here, too, landmarks play a decisive role. Some important basic navigation mechanisms are illustrated in Fig. 11.1. For surveys of the field, cf. Trullier et al. (1997) and Franz & Mallot (2000).

Navigation uses not only vision, but also other sensory modalities such as, for example, the sense of acceleration (vestibular system) and the sense of the posture and motion of the musculature (proprioception). Acoustic signals, too, play a role as "landmarks" or for the estimation of the observer's motion. Finally, navigation to a goal, always presupposes the existence of memory, since, at the very least, the goal must be recognized upon reaching it. We will here examine mostly the visual aspects.

11.1 Path integration

Even in the absence of visual landmarks, many animals and also humans are able to return to the point of departure of an excursion, and by nearly the shortest path. A mechanism which makes this possible is path integration (Mittelstaedt & Mittelstaedt 1980, Müller & Wehner 1988, Maurer & Séguinot 1995, Klatzky et al. 1998). In this process, the observer's motion is continually determined and the current position is calculated on the basis of successive egomotion estimates. In ship navigation, path

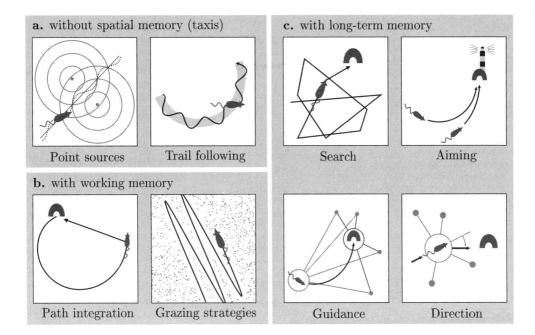

Figure 11.1
Locomotor behavior in space. **a** Without spatial memory, so-called taxes (reflexive orienting reactions in a stimulus field), are operative. Shown are two examples of a "tropotaxis", in which an organism balances the stimuli at its two sensors. (cf. McFarland 1993, p. 273ff). **b.** Spatio-temporal maneuvers and spatial integration require at least a working memory which identifies the current phase of the task. (On search strategies, cf. Bell 1991.) **c.** A prerequisite for recognition of the destination, for example by its visual features, is a long-term memory of these features. The mechanisms of path integration, aiming and guidance are discussed in the text. The dots and circles in panels "Guidance" and "Direction" symbolize the landmark configuration in the observer's visual array.

integration is often called "dead reckoning"*. In robotics, the expression *odometry* is used. The vector from the current position to the starting position, expressed in body coordinates, is called the "home vector".

Various sources can contribute information about the observer's egomotion. The vestibular system provides information about accelerations; motions generated by the observer can be determined through the positioning and motion sense of the musculature (proprioception) or through the control signals themselves ("efference copy"). Among visual information sources, optical flow is the most significant; Chapter 10 gave a thorough description of how the observer's motion can be determined from

---

*This expression is thought to be a corruption of "thread reckoning". The path integration was originally carried out using a thread stretched across a pin-board.

a. Translational step   **b.** Rotational step

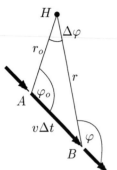

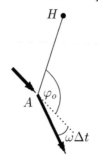

Figure 11.2
Path integration by triangulation. H starting point ("home"); A current position; B new position after translational step; r_o, r distance from starting point; φ_o, φ angle to the starting point relative to the forward direction; v translational velocity; ω rate of rotation; Δt time duration of a step.

optical flow. Insects can in addition use the polarization pattern of the sunlit sky and an internal clock to determine the compass direction (Rossel 1993), so that path integration is used not for body orientation, but rather only for the total distance from the start. For an artificial implementation of the polarization compass, see Lambrinos et al. (1997). The existence of a magnetic compass system has been demonstrated in birds (e.g., Wiltschko & Wiltschko 1995); clearly, magnetic compasses work without the need for an internal clock.

Let us consider the case in which egomotion is described by means of two observer-centered quantities, namely the momentary forward speed v and the momentary rate of rotation ω (see Fig. 11.2). The starting position (home) H is given in polar coordinates relative to the observer, i.e., by the distance r and the angle between the forward direction of the observer and the direction to the starting point, φ. If the observer carries out a purely translational motion, then the resulting values of r and φ can be calculated using elementary trigonometry. The two legs r_o and $v\Delta t$ and the included angle φ_o define the triangle whose three corners are the home position H and the starting and ending points of the momentary motion. Formal expressions may be developed using the sine and cosine laws. The new distance r from the home position may, for example, be determined by applying the law of cosines to the angle φ_o enclosed by the legs r_o and $v\Delta t$:

$$r = \sqrt{r_o^2 + (v\Delta t)^2 - 2r_o\, v\Delta t\, \cos\varphi_o}. \qquad (11.1)$$

To formulate the equation for the new angle $\varphi(t)$, we need the argument function, which extends the arctangent to angles of more than 90 degrees:

$$\arg(x,y) := \begin{cases} \arctan \frac{y}{x} & \text{if } x > 0 \\ \arctan \frac{y}{x} + \pi & \text{if } x < 0, y \geq 0 \\ \arctan \frac{y}{x} - \pi & \text{if } x < 0, y < 0 \end{cases} \qquad (11.2)$$

The new angle φ is calculated by application of the law of sines to $\pi - \varphi$ and $\Delta\varphi$:

$$\varphi = \arg(r_o \cos\varphi_o - v\Delta t,\ r_o \sin\varphi_o) \qquad (11.3)$$

If the motion is a rotation, the distance r does not change; for the angle,

$$\varphi = \varphi_o + \omega \Delta t. \tag{11.4}$$

A Taylor series expansion about the point $t = 0$ leads to the differential representation

$$\frac{dr}{dt} = -v \cos \varphi \tag{11.5}$$

$$\frac{d\varphi}{dt} = \frac{v}{r} \sin \varphi + \omega. \tag{11.6}$$

The equations show that it is possible in theory to determine the current position of the starting point in observer-centered polar coordinates, by continuous updating from the observer's rates of translation and rotation. It is mathematically simpler, but equivalent, to use a formulation relative to a fixed world coordinate system, in which, for example, the starting point is the origin and the x-axis is the direction of the initial motion; the x axis is, then, tangent to the observer's path at the origin. In this world centered coordinate frame, the current (x, y) coordinates of the observer are

$$x(t) = \int_o^t v(t') \cos \left(\int_o^{t'} \omega(t'') dt'' \right) dt' \tag{11.7}$$

$$y(t) = \int_o^t v(t') \sin \left(\int_o^{t'} \omega(t'') dt'' \right) dt'. \tag{11.8}$$

The conversion to the observer-centered polar coordinates is given by $r = \sqrt{x^2 + y^2}$ and $\varphi = \arg(x, y) - \arg(x', y') + \pi$, where, x' and y' are the derivatives of x and y with respect to time.

The mathematics of path integration, which we have analyzed here only in the plane, is essentially an application of the fundamental theorem of local curve theory (cf. do Carmo 1976). This theorem states that curves in space are fully defined by their local curvature and torsion, except for global displacement and rotation of the entire curve. (For explanations of the concepts "curvature" and torsion" cf. Section 10.2.2 and Fig. 10.9.) In the case considered here, in the plane, the torsion is everywhere zero, and the curvature depends on the ratio of v and ω. Path integration in three-dimensional space must also account for roll movements (rotations about the tangent vector of the path) of the observer. If this is done, the fundamental theorem guarantees that path integration is possible in three-dimensional space as well.

Path integration is intolerant of errors, since, errors do not correct themselves as time passes, but instead accumulate. This problem can be avoided only by making use of additional sources of information in navigation. The compass has already been mentioned, and replaces the inner integral in Equations 11.7, 11.8. The information most commonly used for calibrating path integration is provided by landmarks.

11.2 Navigation using landmarks

The concept of *landmarks* is not a precisely defined one. Let us first make a distinction between the function of landmarks—the role they play in navigation—and their identification in the image, i.e. the image computations involved in their recognition.

11.2.1 Functions of landmarks

Some functions of landmarks have already been indicated in Fig. 11.1c. In the simplest case, that of search, the destination is also the landmark. In aiming, the destination is characterized by a landmark visible from a distance, and toward which the observer proceeds. The observer must in this case orient towards the landmark and then proceed in the direction of view. If the destination itself is not marked, but instead is located, for example, in a particular place in a clearing in a forest, then so-called guidance or piloting also comes into use (O'Keefe & Nadel 1978, Trullier et al. 1997). This is motion to a location from which a number of landmarks appear at certain angles (bearings) to one another. A location in the clearing might, for example, be characterized in that the top of the tallest tree is 30 degrees to the left of the top of the second-tallest tree as seen from that point.

A standard experiment in guidance uses a circular basin filled with an opaque liquid. At one location just under the surface, there is a small platform. A rat dropped into the basin learns to swim to the invisible platform by examining the configuration of landmarks visible above the wall of the basin (the Morris water maze, Morris 1981). Analysis of search patterns in honeybees after landmarks have been moved has shown that they possess a similar mechanism (Cartwright & Collett 1982).

For the mechanisms described so far, the landmarks define the ultimate goal of the navigation. In order to construct longer routes from series of aimings or other navigation mechanisms, an additional landmark function, that of direction, or recognition-triggered response, is needed (O'Keefe & Nadel 1978; Trullier et al., 1997). In this case, the landmark is stored in memory, but an action also is stored which is to be carried out when the landmark is recognized, that is, when the location it defines is reached. Such actions can, for example, be decisions about which direction to take, for example "here, turn 50 degrees to the left and proceed." More general types of actions would be, for example, "here, go up the stairs" or "here, follow the wall"; a navigation system for autonomous robots based on this mechanism has been described by Kuipers & Byun (1991). Even when navigation is carried out as a series of guidances, direction plays a part: after each intermediate destination is reached, the landmark information characterizing the next intermediate destination must be retrieved from memory and "loaded" into the guidance mechanism.

11.2.2 Local position information

For the purpose of defining a landmark, all of the receptor signals which can be received at a given location and with a given direction of view are collectively called the *local position information*. At least in first establishing this concept, no distinction

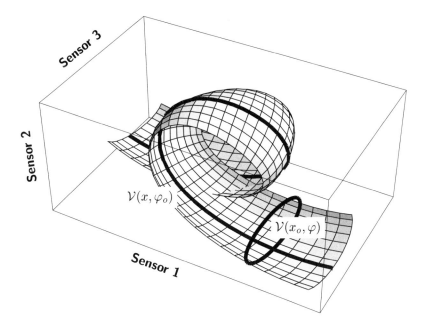

Figure 11.3
Diagram of the image manifold $\mathcal{V}$ for an agent with three point sensors (generating three-pixel "images"), which moves in a straight line and can rotate. The longitudinal curve $\mathcal{V}(x, \varphi_o)$ connects the "images" which the agent sees if it moves in translation while its orientation φ_o remains fixed; the images in the loop $\mathcal{V}(x_o, \varphi)$ appear if the agent rotates while at the fixed location x_o. The manifold's self-intersection indicates that identical images can occur at different locations. The illustration shows only a part of the manifold $\mathcal{V}$; since the image which appears after a full turn of the agent must be the same as at the beginning, the entire surface is closed, like a tube. For agents which can move in a plane, the manifold is three-dimensional, and it can therefore no longer be represented graphically.

is made among the different sensory modalities. The local position information for each location and each direction of view may be described by a data vector whose number of dimensions N corresponds to the number of receptors: if we consider a robot equipped only with a single camera, N is the number of pixels on the camera target. Without excluding other sense modalities, we will call the vector of the local position information a "view", $\mathcal{V}(x, y, \varphi)$. The totality of the views which an earth-bound observer with sensors fixed to its body can have as input within an environment $U \subset \mathbb{R}^2$ forms a three-dimensional manifold (two dimensions for position, one for the direction of view), which can be described by the parameterization

$$\mathcal{V} : U \times S^1 \to \mathbb{R}^N. \tag{11.9}$$

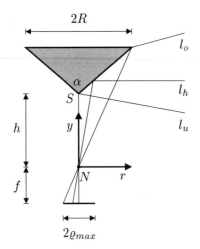

Camera parameters:

R	upper radius of the cone
α	apex angle of the cone
h	distance between S and N
f	focal length
ϱ_{max}	$= fR/(h + R\cot\frac{\alpha}{2})$

Projection formula in cylindrical coordinates,
(r, y), *for* $r \geq 0$, $r\cot\alpha \leq y - h \leq r\cot\frac{\alpha}{2}$:

$$(r, y) \mapsto \varrho$$

$$\varrho = -f\frac{-r\cos\alpha + (y - h)\sin\alpha}{r\sin\alpha + (y - h)\cos\alpha + h}$$

Figure 11.4

Imaging geometry of a conical mirror camera. N camera nodal point; T apex of conical mirror; l_u upper limiting ray; h horizontal ray; l_l lower limiting ray. The conical mirror allows omni-directional images to be captured without rotating the camera. A ring-shaped visual field between l_l and l_u is mapped as a circular disk whose radius is ρ_{max}. The visual field includes the horizon if $\alpha > 90°$ and $R > -h\cos\alpha\tan\frac{\alpha}{2}$.

Here, N is the number of receptors. S^1 represents the unit circle, i.e., the directions of view. Fig. 11.3 illustrates the manifold of images for an observer with three point sensors. In this case, the "views" are points in a three-dimensional space. For real sensors with finite resolution, the image manifold is continuous and differentiable. Curves in the manifold correspond to the optical flow which the observer perceives while traveling along the corresponding curve in the domain of $\mathcal{V}$ (Equation 11.9).

The parameterization of the image manifold by the coordinates of the observer suggests that landmark navigation may be regarded as the deduction of these coordinates from the local position information, i.e., as the inversion of $\mathcal{V}$. However, the observer will not explicitly know this parameterization, though it can be inferred from path integration. Moreover, in purely visual navigation, the aim is to proceed entirely without any knowledge of the external coordinates, and to characterize locations solely on the basis of the local position information. The navigation mechanisms briefly described above—aiming, guidance and direction—are of this type; no knowledge of the coordinates of a location characterized by landmarks is necessary.

The concept of local position information makes it possible to compare the different mechanisms for landmark definition. These mechanisms differ primarily in the degree of invariance in the recognition of a location which has been visited before.

11.2.3   Examples

Snapshots

The simplest way to apply local position information to navigation is to use the captured images or snapshots directly. To suppress noise, uneven illumination or small inaccuracies in the camera alignment, some smoothing operation will always be applied (cf. Chapter 3). Cartwright & Collett (1982) also describe edge detector outputs as "snapshots". An important property of snapshots is that landmarks are not segmented as regions in an image, and that they are not identified as objects.

Navigation using snapshots generally requires the largest possible field of view, while image quality is of lesser importance. A camera system which is especially well adapted to these requirements consists of a camera pointed upward, above which is mounted a conical mirror (Yagi et al. 1995; Chahl & Srinivasan 1996; Franz & Mallot 2000). There appears in the image plane a circular image of the surroundings in all directions. The imaging geometry is shown in Fig. 11.4.

As an example of a snapshot-based algorithm, let us consider the problem of guidance, Fig. 11.1c. If the image at a destination $\vec{z}$ is known, then within a certain distance from $\vec{z}$ it is possible to calculate the direction in which it is necessary to move to reach the destination. The region within which this is possible is called the catchment area of $\vec{z}$. In theory, it is possible to use the algorithms for determining egomotion from optical flow to determine the direction to the destination. This process was described in Chapter 10. First, the displacement vector field between the stored image at the destination and the currently visible image is calculated. Cartwright & Collett (1982) choose for this task a feature-based motion detector, i.e., they solve the correspondence problem for the features of the two images. The result is the flow field for a movement from the destination to the current location. The flow field may include a rotation in addition to a translation, since the current direction of view generally is different from the direction of view when the image at the destination was stored. Once the rotational component is removed, the destination lies in the direction of the point of contraction of the remaining translational field.

An algorithm which avoids the explicit calculation of the displacement field is proposed by Franz et al. (1998b). In this case, too, it is assumed that the snapshot visible at the destination is known. We designate it as $V_{\vec{z}}(\vartheta) := \mathcal{V}(\vec{z}, \vartheta)$. Here, ϑ is the direction of view, i.e., the position on the one-dimensional ring sensor. The idea is to predict how the image will change if the observer proceeds in a specific direction, using the information in the current snapshot $V_{\vec{x}}(\vartheta)$. The movements for which views are predicted are described in terms of their direction α, their distance D and observer rotation ω (cf. Fig. 11.5a). An object which is imaged before the movement at the point ϑ, is imaged after the movement at the location ϑ', given by the transformation $T_{d,\alpha,\omega}$:

$$\vartheta' = T_{d,\alpha,\omega}(\vartheta) := \arg(\sin\vartheta - d\cos\alpha, \ \cos\vartheta - d\sin\alpha) + \omega. \qquad (11.10)$$

Here, $d = D/r$ is the distance traveled relative to the distance from the imaged object, r. The arg-function was defined in Equation 11.2.

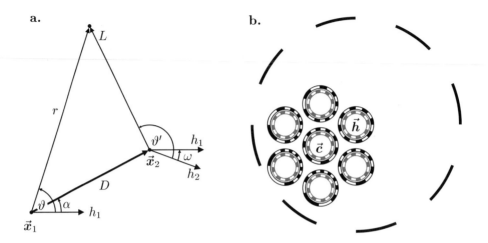

Figure 11.5
Guidance using snapshots. **a.** Diagram showing the trigonometric calculation of
displacement of the image of a landmark L as the observer moves from $\vec{x}_1$ to $\vec{x}_2$ (see
Equation 11.10). h_1, h_2: observer heading. **b.** View-prediction scheme for guidance
proposed by Franz et al. (1998b). The large, outer ring shows a configuration of
landmarks. $\vec{h}$: "home position", at which a snapshot was taken. This snapshot
is stored in long-term memory shown as the inner, gray and white ring for each
observer position. $\vec{c}$: present observer position with the current image (outer, black
and white ring). For each of the other positions, the outer ring shows the image
which is predicted from the current image and the movement from $\vec{c}$ to each point,
using Equation 11.11. The best agreement occurs for the correct movement toward
the upper right.

    This formula makes it possible to predict how the current image $V_{\vec{x}}$ will change
when a motion is carried out. The equation

$$V_{\vec{x}_2}(\vartheta) \approx V_{\vec{x}_1}(T_{d,\alpha,\omega}(\vartheta)) \tag{11.11}$$

applies to this situation. The most important source of error for the approximation
here is the implicit assumption that all landmarks are equally distant from the current
position, and so that the quantity d is the same for all directions of view ϑ.
    Fig. 11.5b illustrates the process. At a starting position ("home") $\vec{h}$, a snapshot
was taken, showing eight wall sections arrayed in a circle. This snapshot $V_{\vec{h}}(\vartheta)$ is
indicated by the inner, gray ring at all illustrated positions. The outer ring at the
position $\vec{c}$ (the current position) represents the snapshot $V_{\vec{c}}(\vartheta)$ which is visible at that
position; this snapshot, and especially its lower part, differs from the stored snapshot.
The views $V_{\vec{c}}(T_{0.4,\alpha,0}(\vartheta))$ predicted by Equation 11.11 for the other positions are
shown; the quantities $d = 0.4$ and $\omega = 0$ have been assigned arbitrarily. It can be
seen that the snapshot predicted for a motion toward the upper right ($\alpha = 30°$) agrees

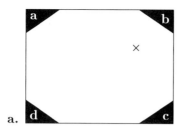 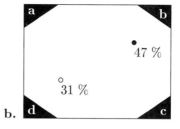

Figure 11.6

Diagram of an experiment by Cheng (1986) indicating that rats use geometrically defined landmarks. A rectangular maze was used whose four corners, here indicated by a, b, c, d, are all easily distinguished from one another visually and by their odors. **a.** The rats find a feeding station at, for example, the location indicated by ×. **b.** After part of the feed has been consumed, the rats are removed from the maze and, after a short time, placed in an identical maze. In 47 out of 100 cases, the rats searched for the feed at the correct position (•); in 31 cases, they searched at the opposite corner (○). At that corner, the geometrical configuration was correct, but the texture and odor were not.

best with the stored snapshot. In a practical applications, the difference E between the stored and expected snapshot is calculated for a number of directions of movement α and distances D, and then the movement which minimizes the difference is chosen:

$$E(d,\alpha) \quad := \quad \min_{\omega} \int (V_{\vec{x}}(T_{d,\alpha,\omega}(\vartheta)) - V_{\vec{h}}(\vartheta))^2 \, d\vartheta \qquad (11.12)$$

$$(d^*,\alpha^*) \quad := \quad \mathrm{argmin}_{(d,\alpha)} E(d,\alpha). \qquad (11.13)$$

This process was tested in real environments with an autonomous robot using the panoramic camera sketched in Fig. 11.4, and produced satisfactory results already with a small number of pixels (about 70 for a ring-shaped image).

Geometry and texture

In addition to the distributions of gray values or colors in snapshots, depth information may also be used as local position information. This depth information can be derived using the processes described in Part III (stereopsis, motion parallax, etc.). In this case, as with snapshots, the landmarks are not necessarily identified as objects. Rather, the "map" of gray values or colors may simply be replaced or supplemented by a map of depth values.

Experimental evidence for the use of geometrical information has been provided in rats (Cheng 1986; cf. Fig. 11.6). Rats were trained to go to a corner of a rectangular box identified by a cue card exhibiting a characteristic visual and olfactory pattern. If the rats' orientation was disturbed by taking them out of the box and replacing them with a random orientation after a period of time, they then looked not only in the corner marked by the card with the correct pattern, but also in another corner which had the correct geometrical configuration: that is, for example, long side of the box on the left of the corner and short side on the right. The geometrical configuration therefore proved to play an important role in this case. Hermer & Spelke (1994) performed similar experiments which show that young children at ages of 18 – 24 months favor geometric information while adults pay more attention to color information.

Identified landmarks

A further processing step consists of identifying objects in images and then recognizing them in images from different points of view. Objects identified in this way will here be called identified landmarks. For navigation in relatively small environments, it is sufficient simply to use salient image features in this way, in which case the problem of identification is reduced to the correspondence problem which we have already examined in connection with stereoscopic vision and motion. In general, however, landmark identification requires that objects be recognized as such.

Barycentric coordinates.   If landmarks are isolated objects standing on a plane, such as trees in a park, it is generally possible to determine the points at which these objects stand. Their height in the image conveys information about their distance from the observer. O'Keefe (1991) assumes that the values of two coordinates of each landmark in observer-centered coordinates are known. It is then possible to describe and store the observer's position in terms of a vector to the average position of the landmarks and the longest axis of the landmark group (the *"slope"*). A generalization of this approach uses *barycentric coordinates* (Prescott 1996). In this approach, every point $\vec{z}$ of the plane is regarded as a weighted average of three reference points which do not lie in a straight line, $\vec{l}_1, \vec{l}_2, \vec{l}_3$:

$$\vec{z} = \beta_1 \vec{l}_1 + \beta_2 \vec{l}_2 + \beta_3 \vec{l}_3 \quad \text{where} \quad \beta_1 + \beta_2 + \beta_3 = 1 \qquad (11.14)$$

Here, $(\beta_1, \beta_2, \beta_3)$ are the barycentric coordinates of $\vec{z}$. Let us assume that $\vec{l}_1$ through $\vec{l}_3$ are the points where identified landmarks are located in the plane and $\vec{z}$ is a destination. If the locations are transformed into homogeneous coordinates (Section 2.3.4), then Equation 11.14 still holds, since $\sum \beta_i = 1$. As was shown in Section 2.3.4, homogeneous coordinates make it possible to describe projection onto a camera at any position as a multiplication by a matrix P. Since this operation is linear, the relationship 11.14 still holds. Therefore, the homogeneous coordinates of the destination, $\tilde{z}$, can be described as a linear combination of the homogeneous coordinates of the landmark points using the unchanged weightings β_i. This approach is clearly valid for all projection matrices P, and so for all points of view from which the three landmarks are visible. If, then, the position of the destination $\vec{z}$ relative to the three landmarks has been learned once in the form of the barycentric coordinates $(\beta_1, \beta_2, \beta_3)$, it is possible to determine the position of the destination from the positions of the landmarks in the image, $\tilde{l}_i$, by means of the relationship $\tilde{z} = \sum \beta_i \tilde{l}_i$. The position of $\vec{z}$ in the image is clearly the value which is relevant in navigation.

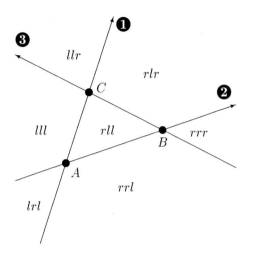

Figure 11.7
Tessellation of the plane into regions by means of three landmarks A, B, C and three directed lines $\overline{AC}$ (1), $\overline{AB}$ (2) and $\overline{BC}$ (3). The central triangle (rll) may, for example, be characterized as being to the right of line 1 and to the left of lines 2 and 3. For the selected directions of the lines, no region with the characteristic lrr exists.

Discrete landmark configurations. Two landmarks A and B, considered once again as points in a plane, define a line dividing the plane into two parts. Let us give the line a direction, (let us say, from A toward B) and say that we are to the right of $\overline{AB}$ if B appears to be to the right of A. If A and B are not simultaneously within view, then we determine whether the angle between A and B is smaller than 180 degrees. In this case, we are also to the right of $\overline{AB}$, and otherwise, to the left. Fig. 11.7 shows how this rule and three landmarks can separate the plane into regions which can each be identified according to the side of each of the three lines on which they lie.

This process and similar ones for the definition of locations using discrete configurations of landmarks were already suggested by Gibson (1979); Penna & Wu (1993) survey the topic. In practice, this approach, like the previous one, is applicable only with difficulty, because the required image processing, namely the identification of the landmarks, is generally complicated. Bachelder & Waxman (1994) avoid this problem by using small lamps as landmarks. In this case, it is possible to guide an autonomous robot using the process illustrated in Fig. 11.7.

The classification of landmarks here, according to their definitions and functions, is clearly not complete. Landmarks can, for example, also function as compasses when they are distant from the observer. An interesting case is the perception of geographical slant, which can be used not only as local position information, but also as a compass, at least when a slant continues for some distance (Mallot et al. 2000). Finally, landmarks are not defined and stored in memory for all locations, but only for those where they are relevant to future navigation needs: in behavior experiments, test subjects perceive changes in landmarks better when they occur near places where paths diverge (Aginsky et al. 1997).

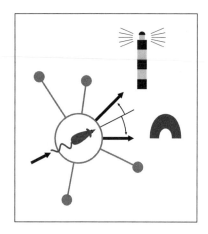

Figure 11.8
Goal-dependent flexibility is the hallmark of cognition. The observer recognizes the current landmark configuration. Recognition does not, however, lead directly to a movement selection, as is the case with a simple recognition-triggered response. Rather, the observer "knows" that it is necessary to turn left to reach the lighthouse, and right to reach the igloo. Therefore, the observer can flexibly choose a direction depending on the pursued goal, even if this goal is not currently visible. The knowledge needed to accomplish this task is called a *cognitive map*.

11.3 Constructed environments

11.3.1 Directions, routes and cognitive maps

Up to this point, we have assumed that a single application of one of the mechanisms presented in Fig. 11.1 is sufficient to reach a destination. In examining guidance, for example, we considered only the case in which the observer is already inside the "catchment area", i.e., within visual range of the stored landmark configuration. In exceptional cases, the distances which can be covered using such mechanisms can be very large; for example, a flight from the equator to the North Pole guided by the pole star involves only a single guidance. Generally, however, this process runs up against its limits very quickly. Clearly, it is not possible to navigate to a neighboring room in a building using the described snapshot process.

A way around this problem is provided by the direction or recognition-triggered response mechanism already illustrated in Fig. 11.1. First, a particular landmark configuration is recognized. In addition to this landmark configuration, memory also holds information on how to proceed from the recognized location to the destination. This information may be directional, such as "turn left here", or may describe more complex sequences of behaviors, such as "follow the street here until you see landmark L." Experimental evidence of such recognition-triggered responses exists, for example, for insects (Collett & Baron 1995) and humans (Mallot & Gillner 2000). Series of recognition-triggered-responses define what are called routes, and are very useful for navigation in complex environments (cf. O'Keefe & Nadel 1978, Kuipers 1978).

Cognitive behavior is that in which an organism is able to react flexibly to the surroundings depending on the intended goal or destination. In this case, the behavior is determined not only by the current inputs to the senses and contents of memory, but also by the organism's goals and by knowledge of how these goals can be reached. For spatial cognition, it is therefore necessary to have knowledge such as "if I want to get from here to destination A, I must turn left, but to get to destination B, I must turn right" (cf. Fig. 11.8). The memory for this type of knowledge is called a *cognitive map* (Tolman 1948, O'Keefe & Nadel 1978). On the level of behavioral tasks, this type of memory makes possible (i) latent learning (as opposed to learning by reinforcement), (ii) goal-dependent flexibility in planning routes and (iii) transfer of knowledge of one route to another which partially overlaps it. In the terminology of neuropsychology, the cognitive map is a declarative memory of space (cf. Squire 1987). Cognitive maps appear to occur within the animal kingdom only in vertebrates; insects can definitely find their way home from different locations by memory, but can not figure out how to travel directly from one of these locations to another. Their memory therefore does not include branching, and is for this reason not cognitive in the sense described above (Collett 1993, Wehner & Menzel 1990).

11.3.2 Topological navigation[*]

On the basis of the directing function of individual landmarks, memory of routes can be understood as a series of individual direction events. Analogously, a cognitive map can be constructed if networks or graphs are considered, instead of only chains of directions or recognition-triggered responses. The nodes of such graphs are recognized landmarks (or locations), while the edges between them correspond to the actions which lead from one location to the next. As is usual in graph theory, the edge therefore contains information about *both* nodes which it connects; the directing function therefore includes not only the action which is to be performed at a given landmark, but also the accompanying expectation of the landmark to which this action will lead. This additional information would not be necessary in the case of pure navigation along a route, but for planning of a route in an actual graph, it is indispensable. Behavior experiments with test subjects suggest that even in navigation along routes, there is knowledge about the next intermediate destination (McNamara et al. 1984). Many ideas in the field of topological navigation are based on the work of Kuipers (1978) and Kuipers & Byun (1991); an up-to-date survey has been provided by Trullier et al. (1997).

Place and view graphs in mazes

How complex must the recognition process be for locations and landmarks in order to allow for the construction of a cognitive map organized as a graph? Fig. 11.9 shows two possibilities (Schölkopf & Mallot 1995). In the first possibility, the nodes of the graph represent locations or places in space. This type of memory organization requires a mechanism which decides where the observer is on the basis of the presently visible landmarks—and independently of the current direction of view. The arrows in the graphs can then describe the movement which is necessary, for example, to get from location p_3 to location p_2, but only in external coordinates: for example, toward

---

[*]In mathematics, *topology* is the study of neighborhoods in sets. In finite sets, arbitrary neighborhoods may be described by graphs.

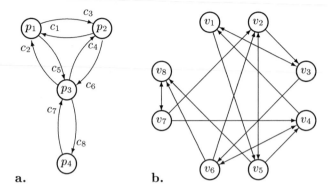

Figure 11.9
a. Illustration of a simple maze with the locations p_i as a directed graph of places. Each corridor between two locations is represented by two arrows c_j pointing in opposite directions. **b.** The corresponding view graph. Each node v_i corresponds to the view when traveling along the corridor c_i with the same subscript i. Further explanations are to be found in the text.

the northeast. The observer must use additional, compass information to arrive at a decision about the direction in which to turn in order actually to arrive at p_2.

A less computationally intensive solution is shown in Fig. 11.9b. Here, the nodes of the graphs represent individual views of the landmarks, or snapshots, as seen when traveling along one of the arrows in the place graph of Fig. 11.9a. Each arrow in the place graph corresponds to a different view and is therefore represented by its own node in the view graph; the example of Fig. 11.9b therefore has eight nodes. The links between the nodes of the view graph, then, reflect the time sequence of the views while traveling through the maze. Two views are connected if they can be seen one after the other without intermediate views. The view graph contains the same information as the place graph, but it has the advantages (i), that recognition is simplified, since the current location need no longer be determined on the basis of the current view, and (ii), that the links between nodes are associated directly with egocentric decisions about movements, so that a compass is no longer necessary.

Graph-based navigation in open environments

The graph-based approach to modeling of cognitive maps works especially well with labyrinths, whose branches and corridors correspond to the nodes and links of the graphs. This approach can, however, be extended to open environments by selecting discrete points and storing them, along with relationships to the neighboring points, as a graph. Considering again the manifold of all possible images within an environment discussed in Section 11.2.2 and Fig. 11.3, this process can be described by sampling the image manifold $\mathcal{V}$ and then approximating its intrinsic geometry, rather than its parameterization, by means of a graph (Fig. 11.10). This will work only if the observer

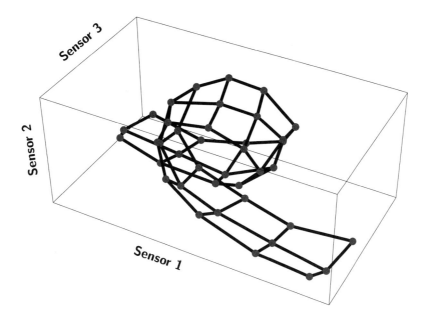

Figure 11.10
Representation of the image manifold of Fig. 11.3 as a graph. At each node, a snapshot is stored. The distances are chosen such that the location at which the snapshot is taken is within the catchment area of all neighboring snapshots. With knowledge of this graph, the robot can plan paths as series of snapshots and can proceed stepwise along these paths using the guidance mechanism described in Fig. 11.5.

is able to find the nodes of the graph reliably. One possible mechanism for achieving this is guidance.

Franz et al. (1998a) describe a navigation system for open environments which combines a view graph of the type shown in Fig. 11.10 with the guidance mechanism using snapshots of Section 11.2.3. A robot begins at a starting point, where it takes a snapshot. Then it travels in a randomly chosen direction while comparing the current view with the stored one. Similarity of views is measured as the maximum of the cross-correlation function. If this falls below a certain threshold, the robot takes a new snapshot. Then it chooses a new direction to explore and continues as before, but comparing the current image with all stored snapshots. The process as described so far permits the robot to learn a series of views and their relationships as neighbors, i.e., a route. The representation becomes a true, cross-linked graph if the robot comes upon a view which is similar to a previously stored snapshot. In this case, the robot attempts to navigate toward the location at which that view was captured, using the homing algorithm sketched in Fig. 11.5. If the attempt succeeds, a cross-link is drawn in the graph.

The described process is dependent only on guidance using snapshots and on rep-

resentation as a graph. Because of the requirement to take new snapshots whenever
the similarity between images sinks below a threshold, the view graph which is constructed samples the image manifold at points which are approximately equidistant
from one another. In spatial coordinates, this means that more snapshots will be
taken in regions where the image changes rapidly, for example in narrow passages.
The coordinates of the space, nonetheless, play no role in the navigation system which
has just been sketched.

11.3.3   Metric and cognitive maps

In geography, a "map" resembles an aerial view, i.e., a two-dimensional representation
of an environment in which angles and scaled distances are maintained as accurately as
possible. Maps of this type are metrically organized; the Euclidean distance between
each two points on the map satisfies a mathematical distance function* which relates
it to a distance in the mapped environment. We therefore call such maps "metric."
Cognitive maps, on the other hand, are characterized by their allowing certain behaviors, such as planning of new paths, to be performed. In the section on topological
navigation, it was shown that that metric representations are not necessarily required
for this task.

Nonetheless, the role of metric information in the cognitive map is of great interest.
Gallistel (1990) points out, for example, that the metric organization of a cognitive
map allows different types of information, such as path integration and landmarks,
to be coordinated. The practical usefulness of metric maps probably consists largely
in their making it possible to plan shortcuts across territory which has not yet been
explored.

Metric information can enter into the representation of location in at least three
ways. Even the simplest type of memory of space, the "home vector" (Section 11.1),
which is defined through path integration, is metric. In topological navigation (Section 11.3.2), distance information can be associated with the links of the landmark
graphs as additional data. Finally, place graphs, along with the local metric information associated with their links, may be embedded into a global metric representation
by multidimensional (here actually two-dimensional) scaling, as used in multivariant
statistics (cf. Mardia et al. 1979). In cognitive psychology, a spatial representation
which is embedded in a global metric frame is known as "survey knowledge".

In conventional robotics, the attempt usually is made from the outset to represent
spatial knowledge as metric maps, for example in the form of a Cartesian point grid
in which objects or obstacles are mapped (an *occupancy grid*). It is of interest that
including a secondary topological component in the representation has proven useful, for example by separating the grid into connected regions and representing the
relationships between neighboring regions in a graph (Thrun 1998).

---

*A distance function d must meet the following four conditions: (i) Distances are not negative
($d(\vec{x}, \vec{y}) \geq 0$); (ii) The distance between two points is zero if and only if the two points coincide
($d(\vec{x}, \vec{y}) = 0 \Leftrightarrow \vec{x} = \vec{y}$); (iii) The distance function is symmetrical ($d(\vec{x}, \vec{y}) = d(\vec{y}, \vec{x})$); and (iv) The
triangular inequality $d(\vec{x}, \vec{z}) \leq d(\vec{x}, \vec{y}) + d(\vec{y}, \vec{z})$ holds.

11.4 Neurophysiology of spatial memory

A structure in the brain which is commonly thought to be involved in the acquisition of spatial memories is the hippocampus. In humans, this function has been demonstrated, for example, by direct observation of brain activity of test subjects solving navigation tasks in a virtual labyrinth (Maguire 1997). Comparative studies in different species of food-storing corvid birds have shown that the size of the hippocampus correlates with the ability to return to food caches (Clayton & Krebs 1995). In rats and some other rodents, finally, electrophysiological recording from individual cells has demonstrated the existence of what are called *place cells* (O'Keefe & Nadel 1978; Eichenbaum 1996). These neurons are active when the rat passes by a particular place, and so they code for location.

Place cells have a number of interesting characteristics which will be summarized here. The location at which a given place cell is active is called the cell's "place field." This somewhat peculiar concept is analogous to that of the receptive field of a sensory neuron. A typical test maze, for example a cross-shaped maze whose greatest length is one meter, is covered by approximately 10 to 20 such place fields. The place fields of different neurons can overlap, and so population coding can occur (Wilson & McNaughton 1993). The arrangement of the place cells in the hippocampus is not topographic: that is, neighboring cells do not generally have neighboring place fields. Possibly related to this finding is another, that one and the same place cell has different place fields if the rat is moved from one maze to another (Wilson & McNaughton 1993). With respect to the cognitive map, two additional characteristics are of particular interest. One is that the activation of the place cells is independent of the destination toward which the rat is currently traveling (Speakman & O'Keefe 1990). This characteristic is required for declarative memory. The other interesting characteristic is that place cells apparently react not only to landmarks, but also to information about egomotion. If, for example, lighting is turned off after the exploration phase, the place fields persist: the place cells therefore know, so to speak, the rat's present location (O'Keefe & Speakman 1987). A model of the interaction of information about landmarks and egomotion in the place cells based on a landmark graph with labels for ego-motions has been proposed by McNaughton et al. (1996).

There is still debate about the significance of the hippocampal place cells in spatial memory. In rats, the head direction cells found in neighboring brain regions also play an important role in navigation. These cells respond to certain head directions of the rat, irrespective of its position; they thus represent compass information (Taube 1998). In primates, no actual place cells have been found so far; instead, there are so-called "view cells", which are specific not to the location of the observer but to the angle of view to a particular object or scene (Rolls et al. 1998). Moreover, the hippocampus is not the only structure in the brain which participates in navigation tasks. In navigating test subjects, activity also occurs in the parietal lobes of the cerebral cortex. More specifically, different regions of the brain participate, depending on whether the test subject is trying to identify landmarks or is envisioning motion along a route (Berthoz 1997).

Part V

Appendix

Glossary of mathematical terms[*]

Angle: For the angle φ which is enclosed by the two vectors $\vec{a}, \vec{b}$, the following relationship holds:

$$\cos \varphi = \frac{(\vec{a} \cdot \vec{b})}{\|\vec{a}\| \cdot \|\vec{b}\|}.$$

Here, $(\vec{a} \cdot \vec{b})$ is the →dot product of $\vec{a}$ and $\vec{b}$. Because $\cos \frac{\pi}{2} = 0$, the formula agrees with the definition of →orthogonality.

A geometric explanation is given in Fig. G.1. Let $\vec{b'}$ be the orthogonal projection of the vector $\vec{a}$ onto the vector $\vec{b}$. Since $\vec{b'}$ is parallel to $\vec{b}$, clearly

$$\vec{b'} = \frac{\|\vec{b'}\|}{\|\vec{b}\|} \cdot \vec{b}.$$

Since we want to calculate the cosine of φ, the projection should naturally be such that $\vec{b'}$ and therefore $\vec{b}$ is orthogonal to $\vec{a} - \vec{b'}$. Therefore,

$$(\vec{b} \cdot (\vec{a} - \frac{\|\vec{b'}\|}{\|\vec{b}\|} \cdot \vec{b})) = 0 \;\; \text{and furthermore} \;\; (\vec{b} \cdot \vec{a}) = \frac{\|\vec{b'}\|}{\|\vec{b}\|} (\vec{b} \cdot \vec{b}).$$

Since $\|\vec{b}\|^2 = (\vec{b} \cdot \vec{b})$, it follows that $\|\vec{b'}\| = (\vec{a} \cdot \vec{b})/\|\vec{b}\|$ and therefore, since $\cos \varphi = \|\vec{b'}\|/\|\vec{a}\|$, the assertion is proven.

Basis: →coordinate system

---

[*]This glossary is intended to serve only as an introduction. A general reference for advanced issues is Korn & Korn (1968). Recommended textbooks on relevant subfields of mathematics include Rudin (1976; analytical calculus), Penna & Patterson (1986; projective geometry), and do Carmo (1976; differential geometry).

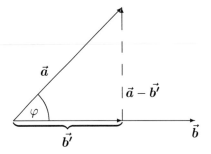

Fig. G.1
Definition of an angle

Bayes formula: Let us consider two overlapping events A, B from the same statistical population Ω ($\rightarrow$probability). If B has already occurred, then

$$P(A|B) = \frac{P(A)}{P(A \cap B)}$$

(read this as "P of A, given B") is the conditional probability of A, given B. The set B thus more or less takes on the role of the statistical population Ω, within which the event $A \cap B$ is considered. The following basic relationship can be determined (the Bayes formula):

$$P(A|B) = \frac{P(B|A)P(A)}{P(B)} = \frac{P(B|A)P(A)}{P(B|A)P(A) + P(B|\neg A)P(\neg A)}.$$

Here, $\neg A = \Omega \backslash A$ is the complement of A. For an application of the formula in the context of this book, see Section 8.4.3.

Cauchy-Schwarz inequality: Consider a vector space with a $\rightarrow$dot product. Then, for any two vectors $\vec{a}, \vec{b}$ in that vector space,

$$(\vec{a} \cdot \vec{b}) \leq \|\vec{a}\| \, \|\vec{b}\|.$$

The equality if obtained if and only if $\vec{a}$ and $\vec{b}$ are parallel and point in the same direction, that is, if a $\lambda \geq 0$ exists such that $\vec{a} = \lambda \vec{b}$.

The projection of a vector onto another is, then, maximized if the two vectors are parallel. As it applies to $\rightarrow$function spaces, the inequality states that the covariance of two functions is smaller than or equal to the product of their standard deviations.

Chain rule: Consider two functions f, g such that the range of g is included in the domain of f. A composition function $h := f \circ g$ can be defined for which $h(x) = f(g(x))$. Then, for the derivative of h,

$$h'(x) = f'(g(x))g'(x).$$

If $f : \mathbb{R}^n \to \mathbb{R}$ is a function of n variables and $g : \mathbb{R}^m \to \mathbb{R}^n$ is a multidimensional transformation, then the chaining $h = f \circ g$ is valid from $\mathbb{R}^m$ to $\mathbb{R}$. For the →gradient of h,

$$\operatorname{grad} h(x_1, ..., x_m) = \operatorname{grad} f(g(x_1, ..., x_m))\ J_g(x_1, ..., x_m).$$

Here, J_g is the →Jacobi matrix of g; it has n rows and m columns.

Complex numbers: are more general than real numbers, and occur in the solutions of algebraic equations. Complex numbers form a two-dimensional plane (the complex plane) which is defined by the axes 1 and $i = \sqrt{-1}$. Each complex number can be represented by two real numbers, either in Cartesian coordinates:

$$z = x + iy$$

in which case x and y are called the real and imaginary parts of z, or in polar coordinates:

$$z = ae^{i\varphi} = a\cos\varphi + ia\sin\varphi.$$

(Euler's formula); a is called the absolute value or modulus and φ, the phase of z. Addition is performed in the usual way, as is multiplication, except that $i^2 = -1$. The polar representation clearly shows that multiplication of complex numbers can be thought of as rotation and scaling in the complex plane.

Continuity: A function is said to be continuous at a point x_o, if, for each series in its domain which converges at the limit x_o, the series of the corresponding function values also converges at the limit $f(x_o)$. Simply stated, this means that it is possible to draw the →graph of the function "without lifting the pencil".

Convolution: For two integrable functions f, g, the function

$$h = f * g; \quad h(x) := \int f(x' - x)\, g(x')\, dx',$$

is the convolution of f and g, if the integral exists (cf. Section 3.3.1). In addition to the examples from image processing discussed in this book, convolution has other applications, for example, in mathematical statistics, where the probability density of the sum of two random variables is the convolution of the individual probability densities. If the input signals are processed through the →Fourier transform, multiplying the results together is the equivalent of convolving the original signals (convolution theorem, Equation 3.22).

If one of the two input functions, let us say f, is fixed, then

$$\varphi \to f * \varphi$$

defines an →operator. In this case, f is called the kernel of the convolution operator.

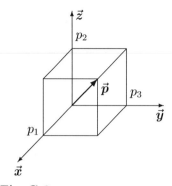

Fig. G.2
Coordinate system in three-dimensional space

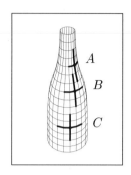

Fig. G.3
Gaussian curvature

Coordinate system: Let us consider as an example the intuitive three-dimensional space shown in (Fig. G.2). A coordinate system is defined by three basis vectors $\vec{x}$, $\vec{y}$, $\vec{z}$. These vectors are of length 1 and are all orthogonal to one another (orthonormal system). Each point in the space can be described by three numbers:

$$\vec{p} = p_1 \vec{x} + p_2 \vec{y} + p_3 \vec{z} =: \begin{pmatrix} p_1 \\ p_2 \\ p_3 \end{pmatrix}.$$

If the column representation of vectors introduced here is applied to the basis vectors themselves, then:

$$\vec{x} = \begin{pmatrix} 1 \\ 0 \\ 0 \end{pmatrix} ; \quad \vec{y} = \begin{pmatrix} 0 \\ 1 \\ 0 \end{pmatrix} ; \quad \vec{z} = \begin{pmatrix} 0 \\ 0 \\ 1 \end{pmatrix}.$$

Correlation: In statistics, the correlation of two random variables X, Y is defined as the quantity

$$cor(X,Y) := \frac{E((X - EX)(Y - EY))}{\sqrt{E((X - EX)^2)E((Y - EY)^2)}}.$$

Here, $E(Z)$ is the expected value of the of the random variable Z ("average of the population"). The numerator of the fraction is called the covariance.

In signal theory, the normalization is usually not performed, and therefore:

$$\varphi_{f,g} := \int f(x)\, g(x)\, dx.$$

Both definitions are identical if it is assumed: that the functions f and g have an average value of zero ($\int f(x)dx = \int g(x)dx = 0$); that the integral of the squared functions is 1 ($\int f^2(x)dx = \int g^2(x)dx = 1$); and that a spatial or time variable x takes the place of the random event in the random variable. The function

$$\Phi_{f,g}(s) := \int f(x+s)\,g(x)\,dx$$

is called the cross-correlation function of f and g.

Cross product: In three-dimensional vector space, a product of vectors can be defined whose result is again a vector. Let $\vec{p}, \vec{q} \in \mathbb{R}^3$ and $\vec{x}$, $\vec{y}$, $\vec{z}$ be the basis vectors; then:

$$\vec{p} \times \vec{q} := \begin{vmatrix} \mathbf{x} & \mathbf{y} & \mathbf{z} \\ p_1 & p_2 & p_3 \\ q_1 & q_2 & q_3 \end{vmatrix} = \begin{pmatrix} p_2 q_3 - p_3 q_2 \\ p_3 q_1 - p_1 q_3 \\ p_1 q_2 - p_2 q_1 \end{pmatrix} \in \mathbb{R}^3.$$

The vector $\vec{p} \times \vec{q}$ is orthogonal to both factors. Its length corresponds to the surface area of the parallelogram described by $\vec{p}$ and $\vec{q}$, $\|\vec{p} \times \vec{q}\| = \|\vec{p}\|\|\vec{q}\| \sin(\angle \vec{p}, \vec{q})$. The direction is defined by the "three-finger rule" where the directions of $\vec{p}, \vec{q}$ and $\vec{p} \times \vec{q}$ are given by the thumb, index, and middle finger of the right hand. The cross product is *not* commutative: $\vec{p} \times \vec{q} = -\vec{q} \times \vec{p}$.

Curvature: The curvature of a plane curve is the inverse of the radius of a circle which approximates the curve at a given point. The center of this circle is called the center of curvature. The curvature of planes is defined by first considering the normal to the surface. Each plane which includes a point on a surface and the normal to the surface at that point intersects with the surface along a plane curve whose curvature is defined as above. The curvatures so defined have a positive sign if the center of curvature is in the direction of the normal, and a negative sign if it is in the opposite direction. The largest and smallest curvatures among these (in terms of magnitude and sign) are the principal curvatures at the point; their product is the Gaussian curvature K.

Fig. G.3 shows three points with different Gaussian curvatures. In A, the centers of curvature for the two principal curvatures lie on different sides of the surface, and so K is negative (hyperbolic point or saddle point). In B, both centers of curvature lie on the same side of the surface, and the curvature is therefore positive (elliptical point). In C, the smallest curvature is 0, and so the Gaussian curvature is zero as well (parabolic point). On smooth surfaces, neighboring areas with negative and positive Gaussian curvatures are separated by lines composed of parabolic points.

The Gaussian curvature is what is called an "intrinsic" characteristic of the surface, which does not depend on the parameters used to describe the surface. Every transformation which changes the Gaussian curvature also changes distances on the surface.

Derivative: The derivative of a function of one variable is the limit value:

$$f'(x) := \lim_{h \to 0} \frac{f(x+h) - f(x)}{h},$$

and exists only if such a limit value exists. We call functions "differentiable" in x, if the derivative exists. The →graph of f then has a unique tangent at $(x, f(x))$, whose slope (tangent of the slope angle) is equal to the derivative.

Functions of more than one variable ("landscapes") can be differentiated with respect to each variable. Or, to express the same concept simply, a cross-section through the map is taken in the direction defined by one of the variables, and the cross-section is differentiated, see Fig. 7.5. If the cross section is taken along one of the coordinate axes, its derivative is called a *partial derivative* of f, for example:

$$\frac{\partial f(x,y)}{\partial x} = f_x(x,y) = \lim_{h \to 0} \frac{f(x+h,y) - f(x,y)}{h}.$$

A cross-section in a general direction $u = ax + by$ is called a directional derivative. It is related to the partial derivatives by:

$$f_u(x,y) = af_x(x,y) + bf_y(x,y).$$

→gradient; →Jacobi matrix.

Determinant: A determinant can be found for every quadratic matrix. The determinant is a number calculated in the following way for 2×2 matrices:

$$\begin{vmatrix} a_1 & a_2 \\ b_1 & b_2 \end{vmatrix} = a_1 b_2 - a_2 b_1.$$

For 3×3 matrices,

$$\begin{vmatrix} a_1 & a_2 & a_3 \\ b_1 & b_2 & b_3 \\ c_1 & c_2 & c_3 \end{vmatrix} = a_1 \begin{vmatrix} b_2 & b_3 \\ c_2 & c_3 \end{vmatrix} - a_2 \begin{vmatrix} b_1 & b_3 \\ c_1 & c_3 \end{vmatrix} + a_3 \begin{vmatrix} b_1 & b_2 \\ c_1 & c_2 \end{vmatrix}.$$

Differential equation: A differential equation is a conditional equation for functions which defines them in terms of the relationships between the values and derivatives of the functions. The highest derivative which is present in the equation is called the order of the equation. If the solution is a function of a single variable, the equation is called an *ordinary* differential equation. If, however, partial →derivatives occur in the equation and the solution is a function of various variables, the equation is called "partial".

Ordinary first-order differential equations can be described as directional fields and then solved graphically. For an equation of the form

$$f'(x) = D(x, f(x))$$

a line whose slope is $D(x, y)$ is drawn which passes through the location (x, y) in a coordinate system. At every such point, solutions of the differential equation must be tangent to the line. An example is shown in Fig. 7.9. A generalization of the directional field to partial differential equations is the Monge cone (Fig. 7.7).

Dimension (of a vector space): The largest number of →linearly independent vectors in a vector space is its dimension. For column vectors of the form

$$\vec{v} = \begin{pmatrix} v_1 \\ \vdots \\ v_m \end{pmatrix},$$

the dimension is m. The three-dimensional space $\mathbb{R}^3$ serves as a model of the intuitive geometrical space.

Dirac impulse, δ: The Dirac impulse $\delta(x)$ was introduced on page 59. It is a distribution or generalized function, as that term is used in functional analysis. The most important characteristic of the Dirac impulse is

$$\int g(x)\,\delta(x)\,dx = g(0).$$

In functional analysis, the set of all $\delta(x - x_o)$ for $x_o \in \mathbb{R}$ provides an orthonormal basis for the (infinitely dimensional) vector space of all functions from $\mathbb{R}$ to $\mathbb{R}$. It is therefore similar to the canonical unit vectors $(0,...0,1,0,...0)^\top$ of a vector space with a finite number of dimensions.

Dot product: The dot product (scalar product, inner product) is a rule for assigning a →scalar to two →vectors. With →orthonormal coordinates $\vec{x} = (x_1, x_2, ..., x_n)^\top$, $\vec{y} = (y_1, y_2, ..., y_n)^\top$,

$$(\vec{x} \cdot \vec{y}) = \sum_{i=1}^{n} x_i y_i.$$

In functional analysis, analogously to the above equation, the quantity

$$\int f(x)\,g(x)\,dx$$

is called the dot product of the functions f and g.

The dot product is commutative $((\vec{x} \cdot \vec{y}) = (\vec{y} \cdot \vec{x}))$ and distributive, but not associative.

If both vectors that contribute to a dot product are of the length (→norm) 1, then the dot product is simply the length of the orthogonal projection of one of the vectors onto the other. In this connection, also see →angle and the related Fig. G.1.

→angle; →Cauchy-Schwarz inequality; →orthogonality

Fourier transform: All continuous, integrable functions (and also some discontinuous functions) can be represented as the limit value of a weighted sum of sinusoidal and cosinusoidal functions. The coefficients constitute the Fourier transform of the function (cf. page 61).

In a →function space, the Fourier transform is an example of an orthogonal coordinate transformation, that is, a rotation.
→spatial frequency

Function: →Mapping

Function space: The set of all functions $f : \mathbb{R} \to \mathbb{R}$ constitutes a →vector space over the field of real numbers. Its dimension is infinite. If, instead of the functions themselves, sampled versions with a number m of sample points are considered, then the space has m dimensions. If $m \to \infty$, this space approximates the function space.

Gradient: The gradient of a function of more than one variable is the vector composed of the first partial →derivatives:

$$\operatorname{grad} f(x,y) = \left(\frac{\partial f(x,y)}{\partial x}, \frac{\partial f(x,y)}{\partial y} \right).$$

In mathematical physics, the gradient is sometimes represented as $\operatorname{grad} f = \nabla f$ (read: nabla f). If the function is described as a landscape, the gradient is the direction of the steepest upslope.

Graph of a function: The graph of a function $f : D \to R$ (→mapping) is the set of points
$$\{(x, f(x)) \mid x \in D,\ f(x) \in R\}.$$

For functions of one variable, the graph is the line which can be drawn in Cartesian coordinates to show the values of the function.

The graph of a function of two variables is a surface without "overhangs." Other surfaces can not be represented as graphs of a function $\mathbb{R}^2 \to \mathbb{R}$, but rather, must be represented parametrically (→parametric surface representation).

Graph (topological graph): A graph is a network composed of *nodes* and *edges* (links) where each edge connects two nodes, or connects one node with itself. In directed graphs, edges have a direction, i.e. one of the nodes connected by each edge is the starting node and the other the ending node. Labeled graphs have an additional mapping assigning a label to each edge. Directed graphs can be represented by an adjacency matrix, for which the value at position (i,j) is the number of edges from node n_i to n_j.

Integral: Intuitively, the integral of a one-dimensional function is the area under the →graph of the function, calculated as the limit of a sum:

$$\int_0^1 f(x)\ dx = \lim_{n \to \infty} \frac{1}{n} \sum_{i=1}^n f\left(\frac{i}{n}\right).$$

The result is a number (definite integral). In this book, an integral without specified limits is the improper integral with the "limits" $\pm\infty$. Multidimensional integrals are defined analogously; the integral of a function of two variables is therefore the volume under the graph of the function.

The fundamental theorem of integral and differential calculus is as follows:

$$\int_a^b f'(x) \; dx = f(b) - f(a).$$

Jacobi matrix: Let us consider a vector valued function of more than one variable:

$$g : \mathbf{R}^n \to \mathbf{R}^m$$

Each of the m components of g can be described as a function of n variables. If g is differentiable, then for each of its m components g_i, the n partial →derivatives

$$g_{i,x_j} = \frac{\partial g_i(x_1, ..., x_j, ...x_n)}{\partial x_j}$$

can be calculated; they describe a →gradient. The matrix of all partial derivatives of g is called the Jacobi matrix:

$$J_g(\vec{x}) = \begin{pmatrix} g_{1,x_1}(\vec{x}) & \cdots & g_{1,x_n}(\vec{x}) \\ \vdots & & \vdots \\ g_{m,x_1}(\vec{x}) & \cdots & g_{m,x_n}(\vec{x}) \end{pmatrix}$$

If, for a fixed point $\vec{x}_o$, this matrix is understood as a →linear mapping, then an approximation of g in the vicinity of $\vec{x}_o$ ("tangent") is obtained; cf. Fig. 8.8.

If $n = m$, then J is quadratic. The →determinant of J is then the local magnification factor of the coordinate transformation g.

Line in space: A line in space is described by a point on the line $\vec{x}_0$ and a directional vector $\vec{g}$ (cf. Fig. G.4). Lines (like other geometric objects) can be considered as sets of points which satisfy a particular equation. In the conditional equation

$$\vec{x} = \vec{x}_0 + \lambda\vec{g} \;\; \text{for } \lambda \in \mathbf{R},$$

$\vec{x}$ passes through all of the points on the line as the parameter λ changes. Clearly, there are other start points and direction vectors defining the same line.

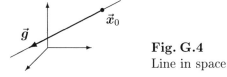

Fig. G.4
Line in space

Linear mapping: A →mapping L is linear if it fulfills the following conditions:

$$L(x+y) = L(x) + L(y)$$
$$L(\lambda x) = \lambda L(x).$$

Here, x and y are any elements in the domain of L and λ is a real number.

In a →vector space with a finite number of dimensions (e.g., $\mathbb{R}^n$), all linear mappings of the space into itself are described by square →matrices with n rows and columns. The mapping is in this case often identified with the matrix, and this is written as $L(\vec{x}) = L\vec{x}$; the right side of the equation indicates a matrix multiplication. All linear mappings of the space onto the underlying number field (in this book, usually the field of real numbers $\mathbb{R}$) are defined by →dot products with a vector element uniquely defined by the mapping.

Linear independence: n vectors $\vec{v}_1, ..., \vec{v}_n$ in a →vector space are linearly independent if it follows from

$$\sum_{i=1}^{n} c_i \vec{v}_i = 0$$

that $c_i = 0$ for all i. A simple way of describing this is that none of the vectors can be represented as a linear combination of the others.

Linear space: →vector space.

Lowpass: A linear filter which passes the low →spatial frequencies of an image, but eliminates the high frequencies. An example is the local averaging in Equation 3.7. Correspondingly, a highpass filter eliminates low spatial frequencies as, for example, in edge sharpening. Filters which cut both the low and the high spatial frequencies but let an intermediate "frequency band" pass through are called bandpass filters.

The terms are applied analogously to temporal signals.

Matrix: An $I \times J$ matrix is an array of real or complex numbers with I rows and J columns, such that:

$$M = \{m_{ij}\}_{i=1,...,I;j=1,...,J} = \begin{pmatrix} m_{1,1} & m_{1,2} & \cdots & m_{1,J} \\ m_{2,1} & m_{2,2} & \cdots & m_{2,J} \\ \vdots & \vdots & & \vdots \\ m_{I,1} & m_{I,2} & \cdots & m_{I,J} \end{pmatrix}.$$

Here, m_{ij} is the component in row i and column j.

If M is an $I \times J$ matrix and N is a $J \times K$ matrix, the product $P = MN$ is defined as follows:

$$p_{ik} = \sum_{j=1}^{J} m_{ij} n_{jk} \quad \text{for} \quad i = 1, ..., I; j = 1, ..., J.$$

Thus, the (i, k)th component of P is obtained by taking the $\rightarrow$dot product of the ith row of M with the jth column of N ("row times column"). If $K = 1$, then N and P are column vectors. The matrix product is not commutative.

$\rightarrow$determinant; $\rightarrow$linear mapping

Mapping: A mapping is a rule for the assignment of a range and a domain. In mathematical symbols:

$$M : D \to R; \quad \text{and} \quad M(d) = r.$$

Here, D and R (which are not necessarily different) are sets and $d \in D$; $r \in R$. If D and R are subsets of the set of $\rightarrow$real numbers, then M is usually called a *function*. The term "mapping" may be used to refer to multi-dimensional as well as one-dimensional domains and ranges.

Norm (length) of a vector: If a $\rightarrow$dot product is defined in a vector space, then the length of a vector is calculated according to the Pythagorean theorem:

$$\|\vec{a}\| := \sqrt{a_1^2 + \ldots + a_n^2} = \sqrt{(\vec{a} \cdot \vec{a})}.$$

This is called the Euclidean norm of a vector. It is sometimes necessary to use the more general p-Norm,

$$\|\vec{a}\|_p := \left(\sum_{i=1}^{n} |a_i|^p \right)^{1/p}.$$

$\|\vec{a}\|_1$ is the sum of the absolute values of the components of $\vec{a}$, sometimes called the "city-block norm". $\| \cdot \|_2$ is the Euclidean norm and $\| \cdot \|_\infty$ is the maximum norm, $\|\vec{a}\|_\infty = \max_i |a_i|$.

Operator: An operator is a $\rightarrow$mapping between $\rightarrow$function spaces. A simple example is the differential operator which assigns the derivative to every function. Another example is the displacement operator which displaces a function by a fixed quantity. For a discussion of the linearity of operators, see $\rightarrow$linear mapping. Translation-invariant operators are those for which a chaining with the displacement operator is commutative. All linear, translation-invariant operators can be described as $\rightarrow$convolutions if the $\rightarrow$Dirac impulse is permitted as a kernel for convolution. In this context, the kernel of a convolution integral is sometimes also called an operator.

Orthogonality: Two vectors are called orthogonal to each other if their $\rightarrow$dot product is zero.

$\rightarrow$angle

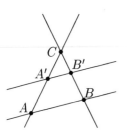

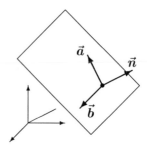

Fig. G.5
Parallel   proportionality
theorem

Fig. G.6
Plane in space (normal representation)

Orthonormal basis: A →coordinate system $(\vec{x}_1, ..., \vec{x}_n)$ of a →vector space is orthonormal if the →norm of the basis vectors is 1 and all pairs of basis vectors are
orthogonal to one another. In the case of a finite number of dimensions, then, it must
be true that:

$$(\vec{x}_i \cdot \vec{x}_j) = \begin{cases} 1 \text{ if } i = j \\ 0 \text{ if } i \neq j \end{cases}.$$

Parallel proportionality theorem: Two lines are given which intersect at C
(Fig. G.5). Let us consider two parallel lines which intersect the first two lines at
A, B and A', B'. The resulting triangles $\triangle ABC$ and $\triangle A'B'C$ are similar, which is
to say that:

$$\frac{\overline{CA}}{\overline{CA'}} = \frac{\overline{CB}}{\overline{CB'}} = \frac{\overline{AB}}{\overline{A'B'}}.$$

Parametric surface representation: A continuous and differentiable →mapping
F from a plane into space can be interpreted in the following way: for each point
(u, v) of the plane, the assigned value $F(u, v) = (x, y, z)^\top$ is a point in space. The
set of all values is a surface for which a (generally curvilinear) coordinate system is
defined by the parameters u and v. Characteristics of such parameterized surfaces
are described by differential geometry.
    Generally, for a mapping $F : \mathbf{R}^n \to \mathbf{R}^m$ with $m > n$, the set of all values of F is
called an n-dimensional manifold in m-dimensional space.
    →plane in space

Plane in space: A plane in space may be described by a normal or a parametric
representation. In the normal representation (Fig. G.6), the plane is defined as the
set of all points whose distance from the origin measured in the direction $\vec{n}$ has the
same value d. Let $\vec{n}$ be a unit vector, and $\vec{x}_0 = d\vec{n}$, the point in the plane which is
closest to the origin (for $d = 0$ this is the origin itself). If $\vec{x}$ is an additional point in
the plane, then $\vec{x} - \vec{x}_0$ is a vector which lies entirely in the plane and which we want

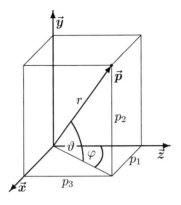

Fig. G.7
Spherical polar coordinates

to be orthogonal to $\vec{n}$. Therefore, $(\vec{n} \cdot (\vec{x} - \vec{x}_0)) = 0$, i.e., $(\vec{n} \cdot \vec{x}) = (\vec{n} \cdot \vec{x}_0)$. Since $\vec{x}_0 = d\vec{n}$ and $\vec{n}^2 = 1$, the normal representation is

$$(\vec{n} \cdot \vec{x}) = d.$$

If it is also required that $d \geq 0$, then the normal representation is unique.

A parametric representation of a plane consists of a point in the plane and two →linear independent vectors in the plane (i.e. →orthogonal to $\vec{n}$):

$$\vec{x} = \vec{x}_0 + \lambda\vec{a} + \mu\vec{b} \quad \text{with} \quad \lambda, \mu \in \mathbb{R}.$$

Each point in the plane is identified here by two numbers λ, μ, and so the parametric representation also defines a coordinate system in the plane. A parametric representation of a plane is not unique.

In psychophysics and computer vision, planes are often described by a point in the plane and two angles. The *slant* is the angle between the normal to the plane and the direction of view of the observer (Fig. 8.6). The *tilt* indicates the direction of the slant, for example, toward the rear or the side. The tilt is defined as the angle between (i) the projection of the direction of view onto the plane and (ii) the intersection of the horizontal plane $(x, z$ plane) of the camera coordinate system with the plane.

Polar coordinates: First, an axis is chosen: for example, the $\vec{y}$ axis of the Cartesian coordinate system. Then at a point $\vec{p} = (p_1, p_2, p_3)^\top$, the three polar quantities (Fig. G.7) are calculated.

$$
\begin{array}{lll}
\text{distance} & r & = \sqrt{p_1^2 + p_2^2 + p_3^2} = \|\vec{p}\| \\[2mm]
\text{azimuth} & \varphi & = \arctan\dfrac{p_1}{p_3} \\[2mm]
\text{elevation} & \vartheta & = \arctan\dfrac{p_2}{\sqrt{p_1^2 + p_3^2}}.
\end{array}
$$

The reverse relations are:

$$\begin{pmatrix} p_1 \\ p_2 \\ p_3 \end{pmatrix} = \begin{pmatrix} r \cos \vartheta \cos \varphi \\ r \sin \vartheta \\ r \cos \vartheta \sin \varphi \end{pmatrix}.$$

If another axis is chosen, then the components must be interchanged accordingly, and/or the formulas given above must be combined with corresponding rotations.

Probability: For a given experiment, such as throwing a dart at a target whose area is 1, let us consider the set Ω of all possible outcomes; in the example, $\Omega = \{(x, y)|x^2 + y^2 < 1/\pi\}$. Each (measurable) subset of $A \subset \Omega$ is called an event; each element of Ω is called an elementary event. If the dart is not aimed, the probability of an event is simply the surface area of the corresponding subset. The probability is denoted by $\mathrm{P}(A)$. It holds that $\mathrm{P}(\Omega) = 1$ and $\mathrm{P}(\{\}) = 0$. For aimed darts, a bell-shaped $\rightarrow$probability density defines the likelihood of hitting each patch of the target.

Probability density function: The density p of the $\rightarrow$probability distribution F of a continuous $\rightarrow$random variable Z describes the contribution which a small interval ("event") of length dz makes to the overall probability:

$$F(z) = \mathrm{P}(Z < z) = \int_{-\infty}^{z} p(z) \ dz.$$

The probability density is therefore the derivative of the probability distribution, wherever this derivative exists. A well-known example of a probability density is the density of the normal distribution whose average is μ and whose variance is σ^2,

$$p(z) = \frac{1}{\sqrt{2\pi}\sigma} \exp(-\frac{(z - \mu)^2}{2\sigma^2}).$$

Probability distribution: For a $\rightarrow$random variable Z, let us consider the event ($\rightarrow$probability) in which the value of Z is smaller than a number z:

$$A_z = \{\omega \in \Omega \mid Z(\omega) < z\}.$$

The $\rightarrow$probabilities of A_z generate a function which depends on z:

$$F(z) := \mathrm{P}(A_z) = \mathrm{P}(Z < z).$$

This function is called the distribution of Z. Here, the expression $(Z < z)$ is an abbreviation of $A_z = \{\omega \in \Omega \mid Z(\omega) < z\}$.

Product rule: Consider two functions f, g with the same domain. It is possible to define a function $h := f \cdot g$ for which $h(x) = f(x) \cdot g(x)$. The derivative of the product function h is as:

$$h'(x) = f'(x)g(x) + f(x)g'(x).$$

Quotient rule: Consider two functions f, g with the same domain. For $g(x) \neq 0$ it is possible to define a function $h := f/g$ for which $h(x) = f(x)/g(x)$. For the derivative of the quotient function h, then:

$$h'(x) = \frac{f'(x)g(x) - f(x)g'(x)}{g^2(x)}.$$

Random variable: Consider a set of possible events which may occur randomly. A random variable is a mapping of the set of possible outcomes of such an experiment into the set of real numbers. If the outcome of the experiment is itself a number (for example, in measuring the height of people), this is in itself also a random variable. An example of a derived random variable is the total number of dots when throwing dice.

Real number: The real numbers $\mathbb{R}$ include, first of all, the integers, and fractions composed of them (rational numbers); then the roots of all of these (solutions to algebraic equations with coefficients which are rational numbers), and finally, the limits of all series whose terms are among the numbers already mentioned.

The real numbers model a one-dimensional continuum. Therefore, between any two real numbers, there is always another—and so there are infinitely many. If $a \in \mathbb{R}$, then the set $\{x \in \mathbb{R} | x < a\}$ has no largest element.

Scalar: A number (in contrast to a vector). More generally, an element of a field (e.g. the real or complex numbers) on which a a →vector space is defined.

Spatial frequency: A spatial sinusoidal function (plane wave) of the form

$$f(x,y) = \cos(\omega_x x + \omega_y y)$$

has the spatial frequency $\vec{\omega} = (\omega_x, \omega_y)^\top$. This is a vector orthogonal to the wavefront. If spatial frequency is considered as a number, then this is the →norm of $\vec{\omega}$.

The →Fourier transform (Equation 3.21) makes it possible to represent any sufficiently continuous function as the sum (super-imposition) of sinusoidal and cosinusoidal functions of various frequencies and amplitudes. The square of the absolute values (→complex numbers) of the Fourier transform $\tilde{g}(\omega)$ in Equation 3.21 is called the power density spectrum of g. This function gives the spatial frequency content in the original function g for each frequency $\vec{\omega}$, but not the phase information..

Sharp, detailed images contain more high spatial frequencies than do blurry images or images with little detail.

Subspace: A (true) subset of a vector space which is itself also a vector space is called a subspace. For example, a plane through the origin is a two-dimensional subspace of the vector space $\mathbb{R}^3$. Lines through the origin are one-dimensional subspaces. The dimension of a subspace is always smaller than that of the space within which it

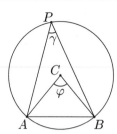

Fig. G.8
Theorem of Thales

exists. In a vector space of n dimensions, $n-1$-dimensional subspaces are sometimes called hyperplanes.

Theorem of Thales: Consider a circle with a chord AB (Fig. G.8) and a point P on the circle. The apex angle $\gamma = \angle APB$ is half the central angle $\varphi = \angle ACB$.

This theorem may be proven simply by dividing the angle γ by extending a line CP and observing the sums of the angles of the two resulting triangles, each of which has two equal legs. If the chord AB is a diameter of the circle, then in this special case the angle in the semi-circle is a right angle.

Transposition: The exchange of columns and rows of a →matrix is called a transposition.

$$\begin{pmatrix} a_1 & a_2 \\ b_1 & b_2 \end{pmatrix}^\top = \begin{pmatrix} a_1 & b_1 \\ a_2 & b_2 \end{pmatrix}.$$

The transposition of a row vector is therefore a column vector.

Vector: Each element of a →vector space is a vector. In the intuitive three-dimensional space ($\mathbf{R}^3$), no distinction is made between points in the space and vectors from the origin to these points. Examples of vector spaces are the n-tuples of →real numbers, corresponding to intuitive geometrical space if $n = 3$. We designate these spaces $\mathbf{R}^n$; their →dimension is n.

The addition of two vectors and the multiplication by a number can be explained one component at a time. If, for example, $\vec{p}, \vec{q} \in \mathbf{R}^3, \lambda \in Reell$, then:

$$\vec{p} + \vec{q} := \begin{pmatrix} p_1 + q_1 \\ p_2 + q_2 \\ p_3 + q_3 \end{pmatrix} \in \mathbf{R}^3$$

and

$$\lambda \cdot \vec{p} := \begin{pmatrix} \lambda p_1 \\ \lambda p_2 \\ \lambda p_3 \end{pmatrix} \in \mathbf{R}^3.$$

For additional rules for calculation, →dot product, →cross product. A vector is multiplied with a →matrix by treating it as a $(1 \times n)$-matrix, i.e. a matrix with just one column.

Vector space: A vector space is a set V of elements $\vec{v}$ which satisfies two groups of requirements. Firstly, addition must be defined within V, with the characteristics

1. *Closure:* For all $\vec{v}, \vec{w} \in V$, $\vec{v} + \vec{w}$ is also in V.

2. *Associativity:* for all $\vec{u}, \vec{v}, \vec{w} \in V$, $(\vec{u} + \vec{v}) + \vec{w} = \vec{u} + (\vec{v} + \vec{w})$.

3. *Neutral element:* There is an element $\vec{0} \in V$ with the characteristic $\vec{0} + \vec{v} = \vec{v}$ for all $\vec{v} \in V$.

4. *Inverse element:* For each element $\vec{v} \in V$, there is an element $(-\vec{v}) \in V$ such that $\vec{v} + (-\vec{v}) = \vec{0}$.

5. *Commutativity:* For all $\vec{v}, \vec{w} \in V$, $\vec{v} + \vec{w} = \vec{w} + \vec{v}$.

Furthermore, multiplication by the elements of a field F (in this book, always the real numbers $\mathbb{R}$) must have the characteristics:

1. *Closure :* for all $\vec{v} \in V$ and $k \in \mathbb{R}$, $k\vec{v} \in V$.

2. *Associativity:* For all $\vec{v} \in V$ and $k, l \in \mathbb{R}$, $k(l\vec{v}) = (kl)\vec{v}$.

3. *Neutral element:* For all $\vec{v} \in V$, $1\vec{v} = \vec{v}$.

4. *Distributivity of multiplication by scalars:* For all $\vec{v} \in V$ and $k, l \in \mathbb{R}$, $(k+l)\vec{v} = k\vec{v} + l\vec{v}$.

5. *Distributivity of multiplication by vectors:* For all $\vec{v}, \vec{w} \in V$ and $k \in \mathbb{R}$, $k(\vec{v} + \vec{w}) = k\vec{v} + k\vec{w}$.

Mathematical symbols and units

$\angle\vec{x},\vec{y}$	Angle between the vectors $\vec{x}$ and $\vec{y}$.
$\circ$	(superscript) Degrees in an angle
$'$	Minutes of arc (1/60 degree)
$''$	Seconds of arc (1/60 minute)
rad	Radian. Unit of measurement for angles; a full circle $= 2\pi$ rad $= 360°$
sr	Steradian. Unit of measurement for solid angles; a complete sphere $= 4\pi$ sr
$\circ$	Chaining of functions; opening operation in mathematical morphology
:= or =:	Definition. The expression on the side with the colon is defined by the expression on the other side
$\equiv$	Equivalence of two functions. $f \equiv g$ means that $f(x) = g(x)$ for all x.
$\|\vec{v}\|$	Norm of a vector $\vec{v}$
$\top$	(superscript) Transposition of a vector or a matrix
∇	(pronounced "nabla"): Gradient in operator notation
f_x	Partial derivative of a function f with respect to the variable x
$\vec{v}_x$	x component of a vector $\vec{v}$
det	Determinant of a matrix
grad$f$	Gradient of f
arg	Argument function; see Equation 11.2
argmin	Argument of the minimum of a function, if well defined. At $x^* = \text{argmin}_x f(x)$, the function $f(x)$ takes the value $\min_x f(x) = f(x^*)$.
exp	Exponential function: $\exp(x) = e^x$; $e \approx 2.718$ is the base of natural logarithms
$\mathbb{N}$	Set of the natural numbers (positive integers) $\{1, 2, 3, ...\}$
$\mathbb{Z}$	Set of all integers $\{... - 2, -1, 0, 1, 2, ...\}$
$\mathbb{R}$	Set of real numbers

Bibliography

Adelson, E. H. and Bergen, J. R. (1985). Spatiotemporal energy models for the perception of motion. *Journal of the Optical Society of America A*, 2:284 – 299.

Adelson, E. H. and Movshon, J. A. (1982). Phenomenal coherence of moving visual patterns. *Nature*, 300:523 – 525.

Aginsky, V., Harris, C., Rensink, R., and Beusmans, J. (1997). Two strategies for learning a route in a driving simulator. *Journal of Environmental Psychology*, 17:317 – 331.

Albright, T. D. and Stoner, G. R. (1995). Visual motion perception. *Proceedings of the National Academy of Sciences, USA*, 92:2433 – 2440.

Aloimonos, J. (1988). Shape from texture. *Biological Cybernetics*, 58:345 – 360.

Anderson, B. L. and Nakayama, K. (1994). Toward a general theory of stereopsis: Binocular matching, occluding contours, and fusion. *Psychological Review*, 101:414 – 445.

Arbib, M. A., editor (1995). *The Handbook of Brain Theory and Neural Networks*. The MIT Press, Cambridge, MA.

Arditi, A. (1986). Binocular vision. In Boff, K. R., Kaufmann, L., and Thomas, J. P., editors, *Handbook of Perception and Human Performance, Vol. 1: Sensory Processes and Perception*. John Wiley & Sons, New York.

Arndt, P. A., Mallot, H. A., and Bülthoff, H. H. (1995). Human stereovision without localized image–features. *Biological Cybernetics*, 72:279 – 293.

Arrowsmith, D. K. and Place, C. M. (1990). *An Introduction to Dynamical Systems*. Cambridge University Press, Cambridge.

Bachelder, I. A. and Waxman, A. M. (1994). Mobile robot visual mapping and localization: A view–based neurocomputational architecture that emulates hippocampal place learning. *Neural Networks*, 7:1083 – 1099.

Bajcsy, R. (1988). Active perception. *Proceedings of the IEEE*, 76:996 – 1005.

Ballard, D. H. (1991). Animate vision. *Artificial Intelligence*, 48:57 – 86.

Ballard, D. H. and Brown, C. M. (1982). *Computer Vision*. Prentice Hall.

Barron, J. L., Fleet, D. J., and Beauchemin, S. S. (1994). Performance of optical flow techniques. *International Journal of Computer Vision*, 12:43 – 77.

Barrow, H. G. and Tenenbaum, J. M. (1981). Interpreting line drawings as three–dimensional surfaces. *Artificial Intelligence*, 17:75 – 116.

Barth, E., Caelli, T., and Zetzsche, C. (1993). Image encoding, labelling and reconstruction from differential geometry. *Computer Vision Graphics and Image Processing: Graphical Models and Image Processing*, 55:428 – 446.

Bell, W. J. (1991). *Searching Behaviour. The behavioural ecology of finding resources*. Chapman and Hall, London etc.

Berger, J. O. (1985). *Statistical Decision Theory and Bayesian Analysis*. Springer Verlag, New York etc., 2nd edition.

Berthoz, A. (1997). Parietal and hippocampal contribution to topokinetik and topographic memory. *Philosophical Transactions of the Royal Society (London) B*, 352:1437 – 1448.

Biederman, I. (1990). Higher–level vision. In Osherson, D. N., Kosslyn, S. M., and Hollerbach, J. M., editors, *Visual Cognition and Action. An Invitation to Cognitive Science Vol. 2*. The MIT Press, Cambridge, MA.

Blake, A. and Bülthoff, H. H. (1990). Does the brain know the physics of specular reflection? *Nature*, 343:165 – 168.

Blake, A. and Bülthoff, H. H. (1991). Shape from specularities: Computation and psychophysics. *Philosophical Transactions of the Royal Society London B*, 331:237 – 252.

Blake, A., Bülthoff, H. H., and Sheinberg, D. (1993). An ideal observer model for inference of shape from texture. *Vision Research*, 33:1723 – 1737.

Blake, A. and Marinos, C. (1990). Shape from texture: Estimation, isotropy and moments. *Artificial Intelligence*, 45:323 – 380.

Blake, A. and Yuille, A., editors (1992). *Active Vision*. The MIT Press, Cambridge, MA, USA.

Blake, A. and Zisserman, A. (1987). *Visual Reconstruction*. The MIT Press, Cambridge, Ma.

Blake, R. and Wilson, H. R. (1991). Neural models of stereoscopic vision. *Trends in Neurosciences*, 14:445 – 452.

Blakemore, C. and Campbell, F. W. (1969). On the existence of neurons in the human visual system selectively sensitive to the orientation and size of retinal images. *Journal of Physiology (London)*, 203:237 – 260.

Borst, A., Egelhaaf, M., and Seung, H. S. (1993). Two–dimensional motion perception in flies. *Neural Computation*, 5:856 – 868.

Braddick, O., Campbell, F. W., and Atkinson, J. (1978). Channels in vision: Basic aspects. In Held, R., Leibowitz, H. W., and Teuber, H.-L., editors, *Perception. Handbook of Sensory Physiology VIII*. Springer Verlag, Berlin.

Brainard, D. H. and Wandell, B. A. (1986). Analysis of the retinex theory of color vision. *Journal of the Optical Society of America A*, 3:1651 – 1661.

Braitenberg, V. (1984). *Vehicles. Experiments in Synthetic Psychology*. The MIT Press, Cambridge, MA.

Bressan, P., Tomat, L., and Vallortigara, G. (1992). Motion aftereffects with rotating ellipses. *Psychological Research*, 54:240 – 245.

Brooks, M. J., Chojnacki, W., and Kozera, R. (1992). Impossible and ambiguous shading patterns. *International Journal of Computer Vision*, 7:119 – 126.

Brooks, R. A. (1981). Symbolic reasoning among 3-D models and 2-D images. *Artificial Intelligence*, 17:285 – 348.

Buchsbaum, G. and Gottschalk, A. (1983). Trichromacy, opponent colours coding and optimum colour information transmission in the retina. *Proceedings of the Royal Society (London) B*, 220:89 – 113.

Bülthoff, H. H., Little, J. J., and Poggio, T. (1989). A parallel algorithm for real–time computation of optical flow. *Nature*, 337:549.

Bülthoff, H. H. and Mallot, H. A. (1988). Integration of depth modules: Stereo and shading. *Journal of the Optical Society of America A*, 5:1749 – 1758.

Bülthoff, H. H. and Yuille, A. (1991). Bayesian models for seeing shapes and depth. *Comments on Theoretical Biology*, 2:283 – 314.

Burt, P. J. and Adelson, E. H. (1983). The Laplacian pyramid as a compact image code. *IEEE Transactions on Communications*, 31:532 – 540.

Cagenello, R. and Rogers, B. (1993). Anisotropies in the perception of stereoscopic surfaces: the role of orientation disparity. *Vision Research*, 33:2189 – 2201.

Campani, M., Giachetti, A., and Torre, V. (1995). Optic flow and autonomous navigation. *Perception*, 24:253 – 267.

Campenhausen, C. von (1993). *Die Sinne des Menschen [The Human Senses]*. G. Thieme Verlag, Stuttgart, 2. edition.

Camus, T. (1997). Real-time quantized optical flow. *Real-Time Imaging*, 3:71–86.

Canny, J. F. (1986). A computational approach to edge detection. *IEEE Transactions on Pattern Analysis and Machine Intelligence*, 8:679 – 698.

Cartwright, B. A. and Collett, T. S. (1982). How honey bees use landmarks to guide their return to a food source. *Nature*, 295:560 – 564.

Chahl, J. S. and Srinivasan, M. V. (1996). Visual computation of egomotion using an image interpolation technique. *Biological Cybernetics*, 74:405 – 411.

Cheng, K. (1986). A purely geometric module in the rat's spatial representation. *Cognition*, 23:149 – 178.

Christou, C. G. and Koenderink, J. J. (1997). Light source dependence in shape from shading. *Vision Research*, 37:1441 – 1449.

Chubb, C. and Sperling, G. (1988). Drift–balanced random stimuli: a general basis for studying non–Fourier motion perception. *Journal of the Optical Society of America A*, 5:1986 – 2007.

Clayton, N. S. and Krebs, J. R. (1995). Memory in food–storing birds: from behaviour to brain. *Current Biology*, 5:149 – 154.

Collett, T. S. (1993). Route following and the retrieval of memories in insects. *Comparative Biochemistry & Physiology*, 104A:709 – 716.

Collett, T. S. and Baron, J. (1995). Learnt sensori–motor mappings in honeybees: interpolation and its possible relevance to navigation. *Journal of Comparative Physiology A*, 177:287 – 298.

Collewijn, H., Erkelens, C. J., and Steinman, R. M. (1997). Trajectories of the human binocular fixation point during conjugate and non-conjugate gaze-shifts. *Vision Research*, 37:1049–1069.

Cornsweet, T. N. (1970). *Visual Perception*. Academic Press, New York.

Cover, T. M. and Thomas, J. A. (1991). *Elements of Information Theory*. Wiley Series in Telecommunications. John Wiley & Sons, Inc., New York.

Coxeter, H. S. M. (1987). *Projective geometry*. Springer Verlag, New York, second edition.

Crowell, J. A. and Banks, M. S. (1996). Ideal observer for heading judgements. *Vision Research*, 36:471 – 490.

Cutting, J. E., Vishton, P. M., and Braren, P. A. (1995). How we avoid collisions with stationary and moving obstacles. *Psychological Review*, 102:627 – 651.

Dacey, D. M. (1996). Circuitry for color coding in the primate retina. *Proceedings of the National Academy of Sciences, USA*, 93:582 – 588.

Dartnall, H. J. A., Bowmaker, J. K., and Mollon, J. D. (1983). Microspectrophotometry of human photoreceptors. In Mollon, J. D. and Sharpe, L. T., editors, *Colour Vision. Physiology and Psychophysics*, pages 69 – 80. Academic Press, London.

Darwin, C. R. (1859). *On the Origin of Species by Means of Natural Selection or the Preservation of Favoured Races in the Struggle for Life*. John Murray, London.

DeValois, R. L. and DeValois, K. K. (1988). *Spatial Vision*. Oxford Psychology Series No. 14. Oxford University Press, Oxford.

DeAngelis, G. C., Ohzawa, I., and Freeman, R. D. (1995). Neuronal mechanisms underlying stereopsis: how do simple cells in the visual cortex encode binocular disparity? *Perception*, 24:3 – 31.

Deseilligny, M. P., Stamon, G., and Suen, C. Y. (1998). Veinerization: A new shape description for flexible skeletonization. *IEEE Transactions on Pattern Analysis and Machine Intelligence*, 20:505 – 521.

Dhond, U. R. and Aggarwal, J. K. (1989). Structure from stereo – a review. *IEEE Transactions on Systems, Man, and Cybernetics*, 19:1489 – 1510.

do Carmo, M. P. (1976). *Differential Geometry of Curves and Surfaces*. Prentice Hall.

Duda, R. O. and Hart, P. E. (1973). *Pattern classification and scene analysis*. John Wiley & Sons, New York.

Dusenbery, D. B. (1992). *Sensory Ecology. How Organisms Acquire and Respond to Information*. W. H. Freeman and Co., New York.

Eastwood, M. (1995). Some remarks on shape from shading. *Advances in Applied Mathematics*, 16:259 – 268.

Eichenbaum, H. (1996). Is the rodent hippocampus just for 'place'? *Current Opinion in Neurobiology*, 6:187 – 195.

Enright, J. T. (1998). Monocularly programmed human saccades during vergence changes? *Journal of Physiology*, 512.1:235 – 250.

Ernst, B. (1976). *The magic mirror of M.C. Escher*. Random House, New York.

Fahle, M. and Poggio, T. (1981). Visual hyperacuity: Spatiotemporal interpolation in human vision. *Proceedings of the Royal Society (London) B*, 231:451 – 477.

Faugeras, O. (1993). *Three–dimensional computer vision. A geometric viewpoint*. The MIT Press, Cambridge, MA.

Feitelson, D. G. (1988). *Optical Computing*. The MIT Press, Cambridge, MA.

Finlayson, G. D. (1996). Color in perspective. *IEEE Transactions on Pattern Analysis and Machine Intelligence*, 18:1034 – 1038.

Fischer, B. (1973). Overlap of receptive field centers and representation of the visual field in the cat's optic tract. *Vision Research*, 13:2113 – 2120.

Flocon, A. and Barre, A. (1987). *Curvilinear perspective: from visual space to the constructed image.* University of California Press, Berkeley, CA.

Foley, J. D., Hughes, J. F., Feiner, S. K., and Phillips, R. L. (1995). *Computer Graphics. Principles and Practice, Second Edition in C.* Addison–Wesley, Reading, MA.

Förstner, W. (1993). Image matching. Chapter 16 of R. M. Haralick and L. G. Shapiro: Computer and Robot Vision. Vol 2. Reading, MA: Addison Wesley.

Forsyth, D. A. (1990). A novel approach to colour constancy. *International Journal of Computer Vision*, 5:5 – 36.

Franz, M. O. and Krapp, H. G. (2000). Wide-field, motion-sensitive neurons and matched filters for estimating self-motion from optic flow. *Biological Cybernetics, in press.*

Franz, M. O. and Mallot, H. A. (2000). Biomimetic robot navigation. *Robotics and Autonomous Systems*, 30:133 – 153.

Franz, M. O., Schölkopf, B., Mallot, H. A., and Bülthoff, H. H. (1998a). Learning view graphs for robot navigation. *Autonomous Robots*, 5:111 – 125.

Franz, M. O., Schölkopf, B., Mallot, H. A., and Bülthoff, H. H. (1998b). Where did I take that snapshot? Scene–based homing by image matching. *Biological Cybernetics*, 79:191 – 202.

Fredericksen, R. E., Verstraten, F. A. J., and van de Grind, W. A. (1994). Spatial summation and its interaction with the temporal integration mechanisms in human motion perception. *Vision Research*, 34:3171 – 3188.

Freeman, W. T. (1996). Exploiting the generic viewpoint assumption. *International Journal of Computer Vision*, 20:243 – 261.

Gallistel, C. R. (1990). *The organization of learning.* The MIT Press, Cambridge, MA, USA.

Gegenfurtner, K. R. and Hawken, M. J. (1996). Interaction of motion and color in the visual pathways. *Trends in Neurosciences*, 19:394 – 401.

Geman, S. and Geman, D. (1984). Stochastic relaxation, Gibbs distribution, and the Bayesian restoration of images. *IEEE Transactions on Pattern Analysis and Machine Intelligence*, 6:721 – 741.

Georgopoulos, A. P., Kalasak, J. F., Caminiti, R., and Massey, J. T. (1982). On the relation of the direction of twodimensional arm movements and cell discharge in primate motor cortex. *The Journal of Neuroscience*, 2:1527 – 1537.

Gibson, J. J. (1950). *The Perception of the Visual World*. Houghton Mifflin, Boston.

Gibson, J. J. (1979). *The Ecological Approach to Visual Perception*. Houghton Mifflin, Boston.

Gillner, W., Bohrer, S., and Vetter, V. (1993). Objektverfolgung mit pyramiden-basierten optischen Flußfeldern. [Object Tracking with Optical Flow Fields Based on Pyramids.] In *3. Symposium, Bildverarbeitung '93*, pages 189–220, Esslingen. Technische Akademie Esslingen.

Goldsmith, T. H. (1990). Optimization, constraint, and the history in the evolution of eyes. *The Quaterly Review of Biology*, 65:281 – 322.

Goldstein, H. (1980). *Classical Mechanics*. Addison-Wesley, 2. edition.

Greenberg, D. P. (1989). Light reflection models for computer graphics. *Science*, 244:166 – 173.

Grimson, W. E. L. (1982). A computational theory of visual surface interpolation. *Philosophical Transactions Royal Society London B*, 298:395 – 427.

Grossberg, S. and Mingolla, E. (1985). Neural dynamics of perceptual grouping: Textures, boundaries, and emergent segmentation. *Perception & Psychophysics*, 38:141 – 171.

Halder, G., Callerts, P., and Gehring, W. J. (1995). New perspectives on eye evolution. *Current opinion in Genetics & Development*, 5:602 – 609.

Hallett, P. E. (1986). Eye movements. In Boff, K. R., Kaufman, L., and Thomas, J. P., editors, *Handbook of Perception and Human Performance. Vol. I: Sensory Processes and Perception*, chapter 10. John Wiley and Sons, Chichester.

Haralick, R. M. and Shapiro, L. G. (1992). *Computer and Robot Vision, 2 Vols.* Addison Wesley, Reading MA.

Harmon, L. D. and Julesz, B. (1973). Effects of two–dimensional filtered noise. *Science*, 180:1194 – 1197.

Hassenstein, B. and Reichardt, W. (1956). Reihenfolgen-Vorzeichenauswertung bei der Bewegungsperzeption des Rüsselkäfers Chlorophanus. [Evaluation of Sequential and Sign Cues in the Motion Perception of the Weevil Chlorophanus.] *Zeitschrift für Naturforschung, Teil B*, 11:513 – 524.

Heeger, D. J. (1987). Optical flow from spatiotemporal filters. In *Proc. First International Conference on Computer Vision*, Washington, D.C. Computer Society Press of the IEEE.

Heeger, D. J., Simoncelli, E. P., and Movshon, J. A. (1996). Computational models of cortical visual processing. *Proceedings of the National Academy of Sciences, USA*, 93:623 – 627.

Heijmans, H. J. A. M. (1995). Mathematical morphology: a modern approach in image processing based on algebra and geometry. *SIAM Review*, 37:1 – 36.

Heitger, F., Rosenthaler, L., von der Heydt, R., Peterhans, E., and Kübler, O. (1992). Simulation of neural contour mechanisms: from simple to end-stopped cells. *Vision Research*, 32:963 – 981.

Helmholtz, H. von (1909 – 1911). *Handbuch der physiologischen Optik. [Handbook of Physiological Optics]*. Voss, Hamburg, 3. edition.

Hermer, L. and Spelke, E. S. (1994). A geometric process for spatial reorientation in young children. *Nature*, 370:57 – 59.

Hershberger, W. (1970). Attached–shadow orientation perceived as depth by chickens reared in an environment illuminated from below. *Journal of Comparative and Physiological Psychology*, 73:407 – 411.

Hildreth, E. C. (1984). Computations underlying the measurement of visual motion. *Artificial Intelligence*, 23:309 – 354.

Hildreth, E. C. (1992). Recovering heading for visually–guided navigation. *Vision Research*, 32:1177 – 1192.

Hildreth, E. C. and Koch, C. (1987). The analysis of visual motion: From computational theory to neuronal mechanisms. *Annual Review of Neuroscience*, 10:477 – 533.

Hine, T. J., Cook, M., and Rogers, G. T. (1997). The Ouchi illusion: An anomaly in the perception of rigid motion for limited frequencies and angles. *Perception & Psychophysics*, 59:448 – 455.

Horn, B. K. P. (1974). Determining lightness form an image. *Computer Graphics and Image Processing*, 3:277 – 299.

Horn, B. K. P. (1986). *Robot Vision*. The MIT Press, Cambridge, Ma.

Horn, B. K. P. and Brooks, M. J., editors (1989). *Shape from Shading*. The MIT Press, Cambridge, Ma.

Horn, B. K. P. and Schunk, B. G. (1981). Determining optical flow. *Artificial Intelligence*, 17:185 – 203.

Horridge, G. A. (1987). The evolution of visual processing and the construction of seeing systems. *Proceedings of the Royal Society (London) B*, 230:279 – 292.

Horridge, G. A. (1992). What can engineers learn from insect vision? *Philosophical Transactions of the Royal Society (London) B*, 337:271 – 282.

Howard, I. P. and Rogers, B. J. (1995). *Binocular Vision and Stereopsis.* Number 29 in Oxford Psychology Series. Oxford University Press, New York, Oxford.

Hubel, D. H. and Wiesel, T. N. (1962). Receptive fields, binocular interaction and functional architecture in the cat's visual cortex. *Journal of Physiology (London)*, 160:106 – 154.

Ikeuchi, K. and Horn, B. K. P. (1981). Numerical shape from shading and occluding boundaries. *Artifical Intelligence*, 17:141 – 184.

Jacobs, G. H. (1993). The distribution and nature of colour vision among the mammals. *Biological Reviews*, 68:413 – 471.

Jähne, B. (1997). *Digital image processing: concepts, algorithms, and scientific applications.* Springer Verlag, Berlin, 4. edition.

Janfeld, B. and Mallot, H. A. (1992). Exact shape from shading and integrability. In Fuchs, S. and Hoffmann, R., editors, *Mustererkennung 1992*, pages 199 – 205, Berlin. Springer-Verlag.

Jenkin, M. R. M., Jepson, A. D., and Tsotsos, J. K. (1991). Techniques for disparity measurement. *CVGIP: Image Understanding*, 53:14 – 30.

Jobson, D. J., Rahman, Z., and Woodell, G. A. (1997). Properties and performance of a center/surround retinex. *IEEE Transactions of Image Processing*, 6:451 – 462.

Johansson, G. (1973). Visual perception of biological motion and a model of its analysis. *Perception & Psychophysics*, 14:201 – 211.

Jordan III, J. R., Geisler, W. S., and Bovik, A. C. (1990). Color as a source of information in the stereo correspondence process. *Vision Research*, 30:1955 – 1970.

Julesz, B. (1971). *Foundations of Cyclopean Perception.* Chicago University Press, Chicago and London.

Julesz, B. (1991). Early vision and focal attention. *Reviews of Modern Physics*, 63:735 – 772.

Kandel, E. R., Schwartz, J. H., and Jesell, T. M., editors (2000). *Principles of Neural Science.* McGraw-Hill, 4. edition.

Kanizsa, G. (1979). *Organization in Vision.* Praeger Publishers, New York.

Klatzky, R. L., Loomis, J. M., Beall, A. C., Chance, S. S., and Golledge, R. G. (1998). Spatial updating of self-position and orientation during real, imagined, and virtual locomotion. *Psychological Science*, 9:293 – 298.

Knill, D. C. and Richards, W., editors (1996). *Perception as Bayesian Inference.* Cambridge University Press, Cambridge, UK; New York.

Koenderink, J. J. (1986). Optic flow. *Vision Research*, 26:161 – 180.

Koenderink, J. J., van Doorn, A. J., and Kappers, A. M. L. (1996). Pictorial surface attitude and local depth comparisons. *Perception & Psychophysics*, 58:163 – 173.

Korn, G. A. and Korn, T. M. (1968). *Mathematical Handbook for Scientists and Engineers.* McGraw–Hill, New York.

Košecka, J., Christensen, H. I., and Bajcsy, R. (1995). Discrete event modeling of visually guided behaviors. *International Journal of Computer Vision*, 14:179 – 191.

Krapp, H. G. and Hengstenberg, R. (1996). Estimation of self–motion by optic flow processing in single visual interneurons. *Nature*, 384:463 – 466.

Krebs, J. R. and Davies, N. B., editors (1993). *Behavioural ecology. An evolutionary approach.* Blackwell Scientific Publications, Oxford, 3. edition.

Krol, J. D. and van de Grind, W. A. (1980). The double-nail illusion: Experiments on binocular vision with nails, needles, and pins. *Perception*, 9:651 – 669.

Kuffler, S. W. (1953). Discharge pattern and functional organization of mammalian retina. *Journal of Neurophysiology*, 16:37 – 68.

Kuipers, B. (1978). Modeling spatial knowledge. *Cognitive Science*, 2:129 – 153.

Kuipers, B. J. and Byun, Y.-T. (1991). A robot exploration and mapping strategy based on a semantic hierarchy of spatial representations. *Journal of Robotics and Autonomous Systems*, 8:47 – 63.

Lambrinos, D., Maris, M., Kobayashi, H., Labhart, T., Pfeifer, R., and Wehner, R. (1997). An autonomous agent navigating with a polarized light compass. *Adaptive Behavior*, 6:131 – 161.

Land, E. H. and McCann, J. J. (1971). Lightness and retinex theory. *Journal of the Optical Society of America*, 61:1 – 11.

Land, M. F. and Fernald, R. D. (1992). The evolution of eyes. *Annual Review of Neuroscience*, 15:1 – 29.

Langer, M. S. and Zucker, S. W. (1994). Shape–from–shading on a cloudy day. *Journal of the Optical Society of America A*, 11:467 – 478.

Langton, C. G., editor (1995). *Artificial Life: an overview.* The MIT Press, Cambridge, Ma.

Lappe, M., Bremmer, F., Thiele, A., and Hoffmann, K.-P. (1996). Optic flow processing in monkey STS: A theoretical and experimental approach. *The Journal of Neuroscience*, 16:6265 – 6285.

Lappe, M., Bremmer, F., and van den Berg, A. V. (1999). Perception of self-motion from visual flow. *Trends in Cognitive Sciences*, 3:329 – 336.

Le Grand, Y. and El Hage, S. G. (1980). *Physiological Optics*. Springer Verlag, Berlin.

Lettvin, J. Y., Maturana, H. R., McCulloch, W. S., and Pitts, W. H. (1959). What the frog's eye tells the frog's brain. *Proceedings of the Institute of Radio Engineers*, 47:1950 – 1961.

Lindeberg, T. (1994). *Scale-Space Theory in Computer Vision*. Kluwer Academic Publishers, Boston, London, Dordrecht.

Lucassen, M. P. and Walraven, J. (1996). Color constancy und natural and artificial illumination. *Vision Research*, 37:2699 – 2711.

Ludwig, K.-O., Neumann, H., and Neumann, B. (1994). Local stereoscopic depth estimation. *Image and Vision Computing*, 12:16 – 35.

Luong, Q.-T., Weber, J., Koller, D., and Malik, J. (1995). An integrated stereo–based approach to automatic vehicle guidance. In *5th International Conference on Computer Vision*, pages 52 – 57, Los Alamitos, CA. IEEE, Computer Society Press.

Mach, E. (1922). *Analyse der Empfindungen [Contributions to the Analysis of Sensations]*. G. Fischer Verlag, Jena.

Maguire, E. A. (1997). Hippocampal involvement in human topographical memory: evidence from functional imaging. *Philosophical Transactions of the Royal Society (London) B*, 352:1475 – 1480.

Mallat, S. G. (1989). A theory for multiresolution signal decomposition: The wavelet representation. *IEEE Transactions on Pattern Analysis and Machine Intelligence*, 11:674 – 693.

Mallot, H. A. (1985). An overall description of retinotopic mapping in the cat's visual cortex areas 17, 18, and 19. *Biological Cybernetics*, 52:45 – 51.

Mallot, H. A. (1997). Spatial scale in stereo and shape–from–shading: Image input, mechanisms, and tasks. *Perception*, 26:1137 – 1146.

Mallot, H. A. (1999). Stereopsis — geometrical and global aspects. In Jähne, B., Haußecker, H., and Geißler, P., editors, *Handbook on Computer Vision and Applications*, volume 2, pages 371 – 390. Academic Press, San Diego etc.

Mallot, H. A., Arndt, P. A., and Bülthoff, H. H. (1996a). A psychophysical and computational analysis of intensity–based stereo. *Biological Cybernetics*, 75:187 – 198.

Mallot, H. A. and Bideau, H. (1990). Binocular vergence influences the assignment of stereo correspondences. *Vision Research*, 30:1521 – 1523.

Mallot, H. A., Bülthoff, H. H., Little, J. J., and Bohrer, S. (1991). Inverse perspective mapping simplifies optical flow computation and obstacle detection. *Biological Cybernetics*, 64:177 – 185.

Mallot, H. A. and Giannakopoulos, F. (1996). Population networks: A large scale framework for modelling cortical neural networks. *Biological Cybernetics*, 75:441 – 452.

Mallot, H. A. and Gillner, S. (2000). Route navigation without place recognition: what is recognized in recognition–triggered responses? *Perception*, 29:43 – 55.

Mallot, H. A., Gillner, S., and Arndt, P. A. (1996b). Is correspondence search in human stereo vision a coarse–to–fine process? *Biological Cybernetics*, 74:95 – 106.

Mallot, H. A., Mochnatzki, H. F., and Steck, S. D. (2000). Geographic slant improves navigation performance in virtual environments. *Investigative Ophthalmology and Visual Science*, 41 Suppl.:S44 (ARVO Abstract 228).

Mallot, H. A., Roll, A., and Arndt, P. A. (1996c). Disparity–evoked vergence is driven by interocular correlation. *Vision Research*, 36:2925 – 2937.

Mallot, H. A., Schulze, E., and Storjohann, K. (1989). Neural network strategies for robot navigation. In Personnaz, L. and Dreyfus, G., editors, *Neural Networks from Models to Applications*, pages 560 – 569, Paris. I.D.S.E.T.

Mallot, H. A., von Seelen, W., and Giannakopoulos, F. (1990). Neural mapping and space–variant image processing. *Neural Networks*, 3:245 – 263.

Maloney, L. T. and Wandell, B. A. (1986). Color constancy: a method for recovering surface spectral reflectance. *Journal of the Optical Society of America A*, 3:29 – 33.

Mamassian, P. and Kersten, D. (1996). Illumination, shading and the perception of local orientation. *Vision Research*, 36:2351 – 2367.

Mamassian, P., Kersten, D., and Knill, D. C. (1996). Categorical local-shape perception. *Perception*, 25:95 – 107.

Mardia, K. V., Kent, J. T., and Bibby, J. M. (1979). *Multivariate Analysis*. Academic Press, London.

Marr, D. (1976). Early processing of visual information. *Proceedings of the Royal Society (London) B*, 275:483 – 519.

Marr, D. (1982). *Vision*. W. H. Freeman, San Francisco.

Marr, D. and Hildreth, E. (1980). Theory of edge detection. *Proceedings of the Royal Society (London) B*, 207:187 – 217.

Marr, D. and Poggio, T. (1976). Cooperative computation of stereo disparity. *Science*, 194:283 – 287.

Marr, D. and Poggio, T. (1979). A computational theory of human stereo vision. *Proceedings of the Royal Society (London) B*, 204:301 – 328.

Marr, D. and Ullman, S. (1981). Directional selectivity and its use in early visual processing. *Proceedings of the Royal Society (London) B*, 211:151 – 180.

Maurer, R. and Séguinot, V. (1995). What is modelling for? A critical review of the models of path integration. *Journal of theoretical Biology*, 175:457 – 475.

Mayhew, J. E. W. and Frisby, J. P. (1981). Psychophysical and computational studies towards a theory of human stereopsis. *Artificial Intelligence*, 17:349 – 385.

McFarland, D. (1993). *Animal Behaviour*. Longman Scientific and Technical, Harlow, UK, 2. edition.

McKee, S. P. and Mitchison, G. J. (1988). The role of retinal correspondance in stereoscopic matching. *Vision Research*, 28:1001 – 1012.

McKee, S. P., Welch, L., Taylor, D. G., and Bowne, S. F. (1990). Finding the common bond: Stereoacuity and other hyperacuities. *Vision Research*, 30:879 – 891.

McNamara, T. P., Ratcliff, R., and McKoon, G. The mental representation of knowledge acquired from maps. *Journal of Experimental Psychology: Learning, Memory, and Cognition*, 10:723 – 732.

McNaughton, B. L., Barnes, C. A., Gerrard, J. L., Gothard, K., Jung, M. W., Knierim, J. J., Kudrimoti, H., Qin, Y., Skaggs, W. E., Suster, M., and Weaver, K. L. (1996). Deciphering the hippocampal polyglot: The hippocampus as a path integration system. *The Journal of Experimental Biology*, 199:173 – 185.

Metzger, W. (1975). *Gesetze des Sehens. [Laws of Vision]*. Senckenberg-Buch 53. Verlag Waldemar Kramer, Frankfurt am Main.

Mingolla, E. and Todd, J. T. (1986). Perception of solid shape from shading. *Biological Cybernetics*, 53:137 – 151.

Mittelstaedt, M.-L. and Mittelstaedt, H. (1980). Homing by path integration in a mammal. *Naturwissenschaften*, 67:566 – 567.

Morris, R. G. M. (1981). Spatial localization does not require the presence of local cues. *Learning Motiv.*, 12:239 – 260.

Mowforth, P., Mayhew, J. E. W., and Frisby, J. P. (1981). Vergence eye movements made in response to spatial–frequency–filtered random–dot stereograms. *Perception*, 10:299 – 304.

Müller, M. and Wehner, R. (1988). Path integration in desert ants, *Cataglyphis fortis*. *Proceedings of the National Academy of Sciences, USA*, 85:5287 – 5290.

Murray, D. W., Du, F., McLauchlan, P. F., Reid, I. D., Sharkey, P. M., and Brady, M. (1992). Design of stereo heads. In Blake, A. and Yuille, A., editors, *Active Vision*. The MIT Press, Cambridge, MA.

Nagel, H.-H. (1995). Optical flow estimation and the interaction between measurement errors at adjacent pixel positions. *International Journal of Computer Vision*, 15:271 – 288.

Nakayama, K. (1985). Biological image motion processing: A review. *Vision Research*, 25:625 – 660.

Nakayama, K. (1996). Binocular visual surface perception. *Proceedings of the National Academy of Sciences, USA*, 93:634 – 639.

Nayar, S. K., Ikeuchi, K., and Kanade, T. (1991). Surface reflection: Physical and geometrical perspectives. *IEEE Transactions on Pattern Analysis and Machine Intelligence*, 7:611 – 634.

Nayar, S. K. and Oren, M. (1995). Visual appearance of matte surfaces. *Science*, 267:1153 – 1156.

Neumann, H. (1996). Mechanisms of neural architecture for visual contrast and brightness perception. *Neural Networks*, 9:921 – 936.

O'Keefe, J. (1991). The hippocampal cognitive map and navigational strategies. In Paillard, J., editor, *Brain and Space*, pages 273 – 295. Oxford University Press, Oxford.

O'Keefe, J. and Nadel, L. (1978). *The hippocampus as a cognitive map*. Clarendon, Oxford, England.

O'Keefe, J. and Speakman, A. (1987). Single unit activity in the rat hippocampus during a spatial memory task. *Experimental Brain Research*, 68:1 – 27.

Oliensis, J. (1991). Uniqueness in shape from shading. *International Journal of Computer Vision*, 6:75 – 104.

Olshausen, B. A. and Field, D. J. (1996). Natural image statistics and efficient coding. *Network: Computation in Neural Systems*, 7:333 – 337.

Olzak, L. A. and Thomas, J. P. (1986). Seeing spatial patterns. In Boff, K. R., Kaufman, L., and Thomas, J. P., editors, *Handbook of Perception and Human Performance. Vol. I: Sensory Processes and Perception*, chapter 7. John Wiley and Sons, Chichester.

Osorio, D. and Vorobyev, M. (1996). Colour vision as an adaptation to frugivory in primates. *Proceedings of the Royal Society (London) B*, 263:593 – 599.

Papoulis, A. (1968). *Systems and Transforms with Applications in Optics*. McGraw–Hill, New York.

Penna, M. A. and Patterson, R. R. (1986). *Projective Geometry and its Applications to Computer Graphics*. Prentice-Hall.

Penna, M. A. and Wu, J. (1993). Models for map building and navigation. *IEEE Transactions on Systems, Man, and Cybernetics*, 23:1276 – 1301.

Pessoa, L. (1996). Mach bands: How many models are possible? Recent experimental findings and modeling attempts. *Vision Research*, 36:3205 – 3227.

Poggio, G. F. (1995). Mechanisms of stereopsis in monkey visual cortex. *Cerebral Cortex*, 5:193 – 204.

Poggio, T., Torre, V., and Koch, C. (1985). Computational vision and regularization theory. *Nature*, 317:314 – 319.

Pokorny, J. and Smith, V. C. (1986). Colorimetry and color discrimination. In Boff, K. R., Kaufmann, L., and Thomas, J. P., editors, *Handbook of Perception and Human Performance, Vol. 1: Sensory Processes and Perception*. John Wiley & Sons, New York.

Pollen, D. A. and Ronner, S. F. (1983). Visual cortical neurons as localized spatial frequency filters. *IEEE Transactions on Systems, Man, and Cybernetics*, 13:907 – 916.

Pratt, W. K. (1991). *Digital Image Processing*. John Wiley & Sons, New York. Second Edition 1991.

Pouget, A. and Sejnowski, T. J. (1994). A neural model of the cortical representation of egocentric distance. *Cerebral Cortex*, 4:314 – 329.

Prescott, T. (1996). Spatial representation for navigation in animals. *Adaptive Behavior*, 4:85 – 123.

Press, W. H., Flannery, B. P., Teukolsky, S. A., and Vetterling, W. T. (1986). *Numerical Recipes. The Art of Scientific Computing*. Cambridge University Press, Cambridge.

Pridmore, T. P., Mayhew, J. E. W., and Frisby, J. P. (1990). Exploiting image-plane data in the interpretation of edge-based binocular disparity. *Computer Vision, Graphics and Image Processing*, 52:1 – 25.

Qian, N. and Mikaelian, S. (2000). Relationship between phase and energy methods for disparity computation. *Neural Computation*, 12:279 – 292.

Ramachandran, V. S. (1988). Perception of shape from shading. *Nature*, 331:163 – 166.

Ramachandran, V. S. and Anstis, S. M. (1985). Perceptual organization in multistable apparent motion. *Perception*, 14:135 – 143.

Ramul, K. (1938). Psychologische Schulversuche. [Student Experiments in Psychology]. *Acta et Commentationes Universitatis Tartuensis (Dorpatensis). B Humaniora*, 34.

Ratliff, F. (1965). *Mach Bands: Quantitative Studies on Neural Networks in the Retina*. Holden–Day, San Francisco, London.

Regan, D. and Beverly, K. I. (1978). Looming detectors in the human visual pathway. *Vision Research*, 18:415 – 421.

Regan, D., Frisby, J. P., Poggio, G. F., Schor, C. M., and Tyler, C. W. (1990). The perception of stereodepth and stereo–motion: Cortical mechanisms. In Spillmann, L. and Werner, J. S., editors, *Visual Perception. The Neurophysiological Foundations*. Academic Press, San Diego etc.

Regan, D. and Vincent, A. (1995). Visual processing of looming and time to contact throughout the visual field. *Vision Research*, 35:1845 – 1857.

Reichardt, W. and Schlögl, R. W. (1988). A two dimensional field theory for motion computation. First order approximation; translatory motion of rigid patterns. *Biological Cybernetics*, 60:23 – 35.

Richards, W. A. (1971). Anomalous stereoscopic depth perception. *Journal of the Optical Society of America*, 61:410 – 414.

Richter, M. (1981) *Einführung in die Farbmetrik [Introduction to Colorimetry]*. de Gruyter, Berlin, 2. edition.

Rogers, B. J. and Bradshaw, M. F. (1993). Vertical disparities, differential perspective and binocular stereopsis. *Nature*, 361:253 – 255.

Rolls, E. T., Treves, A., Robertson, R. G., Georges-François, P., and Panzeri, S. (1998). Information about spatial view in an ensemble of primate hippocampal cells. *Journal of Neurophysiology*, 79:1797 – 1813.

Rosenfeld, A. and Kak, A. C. (1982). *Digital Picture Processing, Vols. 1 and 2*. Academic Press, Orlando, Fla. and London, second edition.

Rossel, S. (1993). Navigation by bees using polarized skylight. *Comparative Biochemistry & Physiology*, 104A:695 – 708.

Rudin, W. (1976). *Principles of mathematical analysis*. McGraw-Hill, New York, 3. edition.

Sanger, T. (1988). Stereo disparity computation using Gabor filters. *Biological Cybernetics*, 59:405 – 418.

Schiller, P. von (1933). Stroboscopische Alternativversuche. [Experiments on Stroboscopic Alternation.] *Psychologische Forschung*, 17:179.

Schölkopf, B. and Mallot, H. A. (1995). View–based cognitive mapping and path planning. *Adaptive Behavior*, 3:311 – 348.

Schor, C. M. and Wood, I. (1983). Disparity range for local stereopsis as a function of luminance spatial frequency. *Vision Research*, 23:1649 – 1654.

Schwartz, E. L. (1980). Computational anatomy and functional architecture of striate cortex: A spatial mapping approach to perceptual coding. *Vision Research*, 20:645 – 669.

Seelen, W. von (1970). Zur Informationsverarbeitung im visuellen System der Wirbeltiere. I. [On Information Processing in the Visual System of Vertebrates I]. *Kybernetik*, 7:43 – 60.

Serra, J. (1982). *Image Analysis and Mathematical Morphology*. Academic Press, London.

Shannon, C. E. (1948). A mathematical theory of communication. *Bell Syst. techn. J.*, pages 379 – 423.

Sharpe, L. T., Stockman, A., Jägle, H., and Nathans, J. (1999). Opsin genes, cone photopigments, color vision, and color blindness. In Gegenfurtner, K. R. and Sharpe, L. T., editors, *Color Vision. From Genes to Perception*, chapter 1. Cambridge University Press, Cambridge UK.

Snippe, H. P. (1996). Parameter extraction from population codes: A critical assessment. *Neural Computation*, 8:511 – 529.

Solomons, H. (1975). Derivation of the space horopter. *British Journal of Physiological Optics*, 30:56 – 90.

Speakman, A. and O'Keefe, J. (1990). Hippocampal complex spike cells do not change their place fields if the goal is moved within a cue controlled environment. *The European Journal of Neuroscience*, 2:544 – 555.

Spillmann, L. and Werner, J. S., editors (1990). *Visual Perception. The Neurophysiological Foundations*. Academic Press, San Diego etc.

Squire, L. R. (1987). *Memory and Brain*. Oxford University Press, New York, Oxford.

Srinivasan, M. V. (1998). Insects as Gibsonian animals. *Ecological Psychology*, 10:251 – 270.

Srinivasan, M. V., Laughlin, S. B., and Dubbs, A. (1982). Predictive coding: a fresh view of inhibition in the retina. *Proceedings of the Royal Society (London) B*, 216:427 – 459.

Stoer, J. and Bulirsch, R. (1992). *Introduction to numerical analysis*. Springer.

Sun, J. Y. and Perona, P. (1996). Preattentive perception of elementary three-dimensional shapes. *Vision Research*, 36:2515 – 2529.

Taube, J. S. (1998). Head direction cells and the neurophysiological basis for a sense of direction. *Progress in Neurobiology*, 55:225 – 256.

Tembrock, G. (1992). *Verhaltensbiologie [Biology of Behavior]*. UTB (Gustav Fischer Verlag), Jena, 2. edition.

Theimer, W. and Mallot, H. A. (1994). Phase–based binocular vergence control and depth reconstruction using active vision. *Computer Vision Graphics and Image Processing: Image Understanding*, 60:343 – 358.

Thompson, P. (1993). Motion psychophysics. In Miles, F. A. and Wallman, J., editors, *Visual Motion and its Role in the Stabilization of Gaze*, Reviews in Oculomotor Research, chapter 2, pages 29 – 52. Elsevier Science Publishers.

Thrun, S. (1998). Learning metric–topological maps for indoor mobile robot navigation. *Artificial Intelligence*, 99:21 – 71.

Tistarelli, M. and Sandini, G. (1992). Dynamic aspects of active vision. *Computer Vision Graphics and Image Processing: Image Understanding*, 56:108 – 129.

Todd, J. T. and Akerstrom, R. A. (1987). Perception of three-dimensional form from patterns of optical texture. *Journal of Experimental Psychology: Human Perception and Performance*, 13:242 – 255.

Todd, J. T. and Mingolla, E. (1983). Perception of surface curvature and direction of illumination from patterns of shading. *Journal of Experimental Psychology: Human Perception and Performance*, 9:583 – 595.

Tolman, E. C. (1948). Cognitive maps in rats and man. *Psychological Review*, 55:189 – 208.

Torre, V. and Poggio, T. (1986). On edge detection. *IEEE Transactions on Pattern Analysis and Machine Intelligence*, 8:147 – 163.

Treisman, A. (1986). Properties, parts, and objects. In Boff, K. R., Kaufman, L., and Thomas, J. P., editors, *Handbook of Perception and Human Performance. Vol. II: Cognitive Processes and Performance*, chapter 35. John Wiley and Sons, Chichester.

Trullier, O., Wiener, S. I., Berthoz, A., and Meyer, J.-A. (1997). Biologically based artificial navigation systems: Review and prospects. *Progress in Neurobiology*, 51:483 – 544.

Tusa, R. J., Rosenquist, A. C., and Palmer, L. A. (1979). Retinotopic organization of areas 18 and 19 in the cat. *The Journal of Comparative Neurology*, 185:657 – 678.

Tyler, C. W. (1974). Depth perception in disparity gratings. *Nature*, 251:140 – 142.

Tyler, C. W. and Clarke, M. B. (1990). The autostereogram. *SPIE Stereoscopic Displays and Applications*, 1258:182 – 196.

Uexküll, J. von (1926). *Theoretical Biology.* Hartcourt, Brace & company, New York.

Uras, S., Girosi, F., Verri, A., and Torre, V. (1988). A computational approach to motion perception. *Biological Cybernetics*, 60:79 – 87.

van Doorn, A. J. and Koenderink, J. J, (1983). The structure of the human motion detection system. *IEEE Transactions on Systems, Man, and Cybernetics*, 13:916 – 922.

van Santen, J. P. H. and Sperling, G. (1985). Elaborated Reichardt detectors. *Journal of the Optical Society of America A*, 2:300 – 321.

Verri, A. and Poggio, T. (1989). Motion field and optical flow: Quantitative properties. *IEEE Transactions on Pattern Analysis and Machine Intelligence*, 11:490 – 498.

Warren, W. H. and Kurtz, K. J. (1992). The role of central and peripheral vision in perceiving the direction of self–motion. *Perception & Psychophysics*, 51:443 – 454.

Wässle, H. and Boycott, B. B. (1991). Functional architecture of the mammalian retina. *Physiological Reviews*, 71:447 – 480.

Wässle, H., Grünert, U., RöhrenbeckJ., J., and Boycott, B. B. (1990). Retinal ganglion cell density and cortical magnification factor in the primate. *Vision Research*, 30:1897 – 1911.

Watt, R. J. (1990). The primal sketch in human vision. In Blake, A. and Troscianko, T., editors, *AI and the Eye*, pages 147 – 180. John Wiley & Sons, Chichester.

Wehner, R. and Menzel, R. (1990). Do insects have cognitive maps? *Annual Review of Neuroscience*, 13:403 – 414.

Weinshall, D. (1991). Seeing "ghost" planes in stereo vision. *Vision Research*, 31:1731 – 1748.

Westheimer, G. (1994). The Ferrier lecture, 1992. Seeing depth with two eyes: stereopsis. *Proceedings of the Royal Society (London) B*, 257:205 – 214.

Westheimer, G. (1999). Gestalt theory reconfigured: Max Wertheimer's anticipation of recent developments in visual neuroscience. *Perception*, 28:5 – 15.

Wheatstone, C. (1838). Some remarkable phenomena of vision. I. *Philosophical Transactions of the Royal Society*, 13:371 – 395.

Wilson, H. R. (1994). The role of second–order motion signals in coherence and transparency. In *Higher–Order Processing in the Visual System*, volume 184 of *Ciba Foundation Symposium*, pages 227 – 244.

Wilson, H. R., McFarlane, D. K., and Phillips, G. C. (1983). Spatial frequency tuning of orientation selective units estimated by oblique masking. *Vision Research*, 23:873 – 882.

Wilson, M. A. and McNaughton, B. L. (1993). Dynamics of the hippocampal ensemble code for space. *Science*, 261:1055 – 1058.

Wiltschko, R. and Wiltschko, W. (1995). *Magnetic orientation in animals.* Springer Verlag, Berlin, New York.

Witkin, A. P. (1981). Recovering surface shape and orientation from texture. *Artificial Intelligence*, 17:17 – 45.

Wyszecki, G. and Stiles, W. S. (1982). *Color Science.* Wiley, New York, 2nd edition.

Yagi, Y., Nishizawa, Y., and Yachida, M. (1995). Map–based navigation for a mobile robot with omnidirectional image sensor COPIS. *IEEE Transactions on Robotics and Automation*, 11:634 – 448.

Yeshurun, Y. and Schwartz, E. L. (1989). Cepstral filtering on a columnar image architecture: A fast algorithm for binocular stereo segmentation. *IEEE Transactions on Pattern Analysis and Machine Intelligence*, 11:759 – 767.

Yuille, A. L. and Poggio, T. (1986). Scaling theorems for zero crossings. *IEEE Transactions on Pattern Analysis and Machine Intelligence*, 8:15 – 25.

Zhang, R., Tsai, P. S., Cryer, J. E. and Shah, M. (1999). Shape from shading: A survey. *IEEE Transactions on Pattern Analysis and Machine Intelligence*, 21:690 – 706.

Zhuang, X. and Haralick, R. M. (1993). Motion and surface structure from time–varying image sequences. Chapter 15 of R. M. Haralick and L. G. Shapiro: Computer and Robot Vision. Vol 2. Reading, MA: Addison Wesley.

Zielke, T., Brauckmann, M., and Seelen, W. von (1993). Intensity and edge–based symmetry detection with application to car–following. *Computer Vision Graphics and Image Processing: Image Understanding*, 58:177 – 190.

Zielke, T., Storjohann, K., Mallot, H. A., and Seelen, W. von (1990). Adapting computer vision systems to the visual environment: Topographic mapping. In Faugeras, O., editor, *Computer Vision – ECCV 90 (Lecture Notes in Computer Science 427)*, Berlin. INRIA, Springer Verlag.

Zrenner, E. (1983). *Neurophysiological studies on simian retinal ganglion cells and the human visual system*, volume 9 of *Studies in Brain Function*. Springer Verlag, Berlin.

Author Index

Subject Index